RAPID REVIEW SERIES

HISTOLOGY AND
CELL BIOLOGY

*Visit our website at **www.mosby.com***

RAPID REVIEW SERIES

Series Editor

Edward F. Goljan, MD

HISTOLOGY AND CELL BIOLOGY

E. Robert Burns, PhD
Course Director, Microscopic Anatomy
Professor of Anatomy
Department of Anatomy and Neurobiology
College of Medicine
University of Arkansas for Medical Sciences
Little Rock, Arkansas

M. Donald Cave, PhD
Professor of Anatomy
Department of Anatomy and Neurobiology
College of Medicine
University of Arkansas for Medical Sciences
Little Rock, Arkansas

Contributor

William D. Meek, PhD
Professor of Anatomy and Cell Biology
Department of Anatomy and Cell Biology
Oklahoma State University Center for Health Sciences
College of Osteopathic Medicine
Tulsa, Oklahoma

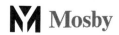 Mosby

An Imprint of Elsevier Science

St. Louis   London   Philadelphia   Sydney   Toronto

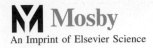
Mosby
An Imprint of Elsevier Science

The Curtis Center
Independence Square West
Philadelphia, PA 19106

NOTICE

Pharmacology is an ever-changing field. Standard safety precautions must be followed, but as new research and clinical experience broaden our knowledge, changes in treatment and drug therapy may become necessary or appropriate. Readers are advised to check the most current product information provided by the manufacturer of each drug to be administered to verify the recommended dose, the method and duration of administration, and contraindications. It is the responsibility of the licensed prescriber, relying on experience and knowledge of the patient, to determine dosages and the best treatment for each individual patient. Neither the publisher nor the editor assumes any liability for any injury and/or damage to persons or property arising from this publication.

The Publisher

International Standard Book Number 0-323-00834-8

Acquisitions Editor: Jason Malley
Managing Editor: Susan Kelly
Developmental Editor: Ruth Steyn
Publishing Services Manager: Patricia Tannian
Project Manager: Richard Hund
Senior Designer: Kathi Gosche
Cover Designer: Melissa Walter
Illustrator: Matt Chansky

GW/CCW

Printed in the United States of America

Last digit is the print number: 9 8 7 6 5 4 3 2 1

To Keith and Sherry, son and daughter, and the two new, bright lights in the Burns' clan: granddaughter Ayla Judith Richardson, born December 16, 1996, and Mary Stuart Lindsey, married April 13, 2000. –ERB

To my wife, Donna, for her support, and to my colleagues who have contributed so much to my life and career. –MDC

To our medical students for constantly challenging us. –ERB and MDC

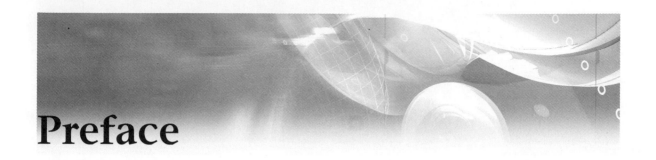

Preface

The *Rapid Review Series* is designed for today's busy medical student who has completed basic science courses and has only a limited amount of time to prepare for the United States Medical Licensing Examination (USMLE) Step 1. With a commitment to meeting the needs of these students, we conducted numerous focus groups throughout the United States, trying to learn what would better prepare students for the Step 1 exam. Each book in the *Rapid Review Series* offers a visually integrated approach to review and is packaged with a CD-ROM to help students practice for the actual USMLE Step 1.

Special Features

BOOK

- **Target topics:** summary of major topics discussed in the chapter
- **Two-color, easy-to-follow outline:** concisely organized need-to-know information integrating basic science and clinical correlations
- **High-yield margin notes:** recall topics most likely tested on Step 1
- **Visual elements:** computer-generated two-color schematics, summary tables, and clinical boxes
- **Bold and color text:** highlights key words and phrases
- **Practice examinations:** two sets of 50 multiple-choice, clinically oriented questions in current USMLE Step 1 format, including complete discussions (rationales) for all options
- **Table of normal laboratory values**

CD-ROM

- **Full-color: 230 clinically oriented multiple-choice questions** in current USMLE Step 1 format and content, approximately 125 color images of gross and pathologic specimens and electron and transmission electron micrographs
- **Test mode:** 60-minute timed test of 50-question block by science, system, or random selection
- **Tutorial (review) mode:** customize review by science, system, or random selection with immediate feedback
- **Bookmark capability**
- **Table of common laboratory values**
- **Scoring function:** instant statistical analysis showing strengths and weaknesses; print capability

Acknowledgment of Reviewers

The publisher wishes to express sincere thanks to the medical students and the resident physician who reviewed both the text and the questions for the book and CD-ROM and provided us with many useful comments and helpful suggestions for improving this product. Our publishing program will continue to benefit from the combined insight and experience provided by your reviews. For always encouraging us to focus on our target, the USMLE Step 1, we thank the following:

Michael W. Lawlor
Loyola University of Chicago
Stritch School of Medicine

Kelly Liang
Jefferson Medical College

Kimberly Liang
Jefferson Medical College

Christopher Lupold
Jefferson Medical College

Tracey A. McCarthy
Loyola University of Chicago
Stritch School of Medicine

Mrugeshkumar K. Shah, MD, MPH
Tulane School of Medicine
Harvard Medical School/Spaulding Rehabilitation Hospital

John K. Su, MPH
Boston University School of Medicine

Acknowledgments

The authors wish to acknowledge the professionalism and the patience of Susan Kelly, Managing Editor, for helping us complete this project. We thank Ruth Steyn, PhD, for her editing skills. Matt Chansky's expertise as an illustrator will be appreciated by every reader. Thanks to the medical students and the resident physician who reviewed the manuscript and the questions—you offered excellent constructive criticism by always focusing the work on the target, the USMLE Step 1.

E. Robert Burns, PhD
M. Donald Cave, PhD

Figure Acknowledgments

Figure 2-3. Adapted from Junqueira LC, J Carneiro: *Basic Histology*, ed 7, East Norwalk, CT, 1992, Appleton-Lange, p. 42, figure 3-17. With permission of The McGraw-Hill Companies.

Figure 2-4. Adapted from Alberts B: *Molecular Biology of the Cell*, ed 3, New York, 1994, Garland Publishing, p. 579, figure 12-33. With permission of Routledge, Inc., part of The Taylor & Francis Group.

Figure 2-5. Adapted from Lodish HA, Berk SL, Zipursky P, Baltimore MD, Darnell J: *Molecular Cell Biology*, ed 4, New York, 2000, W.H. Freeman, p. 698, figure 17-16. Used with permission.

Figure 2-6. Modified from Stevens A, Lowe JS, *Human Histology*, ed 2, London, 1997, Mosby, p. 21, figure 2-16b.

Figure 3-1. Adapted from Junqueira, LC, Carneiro J: *Basic Histology*, ed 7, East Norwalk, CT, 1992, Appleton-Lange, p. 51, figure 3-27. With permission of The McGraw-Hill Companies.

Figure 5-2. Cormack DH: *Ham's Histology*, Philadelphia, 1987, Lippincott, p. 170, figure 7-11. With permission from Lippincott Williams & Wilkins.

Figure 6-4. Lodish HA, Berk SL, Zipursky P, Baltimore MD, Darnell J: *Molecular Cell Biology*, ed 4, New York, 2000, W.H. Freeman, p. 914, figure 21-4a; p. 945, figure 21-35a. Used with permission.

Figure 7-6. Adapted from Ross, RB and EJ Reith, *Histology: a text and atlas*, NY, 1985, Harper & Row, p. 204, figure 10-9 (LD Peachey, 1974).

Figure 17-1. Adapted from Bergman RA, Afifi AK, Heidger Jr PM: *Saunders Text and Review Series Histology*, Philadelphia, 1996, Saunders, p. 284, figure 16-3.

Figure 17-3. Adapted from Randall D, Burggren W, French K: *Eckert Animal Physiology: Mechanisms and Adaptations*, ed 4, New York, 1997, WH Freeman, p. 341, figure 9-32. Used with permission.

Table of Contents

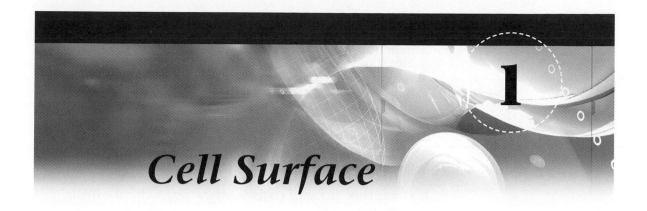

Cell Surface

Target Topics

- Microscopic appearance and molecular organization of phospholipids, proteins, and other components in cellular membranes
- Membrane fluidity
- Mechanisms for transporting molecules in and out of cells
- Ligands, receptors, and overview of cell-cell signaling
- Structure and function of cell junctions
- Cystic fibrosis, hereditary hypercholesterolemia, cystinuria, Graves' disease, toxins that bind to membrane proteins

I. **Introduction: Levels of Anatomic Organization**
   A. **Cells**
   1. **Major cellular components**
      a. **Nucleus** contains the genetic material (**DNA**) and is surrounded by a double membrane.
      b. **Cytoplasm** consists of a fluid portion (**cytosol**), various membrane-bounded **organelles**, inclusions, and **cytoskeletal elements**.
      c. **Plasma membrane** (**plasmalemma**) constitutes the **outer boundary** of a cell, enclosing the cellular contents and separating them from the external environment.
         - In all cells, the plasma membrane also functions in **regulating the intracellular environment** and in **cell-to-cell communication**.
   2. **Essential cell functions that enable life**
      a. Replication (cells arise only from preexisting cells)
      b. Regulation of the intracellular environment
      c. Synthesis of proteins and numerous other molecules
      d. Harnessing and transformation of energy
      e. Differentiation and specialization
      f. Interaction to form larger units

B. Higher levels of organization
   1. Tissues: aggregations of cells and their products specialized to perform a particular function or functions; classified into four major types:
      a. Epithelial tissue
      b. Connective tissue
      c. Nervous tissue
      d. Muscle tissue
   2. Organ: a group of tissues that forms a structural unit and performs a specific function or functions
   3. Organ system: a group of interconnected or interdependent organs that together perform a specific function or functions
   4. Organism: group of systems interacting to form a living economy
C. Dimensions of biological structures and their component molecules are summarized in Figure 1-1.

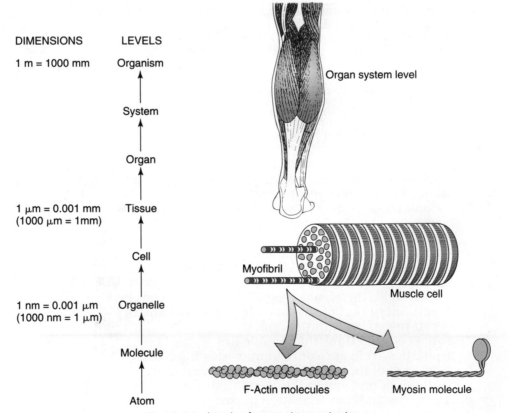

DIMENSIONS   LEVELS

1 m = 1000 mm   Organism

                  System

                  Organ

1 μm = 0.001 mm   Tissue
(1000 μm = 1mm)

                  Cell

1 nm = 0.001 μm   Organelle
(1000 nm = 1 μm)

                  Molecule

                  Atom

Organ system level

Myofibril

Muscle cell

F-Actin molecules

Myosin molecule

Figure 1-1 Levels of anatomic organization.

II. **Structure of the Plasmalemma**
  A. **Trilaminar appearance** in cell sections
   • Transmission electron microscopy of cell sections shows the plasma membrane having **two electron-dense outer layers** (each 3-nm thick) separated by a **less-dense central layer** (3.5-nm thick).
     1. **External (exoplasmic) surface** faces the cell exterior.
     2. **Internal (protoplasmic) surface** faces the cytoplasm.
  B. **Lipid bilayer**
   • The basic structural unit of nearly all cellular membranes is a **bimolecular lipid "sheet"** composed primarily of phospholipids (Figure 1-2).
     1. **Phospholipids** are highly **amphipathic** molecules, containing a **hydrophilic "head" group** and long **hydrophobic "tails"** composed of fatty acids.
       • In membranes, phospholipids are arranged as two sheets (**leaflets**) with their hydrophilic **head** groups facing **outward** and their hydrophobic **tails** facing **inward.**
       a. **Phosphatidylcholine** (lecithin) and **sphingomyelin** are present primarily in the outer leaflet.
       b. **Phosphatidylethanolamine** and **phosphatidylserine** are present primarily in the inner leaflet.
     2. **Cholesterol**, located in both leaflets of the plasma membrane, helps to stabilize membrane structure.
     3. **Glycolipids** have their lipid end inserted into the outer leaflet of the plasma membrane with their carbohydrate moieties extending into the extracellular space.
  C. **Membrane proteins**
   • According to the **fluid-mosaic model**, proteins in cellular

In cells without oxygen, activation of membrane phospholipase by Ca^{2+} leads to irreversible cell injury.

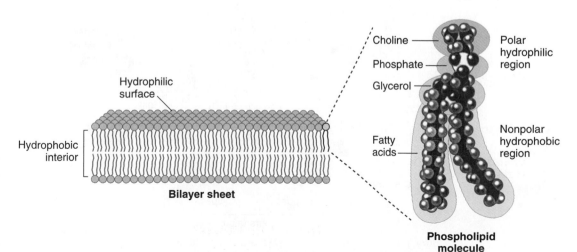

Figure 1-2   Structure of phospholipid bilayer. Hydrophilic heads of the phospholipid molecules face outward, toward the aqueous surroundings.

membranes "float" and move laterally within the lipid bilayer, which acts as a two-dimensional fluid.

- Proteins can associate with the lipid bilayer in various ways (Figure 1-3).

1. Extrinsic (peripheral) proteins are present at membrane surfaces but do not penetrate the lipid bilayer.

- Composed primarily of **hydrophilic amino acids**, extrinsic proteins are held in place by **noncovalent interactions** with other membrane proteins, lipids, or oligosaccharides.

2. Transmembrane intrinsic (integral) proteins span the entire lipid bilayer and generally have covalently linked **carbohydrate residues**, which always project into the extracellular space.

  a. Regions rich in hydrophobic amino acids interact with the nonpolar interior of the lipid bilayer.

    (1) In **single-pass proteins**, the polypeptide chain crosses the membrane once.

    (2) In **multipass proteins**, the polypeptide chain crosses the membrane more than once.

  b. Regions rich in hydrophilic amino acids extend beyond the membrane surfaces, forming **cytosolic** and **exoplasmic domains**.

3. Lipid-anchored intrinsic proteins have a covalently attached lipid group that tethers them to one or the other of the bilayer leaflets.

D. Fluidity of membranes

  1. Lateral movement

   - Phospholipids, glycolipids, and some intrinsic proteins diffuse laterally within the individual leaflets of a membrane.

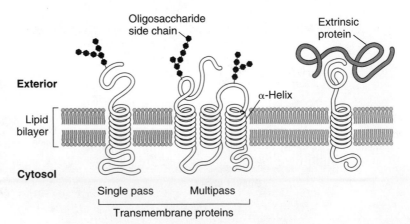

Figure 1-3   Common ways that proteins interact with the lipid bilayer. Hydrophobic, α-helical regions of transmembrane proteins are embedded in the interior of the bilayer. These proteins usually are glycoproteins with oligosaccharide residues covalently attached to the external domain. Extrinsic proteins associate noncovalently with either the external or the cytosolic domain of transmembrane proteins.

2. **Exchange (flip-flop) between leaflets**
   a. Lipids and proteins **do not move spontaneously** between the inner and the outer leaflets of the lipid bilayer.
   b. Phospholipids, which are synthesized in the cytosolic leaflet of the endoplasmic reticulum (ER) membrane, can flip-flop to the other leaflet with the aid of ER-bound enzymes called **phospholipid translocators,** or **flippases.**
3. **Factors affecting membrane fluidity**
   a. **Temperature:** fluidity increases as the temperature rises.
   b. **Phospholipid type:** shorter fatty acid tails and presence of double bonds increase fluidity.
   c. **Cholesterol content:** fluidity decreases as membrane cholesterol increases (e.g., as a result of ethanol intake).
      • Decrease in fluidity of membranes reduces their permeability to small molecules such as water.

Fluidity of cellular membranes affects their functions: temperature and cholesterol content increases fluidity.

E. **Uniformity of cellular membranes**
   1. **Trilaminar appearance and lipid bilayer** molecular organization are characteristic of internal cellular membranes (e.g., nuclear, mitochondrial, and ER membranes) as well as of the plasma membrane.
   2. **Lipid and protein composition** of various cellular membranes differ.
      • **Organelle-specific membrane proteins** confer unique functions on certain organelles.
   3. **Membrane "flow"** refers to the ready exchange of membranes that occurs between cellular compartments.
      a. Plasma membrane → endocytic vesicle
      b. Membrane of secretory vesicle → plasma membrane
      c. ER→ transfer vesicle → Golgi complex → lysosome

F. **Glycocalyx**
   • A **carbohydrate-rich layer,** also known as the **cell coat,** the glycocalyx covers the **external surface** of the plasma membrane of many cells.
   • In contrast to the plasma membrane, the **glycocalyx exhibits extensive variation** in thickness, fuzziness, and general appearance in different cell types.
   1. **Components of the glycocalyx**
      a. **Membrane glycolipids and transmembrane glycoproteins** (exoplasmic domains)
      b. **Extrinsic membrane glycoproteins**
      c. **Proteoglycans** attached to cell surface
   2. **Functions of the glycocalyx**
      • Depending on the cell type and tissue, the glycocalyx may assist in the following:
      a. **Control of cell permeability** by permitting passage of water and small molecules, but not large molecules
      b. **Protection** and **lubrication** of the cell surface
      c. **Cell-cell recognition** and **interaction** (e.g., in lymphocyte recirculation and sperm–egg interaction)
      d. **Localization of extracellular enzymes** to the cell surface

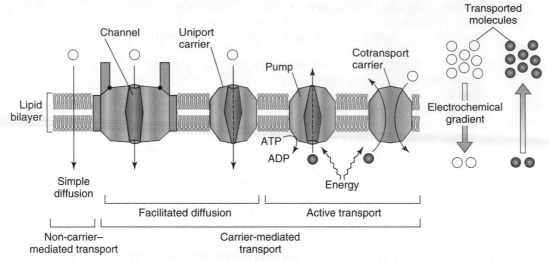

Figure 1-4 Summary of various types of membrane-transport processes. *Open circles* represent molecules that are moving down their electrochemical gradient. *Solid circles* represent molecules that are moving against their electrochemical gradient. Such active transport requires an input of energy.

III. **Movement of Molecules and Ions across Membranes** (Figure 1-4)
- Various multipass transmembrane proteins, called **transport proteins**, mediate passage of most molecules and all ions across the plasma membrane (and internal membranes).
A. **Passive transport:** movement of molecules or ions across the membrane **down** their concentration or electrochemical **gradient; no energy required**
  - Transport proteins exhibit a **high degree of specificity** for the transported molecule or ion and undergo **conformational changes** during the transport process.
  1. **Simple diffusion** occurs without the aid of transport proteins.
     - Small hydrophobic molecules and small uncharged polar molecules (e.g., H_2O, CO_2, O_2, and ethanol) readily diffuse through lipid bilayer membranes.
  2. **Facilitated diffusion** is mediated by channel proteins and certain carrier proteins.
     a. **Channel proteins** form hydrophilic pores that extend across the membrane. When the pores are "open," solutes (primarily ions) flow through them.
     b. **Uniport carrier proteins**, commonly termed **permeases**, transport a single solute (e.g., glucose, particular amino acid) across the membrane in one direction.
B. **Active transport:** protein-mediated movement of molecules or ions across the membrane **against** their concentration or electrochemical **gradient; energy required**
  1. **ATP-powered pumps** have binding sites for ATP (adenosine triphosphate) in their cytosolic domains and **couple ATP**

hydrolysis to transport of ions and small molecules against their gradient.

- **Na⁺/K⁺ pump** moves 3 Na⁺ ions out of and 2 K⁺ ions into the cell, both against their electrochemical gradients, maintaining their typical gradients across the plasma membrane.
- Reduction in ATP synthesis (e.g., in cells without adequate oxygen) causes Na⁺ to move into cells, leading to cellular swelling (hydropic degeneration).

2. Cotransport carrier proteins couple the energy-releasing transport of one solute (e.g., Na⁺) down its gradient to the energy-requiring transport of another solute (e.g., glucose) up its gradient.

- **Na⁺/glucose cotransport protein** mediates transport of glucose from the intestinal lumen into epithelial cells.

C. Bulk movement of materials in and out of cells

1. Exocytosis: the release of large quantities of material from cells by a process that involves fusion of the cytosolic surface of the plasma membrane with the cytosolic surface of secretory vesicle membranes

2. Endocytosis: the uptake of large amounts of material into cells by processes that involve fusion of the external surfaces of the plasma membrane

   a. Phagocytosis is a **nonselective** process whereby large solid particles (e.g., bacteria) are ingested and subsequently degraded.

   b. Pinocytosis is a **nonselective** process whereby small fluid droplets are ingested.

   c. Receptor-mediated endocytosis is a **selective** process whereby specific macromolecules (e.g., antigens, low-density lipoprotein, transferrin) are ingested (Figure 1-5).

D. Disorders involving defective transport

1. Cystic fibrosis is caused by an autosomal recessive mutation in the gene encoding **CFTR protein**, an ATP-powered Cl⁻ channel.

- This genetic defect leads to dysfunction of exocrine glands in the pancreas, respiratory system, and skin.
- Common manifestations are **excess sweat** with electrolytes (basis for the **sweat chloride test**) and excessive amounts of **thick mucus** in the respiratory tract.

2. Cystinuria, an autosomal recessive disease, results from a defect in carrier proteins needed to reabsorb cystine from kidney tubules.

- This condition, marked by excessive excretion of cystine and several other amino acids, may lead to formation of **kidney stones** and the presence of hexagonal cystine crystals in the urine.

3. Hereditary hypercholesterolemia, an autosomal dominant disease, occurs in individuals who lack functional receptors for low-density lipoprotein (LDL).

- LDL, the major carrier of cholesterol in the bloodstream,

Cystic fibrosis, hereditary hypercholesterolemia, and cystinuria result from defects in membrane transport proteins.

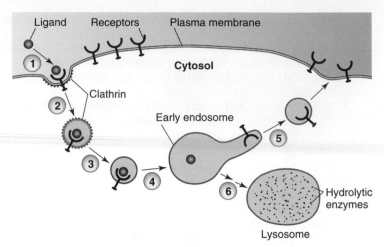

Figure 1-5 Receptor-mediated endocytosis of macromolecular ligands. Ligand molecules bind to their specific cell-surface receptors, which then aggregate over clathrin-coated pits *(1)*. These pits bud off from the membrane *(2)*, forming vesicles that soon shed their coat *(3)*. After uncoated vesicles fuse with endosomes, the low internal pH dissociates the ligand from its receptors *(4)*. The receptors are recycled to the plasma membrane via small vesicles *(5)*, while ligands are moved to lysosomes where they are enzymatically degraded *(6)*.

normally is internalized into cells by receptor-mediated endocytosis.
- Absence of functional LDL receptors causes high blood levels of cholesterol, which contribute to **atherosclerosis** and death due to coronary artery disease and strokes at an early age.
4. **Tetrodotoxin** binds to and inactivates Na^+ channels.
- When ingested by humans, tetrodotoxin from puffer fish and related fish toxins cause dizziness and tingling around the mouth, which may be followed by ataxia, respiratory failure, and death.

IV. **Cell-to-Cell Communication**
- Cells in tissues and organs are continuously bombarded with **signaling molecules**, which carry potentially significant information.
- A cell can respond only to those signaling molecules whose specific **protein receptors** it produces. The **repertoire of receptors** produced by cells **changes during development and differentiation** of various cell types.
A. Sequence of events in cell signaling
   1. **Release of signaling molecules (ligands)** from signaling cell commonly occurs via exocytosis and usually in response to a specific stimulus. Common signaling molecules include:
      a. Neurotransmitters
      b. Hormones
      c. Growth factors
      d. Cytokines

2. **Binding of a ligand** to its specific receptor in a target cell causes **receptor activation.**

3. **Signal transduction** from activated receptor, either directly or indirectly via an intracellular **second messenger**, leads ultimately to **specific cellular responses.** Common second messengers include:
   a. cAMP (cyclic adenosine monophosphate)
   b. cGMP (cyclic guanosine monophosphate)
   c. IP_3 (inositol 1,4,5-triphosphate)
   d. DAG (1,2-diacylglycerol)
   e. Ca^{2+} **ions**
   f. NO (nitric oxide)

B. **Types of signaling**
   1. **Autocrine signaling:** response is elicited in the same cell that produces the signaling molecules.
   2. **Paracrine signaling:** response is elicited in target cells in close proximity to the signaling cell.
   3. **Endocrine signaling:** response is elicited in target cells far removed from signaling cell with hormonal signaling molecule carried in the blood.
      • In **neuroendocrine signaling**, molecules released into the blood from hypothalamic neurosecretory cells act in endocrine fashion on anterior pituitary.

C. **Classification of receptors** (Figure 1-6)
   1. **Intracellular receptors** are located in the cytoplasm or nucleus and bind **lipophilic ligands** (e.g., steroid hormones), which diffuse through the plasma membrane.
      a. Ligand binding alters conformation of the receptor, exposing **DNA-binding domain(s)** in the receptor.
      b. Activated ligand-receptor complex binds to control regions of target genes, **activating transcription** of these genes.
   2. **Cell-surface receptors** are transmembrane proteins that generally bind **hydrophilic ligands.** These receptors can be classified into four major types:
      a. Ion-channel receptors: ligand binding causes the ion channel to open.
         • Examples are **nicotinic acetylcholine (ACh) receptors** in skeletal muscle cells and receptors for other **neurotransmitters** (e.g., serotonin, glutamate) in neurons.
      b. Receptors with inherent enzymatic activity: ligand binding activates the receptor's cytosolic catalytic domain, which acts as a protein kinase, protein phosphatase, or guanylate cyclase.
         • Examples are **insulin receptor** and receptors for many **growth factors.**
      c. Cytokine (tyrosine kinase–linked) receptors: ligand binding activates tyrosine kinases located in the cytosol.
         • Examples are receptors for **cytokines, interferons, human growth hormone,** and **prolactin.**
      d. G protein–linked receptors: ligand binding leads to activation of a membrane-associated trimeric **G protein,**

Steroid hormone receptors are located in the cytoplasm or nucleus. Hormone stimulation normally leads to expression of specific target genes.

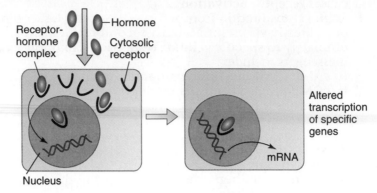

A   **Intracellular receptors**

Receptor-
hormone
complex

Hormone

Cytosolic
receptor

Nucleus

Altered
transcription
of specific
genes

mRNA

B   **Cell-surface receptors**

Surface receptors

Ligands bound to
surface receptors

Ligands

Low concentration
of second messengers

High concentration
of second messengers

Figure 1-6   Signaling mediated by two basic types of receptors. **A,** Lipophilic hormones bind to intracellular receptors, forming complexes that stimulate transcription of specific target genes. **B,** Binding of hydrophilic ligands to cell-surface receptors triggers intracellular signal-transduction pathways that commonly involve a second messenger (e.g., cAMP, DAG, Ca^{2+}). Signaling ultimately modulates the activity or expression of specific proteins.

which in turn activates an **effector protein** that modulates the activity of particular second messengers.

- Examples are **adrenergic receptors**, which bind epinephrine and norepinephrine; **muscarinic ACh receptor;** and receptors for **glucagon, TSH** (thyroid-stimulating hormone), **LH** (luteinizing hormone), and **ACTH** (adrenocorticotropic hormone).

D. GTPase intracellular switch proteins

- These proteins alternate (switch) between an **active state** with bound **GTP** (guanosine triphosphate) and an **inactive state** with bound **GDP** (guanosine diphosphate).
- Examples include **trimeric G proteins**, which directly interact with G protein–linked receptors, and **Ras proteins**, which are indirectly coupled to receptors with tyrosine kinase activity.

E. Role of phosphorylation/dephosphorylation in signal transduction
1. **Protein kinases** add phosphate groups to specific target proteins, causing conformational changes that **modulate protein activity** or **create docking sites** for other proteins.
   - In many signaling pathways, **ligand binding** to the receptor leads to **activation of protein kinases,** whose activity transduces the signal.
2. **Protein phosphatases,** which remove phosphate groups from specific proteins, oppose the effect of protein kinases.
   - In the absence of ligand binding, the constitutive action of phosphatases inactivates intracellular signal transduction induced by many ligands.

F. Disorders involving defective cell-cell signaling
1. **Mutant Ras proteins** are associated with some neoplasms (e.g., **colorectal cancer**).
   - These defective Ras proteins are "turned on" in the absence of normal ligands, leading to **neoplastic transformation** of cells.
2. **Cholera toxin** modifies trimeric G proteins causing them to remain in the active state in the absence of ligand.
   - Resulting prolonged activation of G proteins → **high cAMP levels** → movement of water from the blood across intestinal epithelial cells into the intestinal lumen → **massive diarrhea** with loss of isotonic fluid.
3. **Binding of α-bungarotoxin or curare** to nicotinic ACh receptors in skeletal muscle cells leads to **paralysis.**
4. **Graves' disease** is an autoimmune disease in which **TSH receptors are stimulated** inappropriately by binding of immunoglobulin G (IgG) autoantibodies to the receptor.
   - Manifestations include **decreased levels of TSH, enlarged thyroid gland,** and **hyperthyroidism,** leading to symptoms such as **exophthalmos** (bulging eyes), weight loss, fatigue, hand tremors, and nervousness.

G. Receptor-binding drugs
1. **Agonists** bind to and activate receptors, thereby **mimicking the action of normal ligands.**
2. **Antagonists** (e.g., beta blockers) bind to but do not activate receptors, thereby **inhibiting the action of normal ligands** by competing for binding sites.

V. Specialized Properties of the Plasma Membrane
   - In certain cell types, the plasma membrane has specialized properties that permit it to mediate functions not found in other cell types.

A. Excitability is the ability to respond to stimuli and conduct an action potential.
   - **Neurons** and **muscle cells** are the only cells that exhibit excitability.

B. Specialized attachment areas (cell junctions) are present on cells that are in close contact with other cells.

Receptors for many hormones, neurotransmitters, and other hydrophilic signaling molecules are transmembrane proteins with ligand-binding sites in their extracellular domain.

Defects in signaling can lead to cancer (abnormal Ras proteins) and Graves' disease (overstimulation of TSH receptors by IgG autoantibodies).

Some toxins (e.g., curare) and drugs (beta blockers) bind to cell-surface receptors and inhibit the action of normal ligands.

Cholera toxin acts on intestinal cells causing an increase in cAMP, which leads to massive diarrhea.

1. **Morphological types**
   a. **Zonula (belt-like) junctions** completely encircle cells.
   b. **Fascia (sheet-like) junctions** form broad areas of contact between cells.
   c. **Macula (disk-like) junctions** are like "spot welds" on the cell surface.
2. **General functions of cell junctions**
   a. **Hold cells together** into mechanically coherent tissues (**adherens** and **occludens** type)
   b. **Provide permeability seal** so that tissue as a whole acts as barrier to diffusion (**zonula occludens**)
   c. **Mediate direct communication between cells** so that materials can move from cell to cell without passing through the extracellular space (**nexus**)
3. **Molecular structure of common cell junctions** (Figure 1-7)
   a. **Zonula occludens**, or **tight junction**, is formed by interaction of intrinsic membrane proteins, thereby **fusing the outer leaflets** of the plasma membranes of adjacent cells.
   b. **Macula adherens**, or **spot desmosome**, consists of transmembrane proteins that are anchored in **cytoplasmic plaques** and extend into the intercellular space.
      • Adjacent cell membranes are held together by interlocking of the transmembrane proteins into a fibrous network, leaving a substantial space (15- to 35-nm wide) between the membranes.
      • **Keratin intermediate filaments** (tonofibrils) associate with the cytoplasmic plaques.
   c. **Nexus**, or **gap junction**, is formed by end-to-end associa-

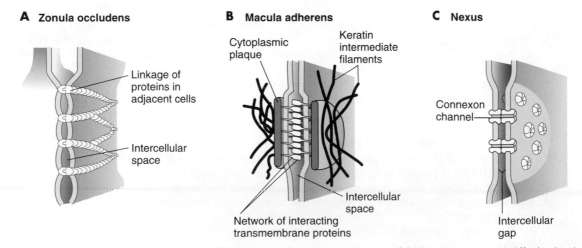

A Zonula occludens

Linkage of proteins in adjacent cells

Intercellular space

B Macula adherens

Cytoplasmic plaque

Keratin intermediate filaments

Network of interacting transmembrane proteins

Intercellular space

C Nexus

Connexon channel

Intercellular gap

Figure 1-7   Structures of three types of cell junctions. **A,** Zonulae occludens, or tight junctions, act as a diffusion barrier (e.g., between the intestinal lumen and extracellular space). **B,** Maculae adherens, or spot desmosomes, mediate cell-cell adhesion. **C,** Nexi, or gap junctions, permit direct movement of small molecules and ions between the cytosol of adjacent cells.

tion of transmembrane **connexon channels** in the interacting membranes.

- Six subunits of the protein **connexin** form each connexon channel.
- Adjacent plasma membranes are separated by a small electron-lucent zone (2- to 3-nm wide) at gap junctions.

2

Cytoplasmic Structures

I. **Introduction**
  • The cytoplasm is composed of a fluid phase (**cytosol**) and three major types of structures: **organelles**, **inclusions**, and the **cytoskeleton.**
  A. Organelles are structural subunits of cell.
    • Each type of organelle has a characteristic appearance and contains organelle-specific proteins that permit it to carry out specific functions (Figure 2-1).
  B. Inclusions are particle-like structures that are often transient, insoluble accumulations of metabolites (e.g., glycogen granules, lipid droplets).
  C. Cytoskeleton is a complex collection of macromolecules that provides structural support for the cell and plays a role in cell movements.
  D. Cytosol, the aqueous portion of the cytoplasm in which organelles and inclusions are suspended, contains numerous **soluble enzymes.**

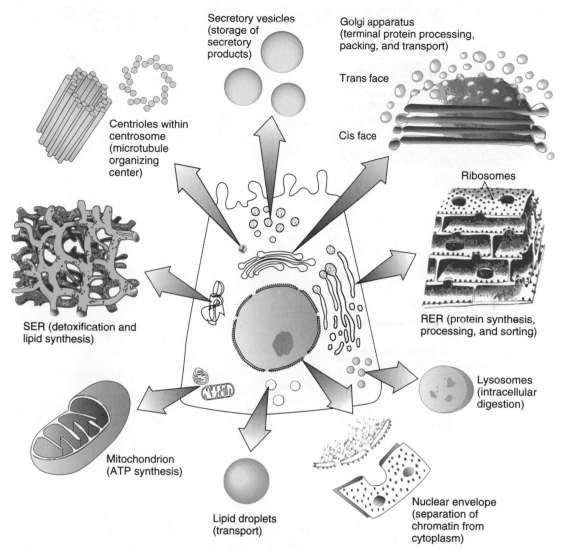

Secretory vesicles (storage of secretory products)

Golgi apparatus (terminal protein processing, packing, and transport)

Trans face

Cis face

Centrioles within centrosome (microtubule organizing center)

Ribosomes

RER (protein synthesis, processing, and sorting)

SER (detoxification and lipid synthesis)

Lysosomes (intracellular digestion)

Mitochondrion (ATP synthesis)

Lipid droplets (transport)

Nuclear envelope (separation of chromatin from cytoplasm)

Figure 2-1 Schematic diagram of "typical" mammalian cell showing major organelles and inclusions. *ATP,* Adenosine triphosphate; *RER,* rough endoplasmic reticulum; *SER,* smooth endoplasmic reticulum.

II. Mitochondria
- In aerobic cells, mitochondria are the principal sites for **synthesis of ATP.**
A. **Mitochondrial structure** (Figure 2-2)
  - Mitochondria are surrounded by **two membranes,** which are structurally and functionally distinct.
  1. **Outer mitochondrial membrane** bounds the organelle and is **freely permeable** to molecules as large as simple sugars.
  2. **Inner mitochondrial membrane** lines the **matrix** and is **relatively impermeable.**

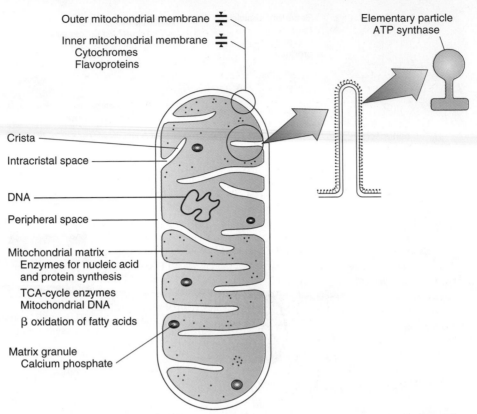

Outer mitochondrial membrane

Inner mitochondrial membrane
Cytochromes
Flavoproteins

Elementary particle
ATP synthase

Crista

Intracristal space

DNA

Peripheral space

Mitochondrial matrix
Enzymes for nucleic acid
and protein synthesis

TCA-cycle enzymes
Mitochondrial DNA

β oxidation of fatty acids

Matrix granule
Calcium phosphate

Figure 2-2 Schematic diagram of mitochondrion showing some of its structural and functional components. Both the inner and outer membranes have the typical phospholipid bilayer structure, similar to the plasma membrane.

> **a. Cristae:** infoldings of the inner mitochondrial membrane that project into the matrix and are more prominent in metabolically active cells than in quiescent cells
> **b. Elementary particles:** small particles (9 nm in diameter) that are attached to the inner membrane by a stalk and project into the matrix
> 3. **Membrane-bound compartments in mitochondrion** (see Figure 2-2)
>   **a. Peripheral (intermembranous) space**
>   **b. Intracristal space**
>   **c. Matrix region**, which contains soluble and insoluble proteins, ribosomes, **mitochondrial DNA**, and electron-dense granules of calcium phosphate.
> **B. Mitochondrial ATP production**
>   1. **Location of required enzymes**
>   **a. Tricarboxylic acid (TCA) cycle enzymes** are located in the matrix or associated with inner membrane.
>   • Catalyze oxidation of acetyl-CoA to CO_2 with generation of reduced coenzymes (NADH and $FADH_2$)

   b. **Cytochromes** and **flavoproteins**, which constitute the **electron-transport system**, are localized on the inner membrane.
   c. **ATP synthase** is localized to the elementary particles associated with the inner membrane.

 2. **Mechanisms of mitochondrial ATP production**
   - ATP is generated during operation of the TCA cycle.
   - Most mitochondrial ATP production involves **oxidative phosphorylation** via a **chemiosmotic coupling mechanism**.

   a. As electrons from reduced coenzymes flow through the electron-transport system, H^+ ions are pumped from the matrix into the intermembranous space **against** their electrochemical gradient.
   b. The reverse movement of H^+ ions into the matrix **down** their electrochemical gradient provides energy for the **coupled synthesis of ATP** from ADP (adenosine diphosphate) and inorganic phosphate (P_i) by ATP synthase.

C. **Biogenesis of mitochondria**
   - Mitochondria arise by division of preexisting mitochondria (not *de novo*) and contain their own **independent genetic machinery**.
   - Most mitochondrial proteins are encoded by nuclear DNA, but a few are encoded by mitochondrial DNA.

 1. **Products encoded by mitochondrial DNA**
   a. A few subunits of the enzymes required for mitochondrial ATP production
   b. Ribosomal RNAs and transfer RNAs required for mitochondrial protein synthesis

 2. **Synthesis of mitochondrial proteins**
   a. **Proteins encoded by mitochondrial DNA** are synthesized within the mitochondrion on ribosomes assembled within the organelle; these proteins remain with mitochondria.
   b. **Nuclear-encoded mitochondrial proteins** are synthesized in the cytosol and imported into the organelle.

 3. **Inheritance of mitochondria**
   - The ovum contributes most of the mitochondrial DNA to the zygote, whereas the sperm contributes little or none (i.e., **maternal inheritance**).

D. **Diseases associated with defective mitochondria** (Box 2-1)

III. **Lysosomes**
   - Lysosomes function as the **cell's digestive system**, degrading many materials taken up by the cell and worn-out cellular constituents (e.g., membranes, organelles).

A. **Lysosomal enzymes**
 1. **Acid hydrolases** present in the lysosomal lumen are **active at acidic pH** of about 5.0.
   - Examples include acid ribonuclease, acid deoxyribonuclease, acid phosphatase, cathepsins, specific glycosidases, and esterases.

BOX 2-1   **Hereditary Mitochondrial Diseases**

Defective mitochondria may exhibit deletions in mitochondrial DNA, defects in enzymes required for ATP synthesis, or crystal-like inclusions. These diseases exhibit **maternal inheritance.** Affected mothers transmit the disease to all their children, whereas affected fathers do not transmit the disease to any of their children. Tissues with high oxygen demand are most affected by mitochondrial dysfunction.

Mitochondrial encephalomyopathies, which usually present in early adulthood, are characterized by malfunctioning muscle mitochondria and involvement of the central nervous system. Groups of structurally abnormal mitochondria may collect just below the sarcolemma of muscle cells, producing **ragged red fibers** marked by an irregular contour and staining pattern. There are three common syndromes:

- **Kearns-Sayre syndrome:** pain in the eyes, degeneration of retinal pigments, progressive weakness of extraocular muscles, and cardiac conduction defect, which may cause death. Ragged red fibers seen on muscle biopsy.
- **MELAS syndrome:** mitochondrial encephalomyopathy, lactic acidosis, and stroke-like episodes.
- **MERRF syndrome:** myoclonus epilepsy with ragged red fibers.

Another mitochondrial disease, **Leber's hereditary optic atrophy,** is caused by a defect in one of the electron-transport complexes. It is characterized by progressive loss of central vision and eventual blindness due to degeneration of the optic nerve. This disease affects more males than females with onset most common in the third decade.

- These enzymes are inactive if released into the cytoplasm (pH 7.0).
  2. **ATP-powered H^+ pump** in the lysosomal membrane pumps H^+ ions into the lysosome maintaining the acid pH of the lumen.
- B. **Types of lysosomal activity**
  1. **Heterophagic function:** digestion of materials exogenous to the cell
  2. **Autophagic function:** digestion of cells and cell components
     - **Autolysis:** self-destruction of entire cells
- C. **Stages in lysosomal digestion** (Figure 2-3)
  1. **Endocytic vesicles** arise by phagocytosis (phagosome), pinocytosis, or receptor-mediated endocytosis (endosome).
  2. **Primary lysosomes** arise by budding from the Golgi apparatus.
  3. **Secondary lysosomes,** the sites where digestion occurs, include two types of digestive vacuoles.
     a. **Heterophagic vacuoles** formed by fusion of primary lysosomes with endocytic vesicles
     b. **Autophagic vacuoles** formed by fusion of primary lysosomes with sequestered cellular constituents

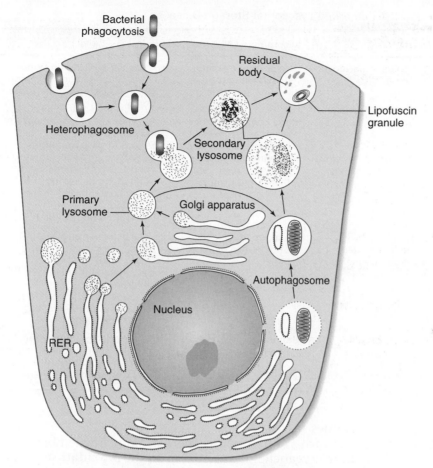

Figure 2-3 Lysosomal digestion of exogenous and endogenous materials. Heterophagic digestion is initiated by phagocytosis of a bacterium *(upper left)* or receptor-mediated endocytosis (see Figure 1-5). Autophagic digestion is initiated by sequestration of cellular components within a membrane *(lower right)*. Residual bodies and lipofuscin granules are remnants remaining after both types of digestion. *RER,* Rough endoplasmic reticulum.

4. **Postdigestive secondary lysosomes**
   a. **Residual bodies:** largely indigestible residues of heterophagic and autophagic activity
   b. **Lipofuscin granules:** large accumulations of lipid-rich material remaining after lysosomal activity in long-lived cells that do not divide
      • Lipofuscin is increased in tissues undergoing atrophy and in tissues damaged by free radicals (solutes with unpaired electrons in their outer orbit).
D. **Lysosomal storage diseases** (Table 2-1)
   • Inherited deficiency of one or more lysosomal enzymes causes **accumulation of materials that normally would be degraded.** Clinical manifestations can involve multiple tissues and organs.

Increased amounts of lipofuscin, an indigestible lipid-rich material within residual bodies, imparts a brown discoloration to tissue. Sometimes called the "wear and tear" pigment, it often is elevated in the elderly.

Lysosomal storage diseases (e.g., Tay-Sachs disease, Pompe's disease) result from defective lysosomal enzymes.

TABLE 2-1 Inherited Lysosomal Storage Diseases

Disorder	Accumulated Material	Clinical Features
Mucopolysaccharidosis	Glycosaminoglycans (GAGs) in many tissues and organs	• Presence of GAGs in urine • Other manifestations depend on which GAGs accumulate (see Box 5-1)
I-cell disease	Many compounds normally degraded in lysosomes (inability to phosphorylate mannose residues that target proteins to lysosomes)	• Absence of lysosomal enzymes in lysosomes • Severe growth impairment, extreme mental and motor retardation, clear corneas • Many dark inclusions in fibroblasts contain many dark inclusions • Onset in young children; fatal
Pompe's disease (type II glycogen storage disease)	Glycogen (deficiency of α-1,4-glycosidase)	• Enlarged liver and heart, hypotonia, mental and motor retardation • Usually fatal in infants and children • In adults, muscle weakness and respiratory problems, but usually not fatal
Tay-Sachs disease	Ganglioside GM_2 in nervous tissue	• Doll-like facies, cherry-red macular spot, seizures, hypotonia, early blindness • Infant onset; death by age 5

IV. **Peroxisomes**
- Also known as **microbodies,** peroxisomes are membrane-bounded organelles that function in the β-**oxidation of long-chain fatty acids** and **catabolism of toxic metabolites.**
  A. **Peroxisomal enzymes**
  1. **Oxidases** metabolize various substrates yielding hydrogen peroxide (H_2O_2), which is toxic to cells.
  2. **Catalase,** present in all peroxisomes, breaks down H_2O_2 to yield H_2O and O_2.
  B. **Peroxisomal disorders**
  1. **Zellweger syndrome** (cerebrohepatorenal syndrome) results from the absence of all peroxisomal enzymes in the brain, liver, and kidneys.
     - Clinical manifestations include craniofacial abnormalities, jaundice, hypotonia, hepatomegaly, and polycystic kidneys.
  2. **Adrenoleukodystrophy (ALD),** a sex-linked recessive disease, is marked by impaired peroxisomal oxidation of very-long-chain fatty acids, leading to lipid accumulation in the brain, spinal cord, and adrenal glands.
     - Clinical manifestations include mental deterioration (aphasia, apraxia), abnormal adrenal function, and loss of vision.

TABLE 2-2 Ribosomal Subunits

Subunit	rRNA*	Functions
Small (40S)	18S	Binds mRNA and aminoacyl-tRNAs Locates AUG start codon
Large (60S)	5S 5.8S 28S	Binds to small subunit after start codon is located Has peptidyl transferase activity

*Each subunit contains one molecule of each rRNA species indicated plus numerous proteins.

V. **Ribosomes**
  - Ribosomes are **particle-like ribonucleoprotein complexes** that function as the cell's **protein-synthesizing machinery**.
  A. **Structure and function of ribosomes**
    - Each ribosome comprises a **small** and **large** subunit, the composition and functions of which differ (Table 2-2).
    1. **Ribosome formation:** small (**40S**) and large (**60S**) ribosomal subunits exist free in the cytoplasm until they associate with an mRNA to form a complete ribosome (**80S**).
    2. **Translation:** an **80S ribosome** moves along the bound mRNA adding individual amino acids to the nascent protein chain one at a time.
      a. **Codons** in the mRNA bound to the **small** subunit sequentially base-pair with **anti-codons** in the corresponding activated tRNA-amino acid complexes (aminoacyl-tRNAs).
      b. **Peptidyl transferase** activity of the **large** subunit sequentially transfers aligned amino acids to the growing peptide chain, and free tRNAs then are released from the ribosome.
    3. **Chain termination:** translation ceases when a ribosome encounters a **stop codon**, causing release of the protein chain and dissociation of the ribosome into its subunits.
  B. **Functional states of ribosomes** (Figure 2-4)
    1. **Polysomes** are extended arrays of individual ribosomes all associated with a single strand of mRNA.
      - The length of a polysome and the number of ribosomes composing it reflect the length of the mRNA.
    2. **Free polysomes in the cytoplasm** carry out synthesis of cytosolic proteins and proteins destined for the nucleus, peroxisomes, and mitochondria.
    3. **Polysomes attached to the endoplasmic reticulum** (ER) carry out synthesis of all other proteins except those encoded by mitochondrial DNA.

VI. **Endoplasmic Reticulum (ER)**
  - The ER is an anastomosing intracytoplasmic membrane system consisting of vesicular, tubular, and broad cisternal profiles often arranged in regular arrays (see Figure 2-1).

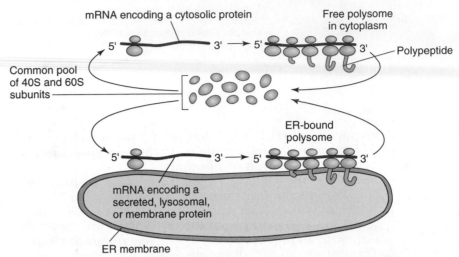

Figure 2-4 Two classes of polysomes. Free (cytosolic) polysomes and polysomes attached to the endoplasmic reticulum *(ER)* are assembled from a common pool of ribosomal subunits. Each class of polysome synthesizes specific types of proteins.

- The membranes of the ER are continuous with the nuclear envelope and are highly pleomorphic.
- **A. Structural and functional elements of the ER**
    1. **Rough endoplasmic reticulum (RER)** has a studded ("rough") appearance due to ribosomes attached to its outer (cytosolic) surface.
        - RER functions in the synthesis and posttranslation modification of the following:
        a. **Proteins secreted from the cell surface**
        b. **Soluble luminal enzymes** within the ER, Golgi apparatus, and lysosomes
        c. **Intrinsic membrane proteins** in the plasma membrane and in ER, Golgi, and lysosomal membranes
    2. **Smooth endoplasmic reticulum (SER)** shows continuities with the RER, but has no attached ribosomes and is not involved in protein synthesis.
- **B. Functions of the SER**
    1. **Lipid metabolism**
        - SER is **most prominent in lipid-metabolizing cells** (see Figure 4-6). Enzymes localized to the SER catalyze synthesis of the following lipids:
        a. **Fatty acids and glycerol**
        b. **Steroid hormones**
        c. **Phospholipids** and **cholesterol**, which are incorporated into the cytosolic side of the ER membrane

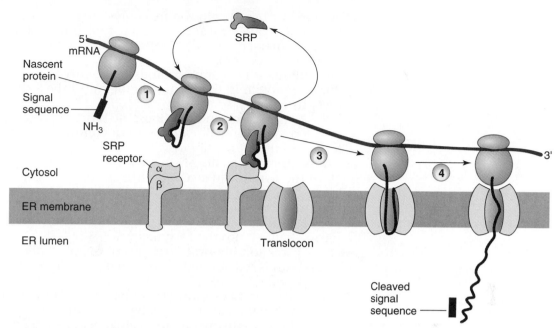

Figure 2-5 Synthesis of proteins containing an endoplasmic reticulum *(ER)* signal sequence. After synthesis of the signal sequence on a free ribosome in the cytosol, the ribosome becomes attached to the ER membrane with the aid of a signal-recognition particle *(SRP)* and SRP receptor *(1 and 2)*. The SRP then dissociates, the ribosome-nascent protein associates with a translocon, and the polypeptide chain enters the open channel in the translocon *(3)*. As translation continues, the elongating polypeptide is translocated into the ER lumen. The signal sequence is subsequently cleaved *(4)*.

- **Phospholipid translocases (flippases)** transfer some of these to the luminal side of the membrane.
2. **Detoxification by cytochrome P450 system**
   - In liver cells, SER enzymes in the cytochrome P450 system **modify** many **toxic substances** (e.g., ingested alcohol, pesticide residues, certain drugs) forming less harmful, water-soluble compounds.
   a. **Enhanced by** certain drugs (e.g., **alcohol**, **barbiturates**, **phenytoin**), leading to increased metabolism of drugs and increased synthesis of γ-glutamyl transferase
   b. **Inhibited by** certain drugs (e.g., **histamine, proton blockers**), leading to drug toxicities
3. **Ca^{2+} storage**
   - Sequestration and release of Ca^{2+} from the SER is critical in regulating the cytosolic Ca^{2+} level, which mediates various cell functions including **muscle contraction**.
4. **Glycogen metabolism**
   - In liver cells, SER enzymes are involved in the **synthesis** and **breakdown of glycogen**.
C. **Protein synthesis on the RER** (Figure 2-5)
   1. **Attachment of ribosomes to ER membrane**
      a. All proteins synthesized on the ER possess an **ER signal sequence** (or signal peptide), typically located at the amino-terminal end.

Cytochrome P450 system within the SER is important in drug metabolism. Its activity is enhanced by alcohol and barbiturates and inhibited by histamine and proton blockers.

b. Protein synthesis begins on free polysomes, but once the signal sequence is formed and extruded from a ribosome, it interacts with a **signal-recognition particle (SRP)** in the cytosol.

c. The SRP-ribosome complex binds transiently to a docking protein in the ER membrane called the **SRP receptor.**

d. The SRP is released and the ribosome-nascent protein is transferred to a **translocator protein complex (translocon)** in the ER membrane.

2. Co-translational translocation

a. Once the signal sequence is inserted into the transmembrane channel of the translocon, translation of the ER-bound mRNA continues.

b. The elongating protein chain moves through the translocon channel into the ER lumen.

(1) Water-soluble proteins: the entire polypeptide chain is translocated into lumen of the RER; signal peptide is cleaved off.

(2) Intrinsic membrane proteins: one or more hydrophobic domains in the polypeptide anchor the protein to the membrane; signal peptide may or may not be cleaved off.

3. Glycosylation of proteins

- Within the RER, a common **N-linked oligosaccharide** is attached covalently to asparagine residues in nearly all newly synthesized proteins.

4. Sorting of RER-synthesized proteins

a. Organelle-specific retention signals direct proteins to their appropriate destinations (default pathways).

- For example, proteins that are to remain in the ER contain an ER retention signal, which keeps them localized within the ER.

b. Transfer (transport) vesicles bud off from **transitional elements** lying between the RER and SER and fuse with the Golgi apparatus.

- All RER-synthesized proteins that lack an ER retention signal move to the Golgi apparatus via transfer vesicles.

c. Recovery pathways

- Proteins that are not sorted to their proper destinations often can be recovered and resorted via various recovery pathways.

In the Golgi apparatus, secreted and membrane proteins undergo processing and are sorted to their final destinations.

VII. Golgi Apparatus

- The detailed morphology and intracellular location of the Golgi apparatus vary among cell types.

A. Structure of the Golgi apparatus

- In the electron microscope, the Golgi apparatus is visualized as stacks of **flattened, disk-shaped saccules** bounded by a typical trilaminar membrane (see Figure 2-1).

1. **Cis (immature) face of the Golgi**, directed toward the ER, consists of forming cisternae and adjacent **transfer vesicles** derived from transitional elements of the ER.
2. **Mid-Golgi region** consists of a few cisternae between the cis and trans faces.
3. **Trans (mature) face of the Golgi**, directed away from the ER, consists of cisternae that bud off to form secretory vesicles and lysosome-bound transfer vesicles.

B. **Functions of the Golgi apparatus**
   1. **Processing of proteins and lipids delivered from the ER**
      • Enzymes localized to the cis, medial, or trans portions of the Golgi catalyze specific modifications (Figure 2-6).
      a. **Removal and addition of sugar residues** to N-linked oligosaccharides
      b. **Formation of O-linked oligosaccharides** by sequential addition of sugar residues to serine and threonine residues
      c. **Phosphorylation** of N-linked oligosaccharides forming **mannose-6-phosphate residues**, which target proteins to lysosomes
         • Mannose-6-phosphate receptors in lysosomes segregate these enzymes into lysosome
      d. **Sulfation** of oligosaccharide side chains on **proteoglycan core proteins** (see Chapter 5)
      e. **Proteolytic cleavage** of some precursor membrane and secreted proteins, releasing the active proteins
      f. **Glycosylation of membrane lipids** delivered to the Golgi from the SER
   2. **Macromolecule sorting from the trans Golgi**
      a. Following their processing in the Golgi, proteins and lipids are incorporated into vesicles that bud off from the trans face of the Golgi.
      b. Each vesicle must take up only appropriate proteins and fuse only with the appropriate target membrane.
   3. **Distribution of oligosaccharides**
      a. The **Golgi and RER enzymes** that form and modify oligosaccharide side chains are localized to the **luminal surface** of these organelles.
      b. Thus **oligosaccharides** in membrane glycoproteins and glycolipids face the lumen of intracellular organelles, but they become located on the **external surface** of the plasma membrane during exocytosis.

VIII. **Cytoskeleton** (Figure 2-7)
   • The three major components of the cytoskeleton—**microtubules, microfilaments,** and **intermediate filaments**—are formed from different proteins, exhibit characteristic structures, and have distinct functions.
   A. **Microtubules** (see Figure 2-7, *A*)
      1. **Structure and polarity of microtubules**

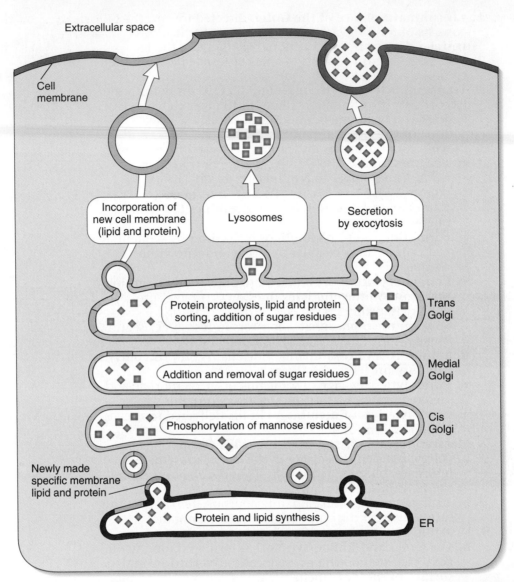

Figure 2-6 Functional regions of the Golgi apparatus. Transport vesicles from the smooth endoplasmic reticulum (SER) and rough endoplasmic reticulum (RER) fuse with the cis Golgi. This region contains enzymes that phosphorylate mannose residues in the N-linked oligosaccharides of proteins destined for lysosomes. Glycosylation of proteins and membrane lipids occurs in the medial Golgi and is completed in the trans Golgi. Vesicles containing specific macromolecules bud from the trans Golgi and eventually fuse with the corresponding target membranes.

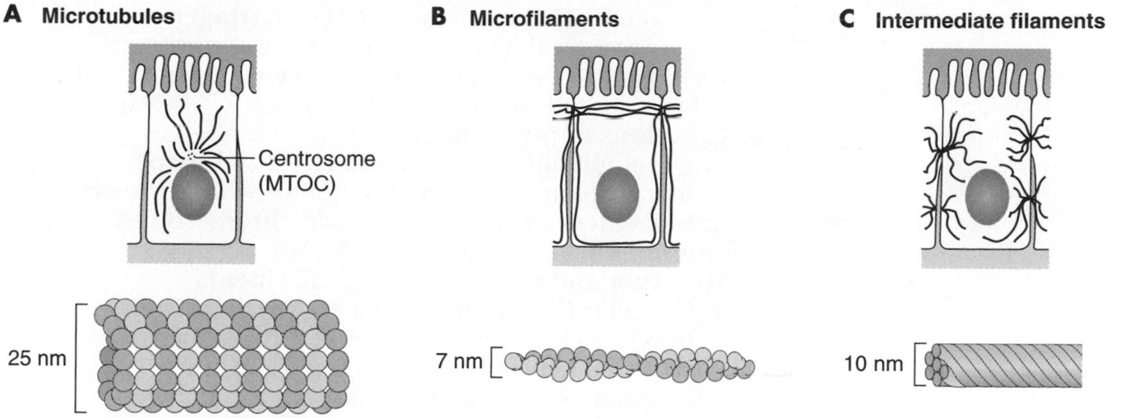

A **Microtubules**   **B** **Microfilaments**   **C** **Intermediate filaments**

25 nm   7 nm   10 nm

Figure 2-7 Comparison of the three major elements of cytoskeleton: **A,** microtubules, **B,** microfilaments, and **C,** intermediate filaments. *MTOC,* Microtubule organizing center.

    a. Each microtubule is a **hollow cylinder** (outer diameter ≈ 24 nm) with a rigid wall composed of 13 **protofilaments**, each of which is a linear polymer of αβ-**tubulin** dimers.

    b. **Plus end** is capable of **rapid growth** by addition of tubulin dimers, a process that requires GTP (guanosine triphosphate).

    c. **Minus end** loses dimers but is stabilized in most cells by association with the **microtubule-organizing center** (MTOC), or **centrosome**.

  2. Microtubule-associated proteins (MAPs)

    a. **Assembly MAPs** function primarily to stabilize microtubules, cross-linking them to each other and to other structures.

    b. **Motor MAPs (motor proteins)** use energy from ATP hydrolysis to walk or slide along microtubules, usually carrying vesicles with them.

      (1) **Dyneins** move toward the **minus end** of microtubules.

      (2) **Kinesins** move toward the **positive end** of microtubules.

  3. Microtubule-containing structures

    • Microtubules are found in the cytoplasm of all cells radiating from the centrosome, or microtubule organizing center (MTOC), which regulates their growth.

    • In addition, microtubules are organized into several specialized structures:

    a. **Mitotic spindle** and **centrioles**, which are found in most cells

    b. **Cilia, flagella,** and **basal bodies**, which have a more limited distribution (see Chapter 4)

      • **Immotile cilia syndrome** is caused by irregular dynein arms, leading to a loss of ciliary movement. This is characteristic of **Kartagener's syndrome**, which also is marked by situs inversus (e.g., heart on the right), bronchiectasis, infertility in men and women, and sinusitis.

Kartagener's syndrome is associated with irregular dynein arms in cilia, leading to a loss of ciliary movement.

   4. **Functions of microtubules**
       a. Development and maintenance of cell shape
       b. Intracellular transport of materials within the cytosol
       c. Movement of cilia, flagella, and chromosomes
   B. **Microfilaments** (see Figure 2-7, *B*)
       1. **Structure and polarity of microfilaments**
           a. Globular **G-actin** monomers polymerize in the presence of ATP to form fibrous **F-actin**, a threadlike, two-stranded helical filament about 6 nm thick.
           b. Monomers are added rapidly to one end (**plus end**) and more slowly to the other end (**minus end**).
           c. **Treadmilling**, the continual addition of monomers at the plus end and loss of monomers from the minus end of a microfilament, results in no change in length.
       2. **Actin-binding proteins**
           • Many functions of microfilaments depend on their association with various proteins. Examples include:
           a. **Anchoring proteins** (e.g., **spectrin** in erythrocytes; **dystrophin** in muscle) link cortical actin network to plasma membrane.
               • Spectrin is important in maintaining the biconcave disk shape of RBCs.
               • **Congenital spherocytosis**, an autosomal dominant disease, is characterized by a defect in spectrin, leading to the formation of spherocytes and a **chronic hemolytic anemia.**
           b. **Cross-linking proteins** (e.g., actinin, filamin) organize actin filaments into fibers, parallel arrays, or networks.

In congenital spherocytosis, a defect in spectrin in the cell membrane results in a chronic hemolytic anemia.

TABLE 2-3   Major Types of Intermediate Filament (IF) Proteins

IF Protein	Location	Function
Desmin	Muscle cells	Helps stabilize sarcomeres
Glial fibrillary acidic protein (glial filaments)	Glial cells of the CNS	Provides structural support
Keratins	Epithelial cells	Form major part of protective outer layer of skin; assist in cell adhesion by attaching to desmosomes (tonofilaments)
Lamins	Nucleus of all cells	Provide supportive network underneath the inner nuclear membrane
NF proteins (neurofilaments)	Axons of mature neurons	Form core of axons and determine their diameter
Vimentin	Fibroblasts, leukocytes, and other cells of mesenchymal origin	Supports cellular membranes; associates with microtubules

    c. Myosins are motor proteins that slide along actin filaments in muscle and nonmuscle cells, generating movement.

  3. Functions of microfilaments

    a. Movements in nonmuscle cells (labile microfilaments)

    b. Contraction of muscle (stable microfilaments)

    c. Support and maintenance of cell shape (cortical actin network)

    d. Control of cell viscosity (sol-gel transformation)

    e. Adhesion to extracellular matrix and other cells

C. Intermediate filaments (see Figure 2-7, *C*)

- Intermediate filaments primarily provide **mechanical support** to cells and **help organize cells into tissues.**
- **Several types of proteins,** exhibiting conserved and variable domains, **form intermediate filaments.**

  1. Structure of intermediate filaments

    a. Protein monomers associate laterally to form dimers with a long **coiled-coil central region;** additional lateral and end-to-end associations generate ropelike 7- to 10-nm–thick filaments.

    b. Unlike microtubules and microfilaments, **intermediate filaments do not continually add and lose monomers** and thus form much more **permanent structures.**

  2. Distribution of intermediate filaments

- Several classes of intermediate filaments exhibit cell type–specific distribution as indicated in Table 2-3.

The origin of some tumors can be determined by identifying which intermediate filament proteins they possess. Tumors of epithelial origin contain keratins and lack vimentin. Tumors of muscle origin contain desmin.

3

Nucleus and Cell Division

Target Topics

▷ Structure of chromatin and packing into chromosomes
▷ Functional elements of chromosomes
▷ Synthesis and processing of mRNA
▷ Role of nucleolus in formation of ribosomal subunits
▷ Cell cycle and its regulation
▷ Comparison of mitosis and meiosis
▷ Drug-induced cell-cycle arrest, psoriasis, tumor-suppressor genes, proto-oncogenes, Down's syndrome, Turner's syndrome, other disorders resulting from abnormal cell division

I. **Nuclear Structures** (Figure 3-1)
- The nucleus serves as a **repository for the genetic material** (DNA), and as the site for **duplication of DNA** and for **transcription of DNA into RNAs.**
   A. **Nuclear envelope:** double membrane consisting of **two trilaminar membranes** with a narrow **perinuclear cisterna** between them
      1. **Outer nuclear membrane** is continuous in places with the RER and is studded with ribosomes on its external surface.
      2. **Inner nuclear membrane** is separated from the nuclear contents by the **nuclear lamina,** a fibrous meshwork composed of **lamin** intermediate filaments.
      3. **Nuclear pores** are found where the inner and outer membranes fuse.

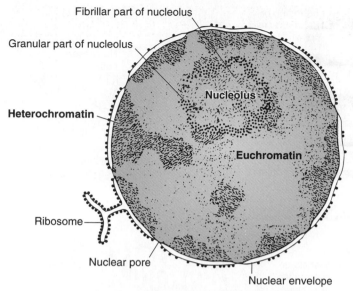

Fibrillar part of nucleolus

Granular part of nucleolus

Nucleolus

Heterochromatin

Euchromatin

Ribosome

Nuclear pore

Nuclear envelope

Figure 3-1 Schematic drawing of the interphase nucleus as visualized by electron microscopy. A narrow space separates the two membranes composing the nuclear envelope. Two types of chromatin are evident: a diffuse form, euchromatin, that is transcriptionally active, and a dense form, heterochromatin, that is largely inactive in transcription. During cell division, the chromatin becomes sufficiently coiled for individual chromosomes to be visible and the nucleolus disappears.

- Multiprotein **nuclear pore complex** associated with each pore actively transports macromolecules in and out of the nucleus.
- Small, water-soluble molecules can diffuse through aqueous channels in the nuclear pore complex.

B. **Nucleoplasm (karyoplasm):** the protoplasm within the nucleus consisting of a fluid portion, proteinaceous matrix, and various ribonucleoprotein particles

C. **Nucleolus:** nuclear region not bounded by a membrane that is involved in the synthesis of **ribosomal RNA** and its assembly into ribosomal subunits

   1. **Granular elements** are 20- to 30-nm particles representing maturing ribosomal precursors.

   2. **Fibrillar elements** may be intermingled or separated to form a fibrillar core and granular cortex (site of rRNA precursor synthesis).

D. **Chromatin and chromosomes:** form in which nuclear DNA exists within cells

- **Chromatin** is a complex of double-stranded **DNA** associated with **histone proteins.**

   1. **Two forms of isolated chromatin** (Figure 3-2, *A–C*):

      a. In **extended beads-on-a-string form,** beadlike **nucleosomes** are separated by a region of linker DNA.

         (1) Nucleosome core contains two molecules each of histones H2A, H2B, H3, and H4.

         (2) DNA is wrapped around each nucleosome core about two turns.

Antibodies against histones are characteristic of drug-induced lupus.

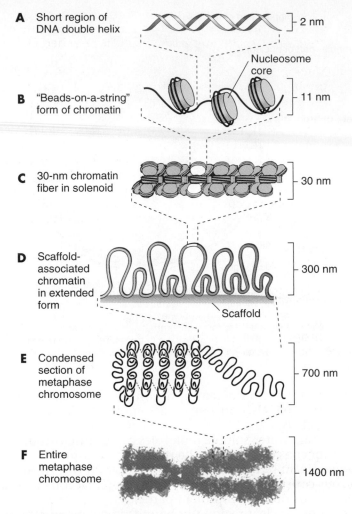

A Short region of DNA double helix — 2 nm

Nucleosome core

B "Beads-on-a-string" form of chromatin — 11 nm

C 30-nm chromatin fiber in solenoid — 30 nm

D Scaffold-associated chromatin in extended form — 300 nm

Scaffold

E Condensed section of metaphase chromosome — 700 nm

F Entire metaphase chromosome — 1400 nm

Figure 3-2 A-F, Model of chromatin packing. A nucleosome core is composed of two molecules: each of four types of histone protein with double-stranded DNA coiled around it twice. An additional histone molecule is associated with the surface of each nucleosome in the 30-nm solenoid form. In interphase chromosomes, long stretches of 30-nm chromatin loop out from a protein scaffold. Further folding of the scaffold yields the highly condensed structure of a metaphase chromosome.

Antibodies against double-stranded DNA and nuclear protein are characteristic of systemic lupus erythematosus (SLE).

b. In compact 30-nm fiber form, the nucleosomes are packed closer together in a **solenoid** arrangement, and a fifth histone (H1) interacts with the DNA between nucleosomes.

2. Metaphase chromosomes
- Extensive packing of chromatin with the aid of nonhistone **scaffold proteins** yields **highly condensed** chromosomes during metaphase (Figure 3-2, *D–F*).

a. Only during metaphase can chromosomes be visualized as separate structures by light microscopy.

   b. Because the chromosomes are duplicated during the S
   phase of the cell cycle, a metaphase chromosome is composed of two **chromatids**, which are attached at a con-
   stricted region, the **centromere.**
   c. Metaphase chromosomes of each species have characteristic sizes, shapes, and banding patterns; the entire set is
   the **karyotype.**
3. **Essential functional components of chromosomes**
   a. Replication origins: unique protein-binding DNA segments required for replication of DNA in chromosomes
   b. Telomeres: regions at the ends of chromosomes that
   prevent their shortening during replication
   c. Centromere: region of metaphase chromosomes from
   which **kinetochore fibers** extend to the spindle pole; required for proper distribution of chromatids to daughter cells
4. **States of chromatin activity** (see Figure 3-1)
   a. Euchromatin: diffuse, lightly staining form of chromatin
   that is **active in RNA synthesis**
   • During interphase, much of the nuclear DNA is
   present as euchromatin.
   b. Heterochromatin: condensed, densely staining form of
   chromatin that is **relatively inactive in RNA synthesis**
   • Some transcriptionally inactive DNA regions are
   permanent and present in all cells; others occur in
   certain tissues or periods of the cell cycle.

> Antibodies against
> the centromere
> are characteristic of
> CREST syndrome.

II. **Transcription of DNA into RNA**
   • A **gene** represents a discrete region of the genome, including a
   coding region and **regulatory sequences**, that is required for
   production of a functional RNA.
   A. **Three types of RNA function in protein synthesis.**
   1. **Messenger RNAs (mRNAs)** direct assembly of amino acids
   into proteins.
   2. **Ribosomal RNAs (rRNAs)** form part of ribosomes, the ribonucleoprotein particles on which protein synthesis occurs
   (see Table 2-2).
   3. **Transfer RNAs (tRNAs)** carry amino acids to the ribosomes
   for incorporation into growing proteins.
   B. **Synthesis of mRNA occurs outside the nucleolus** (Figure 3-3).
   1. **RNA polymerase II** catalyzes transcription of **protein-
   coding genes** into a primary RNA transcript, or **pre-mRNA.**
   2. **Processing to yield functional mRNA** entails three
   basic steps:
   a. 5' capping: addition of methylated guanine nucleotide to
   5' end of pre-mRNA
   b. Polyadenylation: addition of multiple adenylate (A) residues at 3' end of pre-mRNA
   c. Splicing: removal of noncoding introns and joining together of exons by large ribonucleoprotein complexes
   called **spliceosomes**

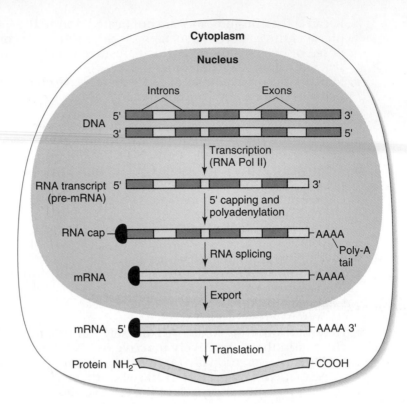

Figure 3-3 Expression of a protein-coding gene. The DNA sequence, containing coding exons and noncoding introns, is transcribed into a primary RNA transcript, or pre-mRNA, by RNA polymerase II (Pol II). Processing of the pre-mRNA yields a functional mRNA, which is translocated through nuclear pores to the cytoplasm, where it is translated into the amino acid sequence of the encoded protein on ribosomes.

C. **Synthesis of rRNA and ribosomal** subunits occurs within the nucleolus.
  1. **Nucleolar organizer DNA** consists of **tandem arrays of 45S rRNA genes** located on several chromosomes in humans.
  2. **RNA polymerase I** catalyzes transcription of pre-rRNA genes within **fibrillar regions** of the nucleolus, yielding **45S RNA precursors.**
  3. **Assembly of ribosomal subunits** occurs within **granular regions** of the nucleolus and involves the following (Figure 3-4):
     a. **Packaging of 45S rRNA precursor** with ribosomal proteins imported from the cytoplasm to form **ribonucleoprotein particles (RNPs)**
     b. **Processing and cleavage of 45S RNA** within RNPs and addition of 5S RNA produced outside the nucleolus
     c. **Separation into large (60S) and small (40S) ribosomal subunits** and their transport through nuclear pores to the cytoplasm

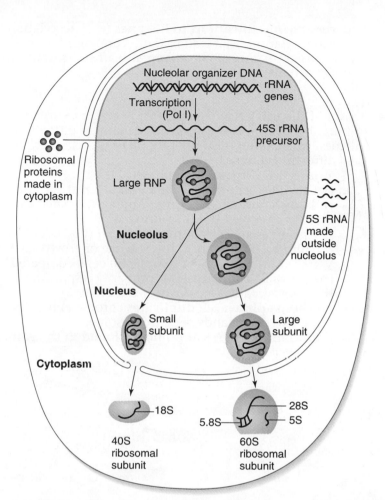

Figure 3-4 Formation of ribosomal subunits. Loops of DNA containing tandem arrays of 45S rRNA genes function as nucleolar organizers. Transcription of these genes by RNA polymerase I (Pol I) yields the 45S rRNA precursor, which associates with ribosomal and nucleolar proteins into a ribonucleoprotein particle (RNP). Processing involves cleavage of 45S rRNA into 18S, 5.8S, and 28S rRNAs; separation of large and small subunits; and incorporation of 5S rRNA (made outside the nucleolus) into large subunits. Nucleolar proteins involved in processing are recycled within the nucleolus. After their transport to the cytoplasm, large and small subunits associate with each other and with an mRNA molecule to form a functional ribosome.

    D. Differential gene expression, the selective production by a cell of only some of the proteins encoded in the genome, results primarily from **regulation of transcription.**

       • Different **cell types express specific sets of genes** related to their unique cellular activities. During development, various genes are turned on and off in highly specific temporal and spatial patterns.

      1. Transcription factors are proteins that bind to regulatory sequences in DNA and modulate expression of the associated genes.

2. Reversible modifications to histones (e.g., acetylation, phosphorylation) that lead to more-condensed or less-condensed packing of chromatin also affect its transcriptional activity.

III. **Cell Cycle**

A. **Phases of the cell cycle** (Figure 3-5)

- Duration of G_1 phase varies considerably in different cell types, whereas duration of other phases is relatively constant in different cell types.

1. **G_1 phase:** cell prepares for S phase.

   a. Cells with a very long G_1 phase, called **resting** (quiescent) **cells**, are considered to have temporarily exited the cell cycle and entered the **G_0 phase.**

      - Examples are cells of the adrenal cortex, liver cells, and cultured fibroblasts in the absence of growth factors.

   b. Variation in G_1 phase of **neoplastic cells** compared with their normal counterparts is primarily responsible for their abnormally long or short cell cycle.

2. **S (synthesis) phase:** cell **duplicates** chromosomal DNA, yielding two chromatids per chromosome.

   a. **C amount of DNA** is the amount found in the **gametes** of a species.

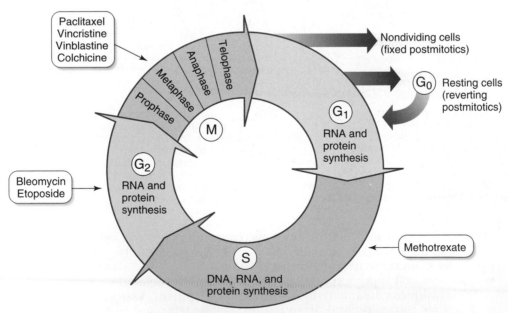

Figure 3-5 The cell cycle in eukaryotic cells. G_1, S, and G_2 constitute interphase, during which synthetic activity takes place. DNA synthesis occurs only during the S phase. The major stages of mitosis *(M)* are indicated. Differentiated cells that no longer divide under any circumstances (e.g., neurons) have left the cycle. Cells that have temporarily stopped dividing (i.e., have very long G_1) but can reenter the cycle are considered to be resting cells in G_0. Certain drugs arrest cells at the indicated stages of the cell cycle.

  b. **Somatic cells** have **2C DNA in G_1** and **4C DNA in G_2** following DNA replication.

  c. **Ploidy** refers to the status of the basic chromosome set characteristic of a species and is indicated by *n*.

   (1) **Haploid cells** = $1n$ = gametes; normal human gametes contain 23 chromosomes.

   (2) **Diploid cells** = $2n$ = somatic cells; normal human somatic cells contain 46 chromosomes, 23 pairs of **homologous chromosomes,** one member of each pair derived from the maternal parent and one from the paternal parent.

 3. **G_2 phase:** cell prepares for division (e.g., synthesis of tubulin, which is necessary for formation of mitotic spindle).

 4. **M (mitotic) phase:** chromatids of duplicated chromosomes segregate toward spindle poles and cytoplasm divides (**cytokinesis**), forming two daughter cells.

  • M phase generally is the **shortest.**

B. **Regulation of the cell cycle**

 1. **Cell-cycle control proteins**

  • Two major classes of proteins regulate progression through the cell cycle.

  a. **Cyclin-dependent protein kinases (Cdks)** phosphorylate various target proteins, thereby modulating their activity at different cell-cycle phases.

  b. **Cyclins** activate Cdks by binding to them.

   • **Concentrations** of various cyclins **rise and fall** throughout the cell-cycle phases, leading to formation of specific **cyclin/Cdk complexes.**

   (1) Cyclin D, synthesized during early G_1, binds to Cdk4, forming a complex that allows the cell to enter S phase.

   (2) **Cyclin A** binds to Cdk1 and Cdk2, forming complexes that allows the cell to progress from S phase to G_2 phase and that induces synthesis of cyclin B.

   (3) **Cyclin B,** synthesized during G_2, binds to Cdk1, forming a complex that allows the cell to enter mitosis (M).

 2. **Cell-cycle checkpoints**

  • Under certain circumstances, **arrest of the cell cycle** at one of several checkpoints **prevents major damage to cells.**

  a. **G_1 checkpoint:** presence of damaged DNA stops cycle before entry into S phase, thus avoiding replication of damaged DNA, which could perpetuate mutations and lead to chromosomal rearrangements.

  b. **G_2 checkpoint:** presence of unreplicated or damaged DNA stops cycle before entry into mitosis.

  c. **M checkpoint:** improper spindle formation stops cycle part way through mitosis, thereby preventing missegregation of chromatids to daughter cells.

3. Role of tumor-suppressor genes in cell-cycle control
   a. Retinoblastoma (Rb) protein, encoded by the *RB* suppressor gene on chromosome 13, inhibits progression from G_1 phase to S phase.
   (1) Phosphorylation of Rb protein by active cyclin D/Cdk4 complex allows cell to enter S phase.
   (2) Inactivation of the *RB* suppressor gene accelerates cell entry into S phase.
   b. p53 Protein, encoded by *p53* suppressor gene on chromosome 17, is stabilized by damaged DNA, leading to its accumulation.
   (1) Inhibition of cyclin D/Cdk4 activity by p53 protein keeps cell in G_1 for DNA repair (G_1 arrest) or apoptosis if damage is too extensive.
   (2) Inactivation of *p53* suppressor gene permits cell to enter S phase continuously.
C. Drugs that target the cell cycle (see Figure 3-5)
   • Many antineoplastic drugs reduce cell proliferation by blocking progression through the cell cycle.
   1. Colchicine inhibits spindle formation, causing arrest in metaphase.
      • Occasionally used in the treatment of **gouty arthritis.**
   2. Vincristine and **vinblastine** block assembly of the mitotic spindle.
   3. Paclitaxel prevents disassembly of the mitotic spindle at the end of mitosis.
   4. Fluorouracil (5-FU) and **methotrexate**, which both inhibit DNA synthesis, primarily inhibit the S phase.
   5. Bleomycin and **etoposide** primarily block the G_2 phase.
D. Classification of cells based on their mitotic activity
   • In the adult organism, cells vary in regard to the frequency with which they undergo mitosis.
   1. Cells that divide continuously
      a. Vegetative intermitotic cells, or **stem cells** (e.g., basal cells in epidermis or intestinal glands; stem cells in the bone marrow)
         • These undifferentiated cells replicate to replace themselves and to provide precursors for specialized cells that are lost or damaged.
      b. Differentiating intermitotic cells (e.g., cells in spinous layer of epidermis)
         • These cells, which arise from stem cells, continue to divide as they differentiate into specialized cells.
   2. Cells that divide infrequently or not at all
      a. Resting cells, or reverting postmitotics (e.g., liver cells, smooth muscle cells, astrocytes)
         • Most resting cells have exited the cell cycle at G_1, entering the so-called G_0 phase (see Figure 3-5).
         • These specialized cells require a loss of tissue (trauma) or stimulation by growth factors or hormones to move them into the G_1 phase and resume replication.

   b. Nonreplicators, or fixed postmitotics (e.g., cells in granu-
      losum or corneum layer of epidermis, neurons, striated
      and cardiac muscle cells)
      • These highly specialized cells, which are **permanently
        incapable of cell division,** can be replaced only from
        an appropriate stem-cell population.
E. Conditions caused by malfunctioning of the cell cycle
   1. Polyploidy results from failure of a cell to undergo cytokine-
      sis (division of the cytoplasm) before entering the next cell
      cycle.
      a. Megakaryocytes normally are polyploid.
      b. Many tumor cells are polyploid, one of the many abnor-
         malities of these cells.
   2. Psoriasis results from failure of replicating cells of the basal
      and spinous layers of the epidermis to differentiate into
      nonreplicating cells of the keratinized layer.
      • Continued proliferation of these cells (hyperplasia) leads
        to formation of the **erythematous plaques** characteristic
        of psoriasis.
   3. Development of many cancers has been associated with
      mutations in two types of genes that regulate cell growth
      and proliferation (Box 3-1).

Oncogenes (e.g., *ras, erbB₂*) can cause transformation of normal cells into cancer cells. Most oncogenes are mutant, unregulated forms of normal genes encoding proteins that promote cell growth or proliferation.

Tumor-suppressor genes (e.g., *RB, p53*) normally encode proteins that inhibit cell proliferation. Inactivating mutations in such genes lead to unrestricted cell growth and potential for cancer.

| **BOX 3-1** | **Properties and Classification of Neoplasms** |

Benign neoplasms are relatively slow growing, commonly circular, and usually encapsulated. Few mitotic figures, which have a normal structure, are seen. The cells are well differentiated, resembling the cell/tissue from which the neoplasm arose.

Malignant neoplasms, or **cancers,** are fast growing, not usually encapsulated, and invade local tissue. Many mitotic figures with some showing abnormalities (e.g., tripolar metaphase) are seen. The cells are in various stages of dedifferentiation and may change so much (**anaplasia**) that the cell/tissue of origin cannot be determined. Cancers are categorized as carcinomas or sarcomas.

A **carcinoma** is any malignant neoplasm that originates in an epithelium (membranous or glandular) regardless of the embryonic germ layer from which the epithelium is derived. For example:
• Squamous cell carcinoma of the epidermis (ectodermal derivative)
• Transitional cell carcinoma of the bladder (mesodermal derivative)
• Adenocarcinoma of the colon (endodermal derivative)
• Carcinoma of the kidney (mesodermal derivative)

A **sarcoma** is any malignant neoplasm that originates in nonepithelial (mesenchymal) tissue. For example:
• Rhabdomyosarcoma (skeletal muscle origin)
• Leiomyosarcoma (smooth muscle origin)
• Liposarcoma (adipose cell origin)
• Fibrosarcoma (fibroblast origin)
• Osteogenic sarcoma (bone origin)

- Usually **several mutations** are required to transform a normal cell into a cancerous cell.
  a. **Tumor-suppressor genes** (e.g., *RB* and *p53*) encode proteins that normally inhibit cell proliferation.
     - Mutations leading to inactivation of these genes contribute to development of **retinoblastoma, pancreatic** and **colon cancers**, and some **breast cancers.**
  b. **Proto-oncogenes** (e.g., *ras* and *erbB₂*) encode proteins that normally promote cell growth and proliferation.
     - Mutations leading to overexpression, amplification, or translocation of these genes contribute to development of **bladder, colon, breast, skin,** and **lung cancers.**

> A neoplasm, or tumor, is any new, abnormal growth of tissue.

IV. **Mitosis and Meiosis**
  A. **Mitosis:** cell division in which diploid **somatic cells** give rise to diploid daughter cells (Figure 3-6, *A*)
     1. **Entering mitosis:** each duplicated chromosome = 2 chromatids; cell contains 92 chromatids = 4C DNA.
     2. **At metaphase:** each duplicated chromosome aligns individually along the equatorial plate.
     3. **At anaphase:** chromatids of each chromosome are pulled toward opposite spindle poles leading to **equational division.**
     4. **Following mitosis and cytokinesis:** each daughter cell receives 46 chromatids corresponding to 23 pairs of homologous chromosomes = 2C DNA.
     5. **During the next S phase:** chromosomes duplicate so that there are 92 chromatids at the beginning of the next mitosis.
  B. **Meiosis:** special form of cell division in which diploid developing **germ cells** give rise to haploid gametes (Figure 3-6, *B*).
     1. Meiosis I (reductional division)
        a. **Pairing of duplicated homologous chromosomes** (4C DNA) at equatorial plate occurs during first meiotic division.
        b. **Crossing over and recombination** between maternal and paternal chromatids leads to new combinations of genes on the chromosomes.
        c. **Chromatids** of each chromosome **do not separate** during anaphase, and maternally and paternally derived chromosomes are randomly segregated to daughter cells.
        d. Both the number of chromosomes and DNA content is halved by this **reductional division,** yielding daughter cells with 23 chromosomes (1*n*), or 46 chromatids = 2C DNA.
     2. Meiosis II (equational division)
        a. Daughter **cells** from meiosis I soon **undergo a second division without any intervening DNA synthesis.**
        b. The chromatids separate at anaphase, similar to mitosis.
        c. Each daughter cell (**gamete**) receives 23 chromosomes (23 chromatids); the haploid chromosome number (1*n*) = 1C DNA.

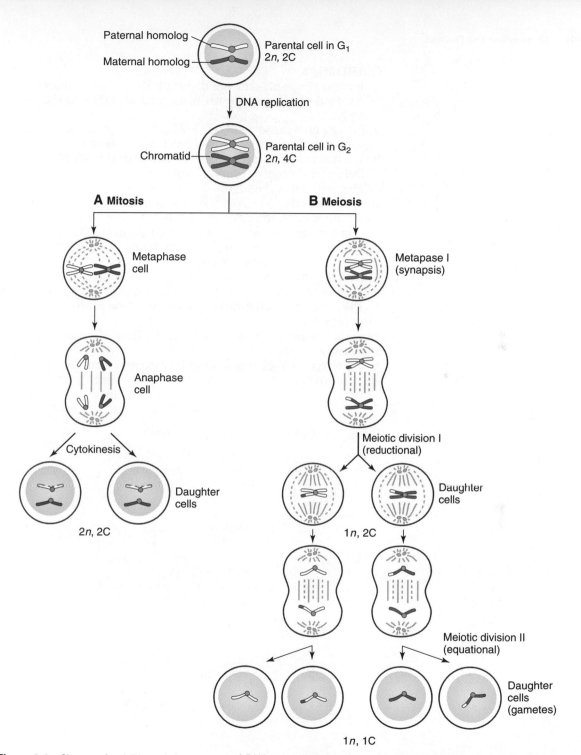

Figure 3-6 Changes in ploidy and the amount of DNA per cell during the cell cycle and mitotic or meiotic division. A normal diploid (2n) cell has 2C of nuclear DNA in G_1. During the S phase, the amount of DNA is precisely doubled to 4C. **A,** Mitosis occurs in somatic cells. The 4C in a G_2 cell is halved, but the number of chromosomes remains the same (2n) in the daughter cells. **B,** Meiosis occurs during formation of gametes. A diploid germ-cell precursor in G_2 with 4C DNA goes through two divisions without intervening DNA synthesis. Meiosis I (reductional division) produces daughter cells (secondary spermatocytes or oocytes) that are haploid (1n) and contain 2C DNA. Meiosis II (equational division) produces gametes (spermatids or ootids), which are haploid (1n) and contain 1C DNA. Because of recombination at synapsis of metaphase I and random segregation of maternal and paternal chromosomes during the first meiotic division, each gamete has a unique genetic constitution.

3. **Fertilization**
   - Fusion of sperm and egg during fertilization **restores the diploid chromosome number and 2C DNA in the zygote.**
   - **a.** 23 egg chromosomes (1C) + 23 sperm chromosomes (1C) = 46 zygote chromosomes ($2n$, 2C).
   - **b.** DNA synthesis restores the G_2 amount of DNA (4C) before the zygote enters mitosis.

C. **Sex determination** (Figure 3-7)
   1. **Human females** produce a **single type of gamete (ovum)** containing 22 autosomes and an X chromosome (**23,X**).
   2. **Human males** produce **two types of gametes (sperm):** one has 22 autosomes and an X chromosome (**23,X**); the other has 22 autosomes and a Y chromosome (**23,Y**).
   3. **Male offspring** results from fertilization of an ovum by a Y-bearing sperm.
      - **Presence of Y chromosome in zygote = male phenotype.**
   4. **Female offspring** results from fertilization of an ovum by an X-bearing sperm.
      - **Absence of Y chromosome in zygote = female phenotype.**

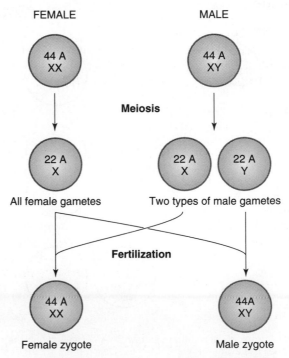

Figure 3-7   Sex determination in humans. *A,* Autosomes; *X* and *Y,* sex chromosomes. The male parent produces two types of gametes and determines the sex of the zygote, which must have a Y chromosome to exhibit the male phenotype.

D. Sex chromatin in females
- In all somatic cells of females, one of the X chromosomes is permanently in condensed heterochromatin form, known as a **Barr body**, which is visible during interphase.
- Presence or absence of Barr bodies permits **identification of the chromosomal sex** of an individual even when the external genitalia are ambiguous. **The number of Barr bodies = number of X chromosomes minus 1.**

Barr body (sex chromatin): permanent heterochromatin mass in female cells corresponding to a single, inactive, condensed X chromosome.

V.   **Abnormalities of Cell Division**
   A. Differences in effects of similar abnormalities
   - Clinical manifestations of cell-division abnormalities vary depending on whether abnormalities occur during mitosis or meiosis and on which chromosomes are affected.
      1. Abnormalities during mitosis result in some somatic cells with the aberration and others that are normal, a condition called **mixoploidy,** or **chromosome mosaicism.**
      2. Abnormalities during meiosis produce aberrant gametes. Fertilization of an aberrant gamete with a normal gamete results in offspring in which virtually all of the cells carry the aberration.
   B. Major causes of cell-division abnormalities
      1. Nondisjunction: failure of a single pair of chromosomes (meiosis I) or a single pair of chromatids (meiosis II or mitosis) to separate at cell division.
      - One daughter cell receives two of the chromosomes or chromatids affected; the other daughter cell receives none.
      2. Anaphase lagging: lagging of a chromosome (meiosis I) or a chromatid (meiosis II or mitosis) behind the remainder of the chromosomes so that it is not included in one of the daughter cells.
      - One daughter cell is normal; the other daughter cell lacks the affected chromosome.
      3. Deletion: a fragment of a chromosome breaks off.
      - If the fragment lacks a kinetochore, that portion of the chromosome is lost at cell division and is missing from one of the daughter cells.
      4. Translocation: a piece of chromosome is broken off of one chromosome and is attached to another chromosome that is not its homologue.
   C. Specific disorders caused by abnormal meiosis
      1. Down's syndrome generally results from nondisjunction.
         a. Affected individuals have **one extra chromosome 21 (trisomy 21)** in all their cells.
         b. Clinical manifestations include **mental retardation, atrial septal defect** (ASD), short stature, anteroposteriorly flattened skull with short flat-bridged nose, epicanthal fold, stubby appendages, and simian crease in the hands.
      2. Turner's syndrome results from nondisjunction or anaphase lagging.

Nondisjunction during meiosis results in some gametes with an extra copy of one chromosome (e.g., 23) and some gametes lacking that chromosome.

Down's syndrome: one extra chromosome 21 (trisomy 21).

Turner's syndrome: lack of all (45,XO) or a portion of one sex chromosome; female phenotype; no Barr bodies.

Klinefelter's syndrome: extra X chromosome in males (47,XXY); one Barr body.

    a. Affected individuals **lack one sex chromosome (monosomy)** in all their cells (most commonly **45,XO** with no Barr bodies).

    b. Clinical manifestations include **short stature, undifferentiated gonads,** web neck, aortic coarctation, and sterility.

  3. Klinefelter's syndrome usually results from nondisjunction.

    a. Affected individuals have an **extra X chromosome** in all their cells (most commonly **47,XXY** with one Barr body).

    b. Clinical manifestations include **tall stature with disproportionately long arms and legs, small testes, eunuchoid body habitus,** gynecomastia, and infertility.

  4. Cri du chat syndrome results from a deletion during meiosis.

    a. Affected individuals have a normal number of chromosomes but **lack short arm of chromosome 5** in all their cells.

    b. Clinical manifestations include **severe mental deficiency, ventricular septal defect,** microcephaly, hypertelorism, and a **plaintive catlike cry.**

D. Specific disorders caused by abnormal mitosis

  1. Chronic myelogenous leukemia results from a reciprocal translocation during hematopoiesis in the bone marrow.

    • Blood cells and their precursors contain a shortened **chromosome 22 (Philadelphia chromosome)** and an abnormal **chromosome 9** that carries the *bcr-abl* oncogene formed by the translocation.

Philadelphia chromosome: shortened chromosome 22 (22q⁻) due to translocation with chromosome 9 (9q⁺). It is present in marrow and blood cells of those with chronic myelogenous leukemia.

  2. Aniridia (absence of the iris) results from deletion of a portion of **chromosome 11** during embryonic development of the eye.

    • Individuals with this disorder have a high incidence of **Wilms' tumor of the kidney.**

Epithelial Tissue

4

Target Topics

▸ Cellular structure of various types of epithelia and their distribution in the body

▸ Specialized structures of apical, lateral, and basal surfaces of epithelial cells

▸ Microvilli, cilia, and cell junctions

▸ Turnover of epithelia

▸ Exocrine gland secretions

▸ Epithelial cell tumors, immotile cilia syndrome, Kartagener's syndrome, bullous pemphigoid

I. **Introduction**
   A. **Major types of epithelia**
      1. **Membranous epithelia** are sheetlike tissues that cover or line the surfaces, cavities, and organs of the body.
      2. **Glandular epithelia** perform secretory functions and form the parenchyma of glands.
   B. **Characteristic properties**
      1. **Polarity:** the cells composing many epithelia have distinct **apical, lateral,** and **basal domains** that are structurally and functionally different.
      2. **Absence of blood vessels:** epithelia are **avascular tissues** that receive nourishment from associated vascularized connective tissue.
      3. **Separation from surrounding tissue:** the **basement membrane** separates epithelia from the underlying connective tissue (see Chapter 5, section V).

II. **Classification of Membranous Epithelia** (Figure 4-1; Table 4-1)
   A. **Simple epithelia** are composed of a **single layer** of cells, all of which contact the basement membrane.

TABLE 4-1   Membranous Epithelia

Type	Surface Layer	Common Locations
Single Layer		
Simple squamous	Flattened cells	• Endothelium (lining of blood vessels) • Mesothelium (lining of peritoneum and pleura) • Lining of alveoli • Renal corpuscles
Simple cuboidal	Cuboidal cells	• Terminal bronchioles • Uriniferous tubules • Ducts of many glands
Simple columnar	Columnar cells	• Epithelial lining of stomach and intestines
Pseudostratified columnar	Columnar cells and basal cells (both contact basement membrane)	• Epithelial lining of large conducting airways (respiratory epithelium)
Multiple Layers		
Stratified squamous (keratinized, dry, cornified)	Flattened anucleated cells filled with many keratin filaments	• Epidermis of skin
Stratified squamous (nonkeratinized, wet, noncornified)	Flattened nucleated cells containing some keratin filaments	• Epithelial lining of mouth, esophagus, and vagina
Stratified cuboidal	Cuboidal cells	• Ducts of sweat glands
Stratified columnar	Columnar cells	• Larger ducts of salivary and mammary glands
Transitional (uro-epithelium)	Large, flattened cells when stretched; thicker, dome-shaped cells when relaxed	• Lining of ureters and bladder

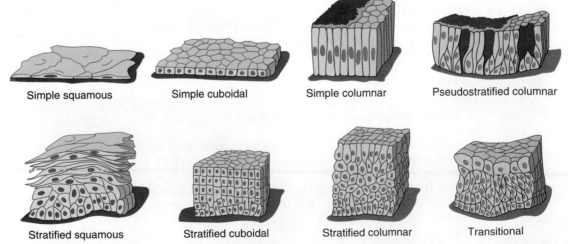

Simple squamous   Simple cuboidal   Simple columnar   Pseudostratified columnar

Stratified squamous   Stratified cuboidal   Stratified columnar   Transitional

Figure 4-1   Membranous epithelia. The number of cell layers in an epithelium and the shape of the surface cells provide the basis for classifying epithelia.

B. Stratified epithelia are composed of **multiple layers** of cells with only cells in the deepest (**basal**) layer contacting the basement membrane.

C. Shape of surface cells is basis for classifying epithelia as **squamous, cuboidal,** or **columnar.**

III. Specializations of the Epithelial Cell Surface

 A. **Apical Epithelial Surface**

  1. **Microvilli** are **short, nonmotile** finger-like projections of the plasma membrane (about 1.5 μm long and 0.1 μm in diameter).

   a. "**Brush**" or "**striated**" **border** visible by light microscopy consists of numerous microvilli extending from the apical surface of an epithelium into a lumen.

   • Prominent in **intestine** and **proximal convoluted tubule** of kidney

   b. **Actin microfilaments** fill the core of microvilli.

   c. **Terminal web,** composed of keratin-like **intermediate filaments,** lies at the base of each microvillus, anchoring it to the cytoskeleton.

  2. **Cilia** are **long, motile** processes extending from cell surface (5 to 15 μm long and 0.2 μm in diameter).

   a. **Axoneme,** or core, of each cilium has **9 + 2 pattern** consisting of 9 radially arranged **doublet microtubules** and 2 **central singlet microtubules** (Figure 4-2).

   b. **Basal body,** containing 9 radially arranged **triplet microtubules,** lies at the base of a cilium and functions to anchor it to the cell.

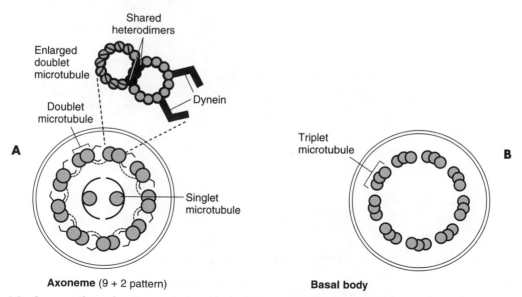

Axoneme (9 + 2 pattern)   **Basal body**

Figure 4-2 Cross sections of a cilium and a basal body. **A,** The axoneme, which forms the core of a cilium, contains two central singlet microtubules surrounded by nine doublet microtubules. **B,** A basal body, the anchoring structure of a cilium, contains a ring of nine triplet microtubules.

c. Ciliary beating propels surrounding fluid or particles along the surface in one direction.

- **Dynein** side arms, which extend between adjacent doublets, **hydrolyze ATP** to generate a sliding force that results in a bending movement responsible for beating of cilia (Box 4-1).

3. Stereocilia are **long, nonmotile** projections similar in structure to microvilli (not cilia).

- Found in the epithelial lining of the **epididymis** and **vas deferens**, where they increase the absorptive surface area
- Also present on **hair cells of the inner ear**, where they have a sensory function (see Chapter 19)

B. **Lateral epithelial surfaces** (Figure 4-3)

BOX 4-1 **Immotile Cilia Syndrome**

Defects in the dynein arms that affect the ability of cilia to beat cause several hereditary disorders collectively termed *immotile cilia syndrome*. These disorders are characterized by delayed or absent clearance of debris and microbes from the airways, leading to **recurrent infection of the lower respiratory tract**. Frequently, sperm motility also is impaired.

Kartagener's syndrome involves a combination of **situs inversus** and immotile cilia syndrome marked by **bronchiectasis** and **sinusitis**. It is transmitted as an autosomal dominant trait.

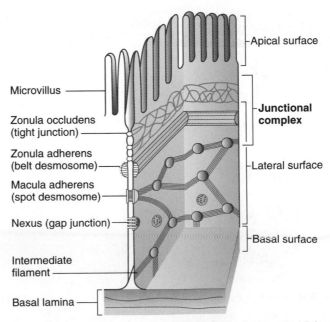

Figure 4-3   General structure of absorptive epithelial cells in the intestinal lining. These polarized cells exhibit numerous apical, lateral, and basolateral specializations. Also see Figure 1-7.

1. **Junctional complex:** three closely associated **cell junctions** generally found on the lateral surfaces of **columnar epithelial cells**
   a. **Zonula occludens,** or **tight junction,** forms a permeability barrier just below apical surface.
   b. **Zonula adherens,** or **belt desmosome,** encircles entire cell periphery forming a broad region of adhesion just basal to zonula occludens.
   c. **Maculae adherens,** or **spot desmosomes,** are disklike adhesive junctions located basal to zonula adherens.
2. **Nexus,** or **gap junction:** protein-lined channel through which ions and small molecules can pass between adjacent cells

C. **Basal epithelial surface**
   1. **Hemidesmosomes:** specialized adherens junctions in the basal plasmalemma that link cells to the underlying **basal lamina** (see Chapter 5)
      - **Bullous pemphigoid** is an autoimmune disease characterized by **chronic blisters (bullae)** in the skin mainly on the thighs, arms, and abdomen. It is associated with IgG autoantibodies against hemidesmosomes and usually seen in the elderly.
   2. **Basal striations:** infoldings of the basal plasma membrane found in epithelia engaged in active transport (e.g., proximal and distal convoluted tubules of the kidney, ducts of certain glands)

IV. **Glandular Epithelia**
   - Glandular epithelial cells are organized into **secretory units,** which in some cases are connected to the surface by **ducts.**
   - The **secretory products** synthesized and released by glandular epithelial cells include proteins, steroid hormones, and mucus.

A. **Exocrine glands** deliver their secretion **externally** to a surface either directly or through a duct system.
   1. **Exocrine glands with ducts** are classified in terms of the **branching** of their ducts (simple, compound) and **shape** of their secretory units (tubular, acinar, alveolar) (Figure 4-4, *A*).
      - These glands include **salivary, sebaceous,** and **gastric glands** as well as the exocrine portions of the **pancreas** and **liver.**
   2. **Exocrine glands without ducts** are part of a membranous epithelium (Figure 4-4, *B*).
      a. **Unicellular glands** (e.g., **goblet cells** in intestinal and respiratory epithelia)
      b. **Intraepithelial gland** (e.g., urethral glands)
   3. **Mechanisms of exocrine secretion**
      a. **Holocrine secretion:** secretory cells in their entirety, along with their contents, are released (e.g., sebaceous gland).
      b. **Apocrine secretion:** apical portion of secretory cells is released with the contents (e.g., mammary gland epithelium).

Bullous pemphigoid (pemphigus vulgaris): chronic blistering of skin and mucous membranes resulting from defective adhesion of epithelia to underlying matrix.

Glandular epithelial cells release secretory products by holocrine, apocrine, or merocrine secretion.

Exocrine glands: secretory product released externally to an internal or external surface; may or may not have ducts.

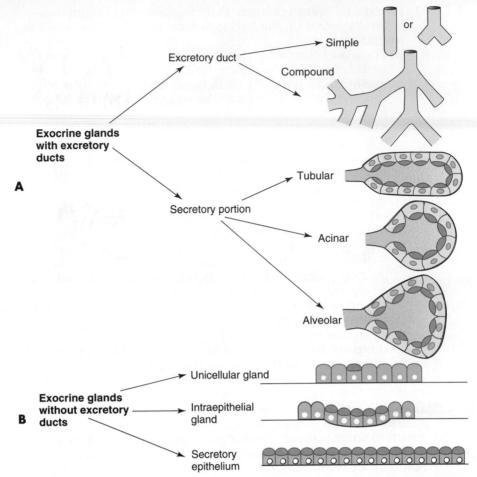

Figure 4-4 Exocrine glands. Glands with ducts are classified as simple or compound based on the branching of their duct system. These glands are further classified according to the morphology of their secretory units.

    c. Merocrine secretion: contents of **secretory granules**, or vesicles, are released from the cells by **exocytosis** (e.g., pancreatic exocrine cell).

B. Endocrine glands do not have ducts and deliver their secretions **internally** into the bloodstream (see Chapter 18).
- Scattered hormone-producing cells present in various epithelia (e.g., in the GI tract) function as **unicellular** endocrine glands.
- Most endocrine glands (e.g., thyroid gland) are **multicellular.**

Endocrine glands: secretory product released internally to bloodstream; no ducts.

V. Turnover of Epithelia
- **Surface epithelial cells,** which constantly undergo cell death or suffer damage, are **replaced on a continuous basis.**

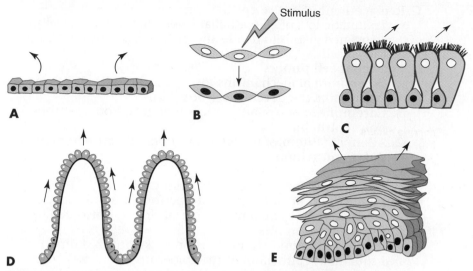

Figure 4-5 Turnover of epithelial cells. **A** and **B,** Epithelia lacking specialized cells. **C-E,** Epithelia containing postmitotic specialized cells and continuously replicating cells. In cells capable of cell division the nucleus is black; in other cells the nucleus is white.

- Various regulatory mechanisms normally control the generation of replacement cells to balance the loss of cells.
A. In simple epithelia consisting of relatively nonspecialized cells
  1. Virtually all the cells either constantly divide and replace themselves (e.g., cuboidal epithelium in bronchioles).
  2. When stimulated by trauma or other signals (e.g., capillary endothelium) (Figure 4-5, *A, B*).
B. In epithelia containing specialized cells
  - Postmitotic **differentiated surface cells,** which have lost the ability to divide, are continually sloughed off and are replaced from a population of **continuously replicating stem cells**.
  1. Pseudostratified epithelium (e.g., respiratory epithelium)
     - **Basal cells** constantly divide; some of their progeny differentiate into glandular or ciliated cells (Figure 4-5, *C*).
  2. Gland-containing columnar epithelium (e.g., intestinal epithelium)
     - **Cells in the necks of glands** constantly divide; some of their progeny differentiate and migrate to the surface where they replace the surface cells (Figure 4-5, *D*).
  3. Stratified epithelium (e.g., epidermis, lining of ducts)
     - **Basal cells** replicate continuously; some of their progeny migrate into the intermediate layers.
     - **Cells in intermediate layers,** adjacent to the basal layer, differentiate and migrate to the surface and may continue to replicate and divide.
     - Cells on the surface are postmitotic cells that have lost the ability to replicate or divide.

The constant turnover of epithelial cells makes epithelia common sites for tumor development.

C. Replacement of entire epithelium

- Traumatic loss of all epithelial layers may stimulate cells in associated glands to divide and differentiate into surface epithelial cells.

D. Epithelial cell tumors

- When normal mechanisms for regulating epithelial turnover fail, tumors can develop (see Box 3-1).
    1. **Carcinomas:** malignant tumors that arise from **membranous epithelia**
    2. **Adenocarcinomas:** malignant tumors that arise from **glandular epithelium**

VI. Functional Specializations of Epithelial Cells

- The ability of different epithelia to perform various functions depends on their numerous specializations, as illustrated by the following examples:

A. Protection from injury and abrasion by keratinized (dry) stratified squamous epithelium of the epidermis

1. **Flattened shape** of surface cells provides maximal strength.
2. **Abundant macula adherens** permit strong adhesion between cells.
3. **Keratinized surface cells** resist water loss.

B. Absorption by intestinal epithelial cells (see Figure 4-3)

1. **Junctional complex** maintains integrity of tissue.
2. **Numerous microvilli** (brush border) increase surface area for absorption.

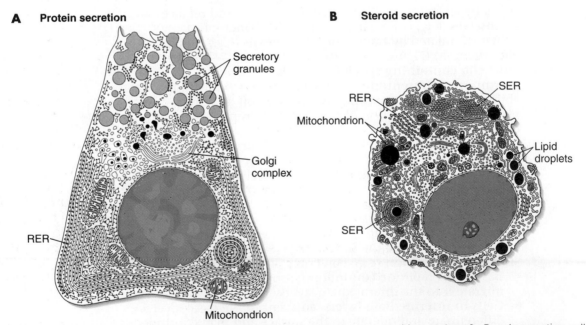

Figure 4-6 Glandular epithelial cells specialized for protein secretion or steroid secretion. **A,** Protein-secreting cells exhibit extensive rough endoplasmic reticulum *(RER)* and Golgi complex as well as many secretory granules in the apical region. **B,** Steroid-secreting cells exhibit well-developed smooth endoplasmic reticulum *(SER)* and numerous lipid droplets throughout the cell. All secretory cells possess abundant mitochondria, which produce ATP for synthetic reactions.

3. **Filamentous glycocalyx** binds digestive enzymes.
4. **Tight junctions** (zonulae occludens) act as a diffusion barrier.
5. **Transport proteins** in apical and basal membranes mediate movement of specific substances across surfaces (see Chapter 1, section III).
6. **Polarization of cells** permits directed transport of nutrients from the apical (luminal) surface to the basal surface.

C. **Transport over the surface of epithelia**
   • **Beating of cilia** on respiratory epithelium **moves debris-filled mucus toward the oral cavity,** helping to prevent microorganisms, dust, and other materials from reaching the lungs (see Box 4-1).

D. **Transport across capillary endothelia**
   1. **Thin, flattened cell shape** provides maximal surface area.
   2. Well-developed **basal lamina** impedes diffusion.
   3. Many **pinocytotic vesicles** aid in transporting material from one side of cells to the other side.
   4. **Fenestrae (pores)** in some capillary endothelial cells increase their permeability to most substances.

E. **Secretion by glandular epithelia** (Figure 4-6)
   1. **Protein-secreting cells** are marked by a well-developed **rough endoplasmic reticulum,** extensive **Golgi apparatus,** and numerous **secretory granules** (vesicles) in apical region of the cell.
   2. **Steroid hormone-secreting cells** are marked by well-developed **smooth endoplasmic reticulum** and numerous **lipid droplets.**

Kartagener's syndrome: situs inversus + immotile cilia syndrome.

Connective Tissue

5

Target Topics

▷ Permanent and migratory connective tissue cells
▷ Major collagen types and their body locations
▷ Overview of collagen structure and synthesis
▷ Structure and distribution of glycosaminoglycans and proteoglycans
▷ Structure and function of the basement membrane
▷ Hurler's syndrome and other types of mucopolysaccharidosis (MPS), scurvy, Ehlers-Danlos syndrome, homocystinuria, Marfan syndrome, lathyrism, Alport's syndrome

I. **Introduction**
    • **Connective tissue** is distributed **throughout all the systems and organs** of the body.
    A. **Functions**
       1. **Structural support** is the primary function of connective tissue.
          • Organs contain a **stroma** of connective tissue, which supports and nourishes the functional elements, or **parenchyma** (e.g., secreting cells in glands, myofibers in muscle).
       2. **Transport, storage, and protection** are specialized functions performed by connective tissue in certain body locations.
    B. **Basic components**
       1. **Cells**
       2. **Extracellular matrix (ECM)**, which consists of **ground substance** and **fibers**
    C. **Classification** (Figure 5-1)
       1. **Loose (areolar) connective tissue:** high proportion of cells and ground substance to fibers (Figure 5-2)

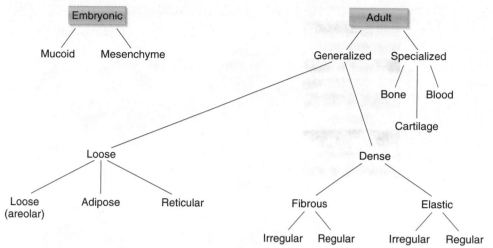

Figure 5-1 Classification of connective tissue. All connective tissues are composed of cells, fibers, and ground substance. They are classified based on the relative amounts and organization of these components.

    2. Dense connective tissue: high proportion of fibers to cells

II.   **Cells of Generalized Connective Tissue**
    A. Permanent residents are formed locally from undifferentiated mesenchymal cells and remain within the connective tissue.
        1. Fibroblasts synthesize connective tissue fibers and the constituents of the ground substance.
            a. Active fibroblasts: synthetically active state containing well-developed rough endoplasmic reticulum (RER) and Golgi complex
            b. Fibrocytes: synthetically inactive state that may revert to the active form during wound healing
        2. Adipose cells store lipid triglycerides in their cytoplasm.
            a. Unilocular (white) adipocytes: one large fat vacuole; the most common form in **adults**
            b. Multilocular (brown) adipocytes: large number of lipid droplets; common in **embryos** and **newborn infants**
        3. Pericytes are **flattened cells** that lie adjacent to capillary endothelium and are enclosed within its basal lamina.
    B. Migratory (transient) residents are formed primarily in the bone marrow and migrate from the blood into connective tissue.
       • These cells, which are most numerous during infection and at inflammatory sites, play an **important role in the body's defense system** (see Chapter 13).
       1. Macrophages, which arise from circulating monocytes, are the **most abundant phagocytic cells** in connective tissue.
          • Some macrophages are **fixed** to fibers; others migrate throughout connective tissues.

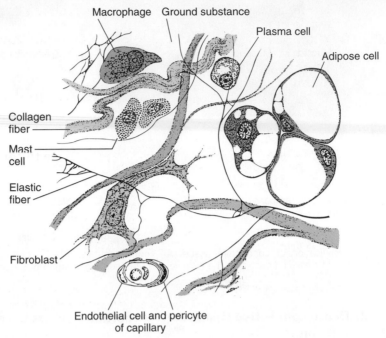

Macrophage Ground substance

Plasma cell

Adipose cell

Collagen fiber

Mast cell

Elastic fiber

Fibroblast

Endothelial cell and pericyte of capillary

Figure 5-2 Sketch of the cells and fibers of loose connective tissue as seen with the light microscope. The visible components lie in the optically homogeneous ground substance.

   2. Mast cells are filled with membrane-bound granules containing various biological mediators including **histamine, heparin,** and platelet-activating factor (PAF).
   - Release of these substances leads to an **immediate (type I) hypersensitivity reaction** (see Figure 13-5).
   3. T and B lymphocytes accumulate in large numbers during chronic infection.
   4. Plasma cells, which produce **secreted antibodies,** are commonly found where microorganisms and toxins can penetrate epithelial surfaces of the body.
   5. Granulocytes (see Chapter 12)
      a. Neutrophils are highly phagocytic cells found at sites of acute infections.
      b. Eosinophils increase in number during parasitic infection and at sites of allergic reactions.

III. **Ground Substance**
   - This optically homogeneous material, filling the space between connective tissue cells and fibers, consists of a complex scaffold of **macromolecules** bathed in **tissue fluid.**
   A. **Glycosaminoglycans (GAGs)** are **unbranched** polysaccharides composed of repeating **disaccharide subunits.**
      1. Common properties of GAGs
         a. All GAGs have regularly spaced **negatively charged**

groups and exhibit **metachromasia** (i.e., they stain red with a blue dye).

b. With the exception of hyaluronic acid, GAGs are **covalently attached to core proteins** and contain covalently attached sulfate groups.

2. Hyaluronic acid

a. This very large, highly coiled molecule (MW $\approx 10^6$ Da) is synthesized by enzyme complexes embedded in the plasma membrane of fibroblasts.

b. It can bind many water molecules, forming a **viscous hydrated gel** that imparts stiffness and resilience to connective tissues.

- Is the lubricant in **synovial fluid**

c. Hyaluronic acid interacts with itself and with proteoglycans to provide **a barrier to spread of bacteria, tumor cells, and large molecules.**

- Is degraded by **hyaluronidase**, an enzyme produced by some bacteria and many tumor cells

3. Major sulfated GAGs

a. Chondroitin sulfate (cartilage, bone, blood vessels)

b. Dermatan sulfate (skin, blood vessels, heart valves)

- Is present in increased amounts in **mitral valve prolapse**

c. Heparan sulfate (basal laminae, plasma membranes)

- Imparts negative charge to **glomerular basement membrane**

d. Keratan sulfate (cornea, cartilage)

B. Proteoglycans are a diverse group of molecules composed of a **core protein** from which covalently attached **GAG side chains** extend.

- **Most proteoglycans** are secreted into the **extracellular matrix** after their synthesis, but some remain attached to the plasma membrane by a transmembrane domain (e.g., **syndecans**).

1. Proteoglycan aggregates consist of a **central hyaluronic acid molecule** to which ≈ 100 **proteoglycan monomers** are bound (Figure 5-3).

- These large aggregates are particularly **abundant in cartilage.**
- Aggregates are assembled in extracellular space from hyaluronic acid and proteoglycan monomers.

2. Synthesis and turnover of proteoglycans

a. Core protein is synthesized on the RER of fibroblasts.

b. GAG side chains are assembled on the core protein one sugar at a time in the RER and Golgi complex.

c. Certain **lysosomal enzymes** degrade proteoglycans, accounting for their turnover in connective tissue.

- **Mucopolysaccharidoses** are characterized by hereditary defects in various lysosomal enzymes (Box 5-1).

3. Functions of connective tissue proteoglycans

a. Act as supporting matrix for cells and fibers

Hyaluronic acid: large, abundant, hydrated glycosaminoglycan that impedes spread of bacteria and tumor cells through extracellular matrix; joint lubricant.

Invasion of connective tissue by some bacteria (e.g., group A streptococci) and many tumor cells is promoted by hyaluronidase, which is produced by these invaders.

Hurler's syndrome and other forms of MPS result from defective degradation of glycosaminoglycans in lysosomes, leading to their accumulation in various tissues and excretion in urine.

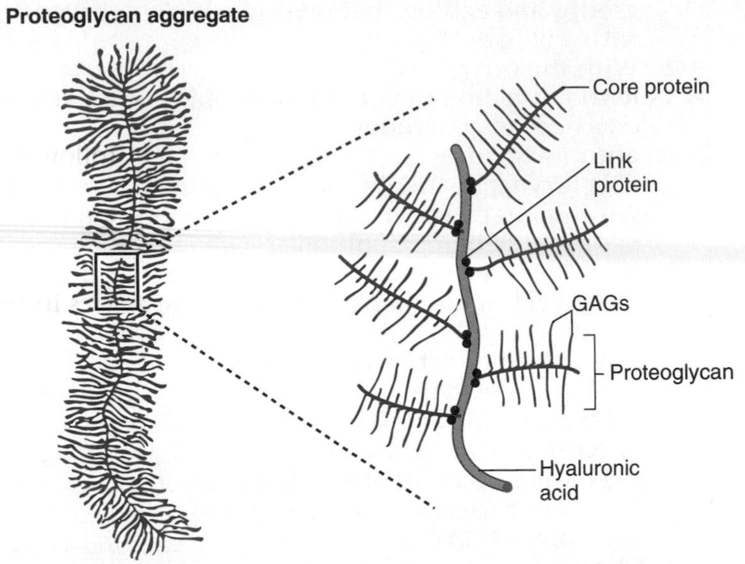

Proteoglycan aggregate

Figure 5-3 Proteoglycan aggregate. Proteoglycans are attached at regular intervals to a central hyaluronic acid molecule *(left)*. These aggregates may attain a molecular weight of 10^8 and occupy a volume equivalent to that of a bacterium. Each proteoglycan consists of a central core protein and numerous covalently bound glycosaminoglycans *(GAGs)*, as shown in enlarged view *(right)*.

BOX 5-1	Mucopolysaccharidoses (MPS)

Defects in lysosomal degradation of **glycosaminoglycans (GAGs)** leads to excretion of GAGs in the urine and their accumulation in many tissues. These defects usually are **autosomal recessive** and cause various clinical syndromes, which constitute one type of lysosomal storage disease.

Hurler's syndrome (MPS I H): prototype mucopolysaccharidosis. Most severe of three allelic forms of MPS I. Progressive **corneal clouding**, severe mental retardation, **gargoyle-like facies** (low forehead, widely spaced teeth, large tongue), short neck and trunk, joint contractures, enlarged liver and spleen. Dermatan sulfate and heparan sulfate in the urine. Early death usually from respiratory infection or heart failure.

Hunter's syndrome (MPS II): severe form is marked by mental retardation, dwarfism, deafness, hernia, **claw hand,** and **valvular heart disease.** Dermatan sulfate and heparan sulfate in the urine. Only X-linked MPS. Death before age 15, usually from heart disease.

Morquio's syndrome (MPS IV): normal intelligence, dwarfism, hunchback, knock-knees, progressive deafness, mild corneal clouding. Keratan sulfate in the urine.

b. Attract and hold tissue fluid
c. Permit diffusion of small molecules in solution
d. Obstruct the movement of large molecules
e. Bind fibroblast growth factor (FGF) and other growth factors in the ECM, protecting them from degradation and presenting them to cell-surface receptors

C. Matrix adhesive (structural) proteins are large **glycoproteins** that cross-link other ECM components with specific cell-surface proteins.

   1. **Fibronectins** play an important role in **cell migration** during development and in **wound healing.**
      a. Specific domains in fibronectins bind the following:
         (1) **Collagen** and **heparan sulfate** (ECM components)
         (2) **Fibrin** (major component of blood clots)
         (3) **Integrins** (intrinsic membrane proteins)
      b. **Fibroblasts** produce connective-tissue fibronectins.
      c. **Liver cells** produce fibronectin that circulates in the blood.
   2. **Laminins** promote adhesion of epithelial cells to the underlying connective tissue.
      a. All **basal laminae** contain laminins.
      b. Specific domains in laminins bind the following:
         (1) **Type IV collagen** and **perlecan** (a heparan sulfate proteoglycan), both components of basal laminae
         (2) **Integrins** in the plasma membrane of epithelial cells

D. Tissue fluid, the fluid part of the ground substance, provides a **medium for diffusion** of metabolites in the intercellular space.
   • It is constantly being **formed from the blood** as it passes through arterioles and **resorbed** into venules and lymphatic vessels.

> Fibronectins and laminins bind to other ECM components and to cell-surface proteins, linking cells to the ECM. Important in wound healing and tumor invasion.

IV. Extracellular Fibers

A. Collagen fibers are inelastic, flexible fibers (1–12 μm in diameter) with **high tensile strength** that constitute the major fibrous component of connective tissue.
   • A single collagen fiber consists of aggregations of long, thin **fibrils** (20–100 nm in diameter) composed of **tropocollagen** molecules.
   • **Turnover of collagen** in adult tissues is much slower than that of most intercellular proteins (e.g., collagen molecules persist for years in bone).

   1. **Tropocollagen** (Figure 5-4)
      a. A long, rigid molecule (MW = 300 kDa), tropocollagen is composed of three polypeptide chains (**α chains**) coiled about one another, forming a **triple helix.**
      b. **Unusual amino acid composition** of tropocollagen (30% **glycine** and 25% **proline + hydroxyproline**) contributes to its rigidity and assembly into fibrils.
   2. **Collagen fibrils**
      a. Triple-helical **tropocollagen molecules,** which have distinct head and tail regions, are assembled into fibrils **all oriented in the same direction.**
      b. **Dark and light periodicity** (every 64–67 nm, depending on the preparation) of many native collagens reflects the highly organized, packing of tropocollagen subunits into fibrils.
   3. **Collagen formation—intracellular events** (Figure 5-5)
      a. **In RER**

(1) Synthesis of **pro-α chains**
(2) Hydroxylation of proline and lysine in pro-α chains (requires ascorbic acid) and addition of carbohydrate
(3) Assembly of three-stranded **procollagen** stabilized by intrachain disulfide bonds in the nonhelical **propeptides** at both ends
b. Transfer to Golgi complex, where oligosaccharide side chains on procollagen are completed
c. Transfer to secretory vesicle, which then move to the cell surface

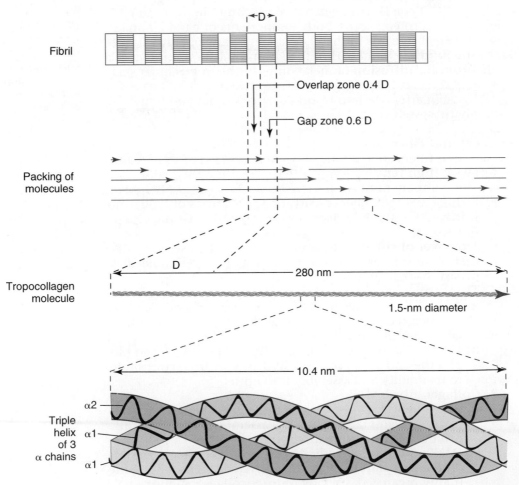

Figure 5-4   Organization of tropocollagen in collagen fibrils that display a characteristic periodicity of 64 nm *(D)*. In these fibrils, tropocollagen molecules are organized in a quarter-staggered array (i.e., the ends of adjacent molecules are displaced about one quarter of the length on one molecule). Each tropocollagen molecule is a triple helix of three interwoven α chains, which may be identical or different.

    d. At surface of cell, exocytosis of procollagen and removal of peptides at amino and carboxyl ends by proteases on the cell surface to yield tropocollagen

4. Collagen formation—extracellular events
    a. Self-assembly of tropocollagen to form collagen fibrils
    b. Formation of cross-links
- **Lysyl oxidases** deaminate hydroxylysine and lysine to form highly reactive aldehyde groups, which spontaneously form covalent bonds within and between tropocollagen molecules, **stabilizing the fibrils.**

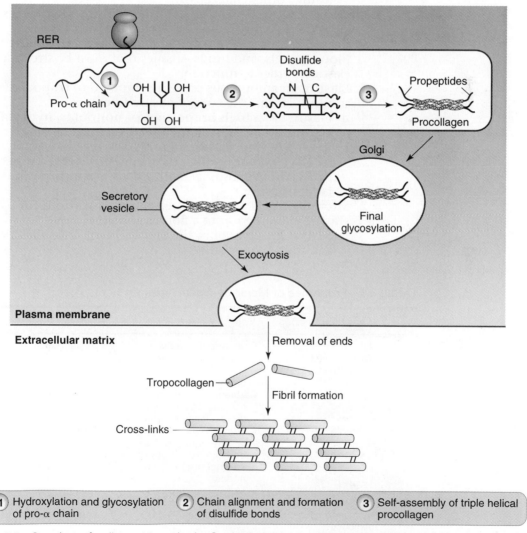

Figure 5-5 Overview of collagen biosynthesis. Synthesis begins in the rough endoplasmic reticulum *(RER)* and is completed outside the cell with cleavage of the ends to yield tropocollagen, which assembles into cross-linked fibrils. Side-by-side aggregation of fibrils produces large collagen fibers.

- Cross-linking increases as collagen ages, so that it becomes more insoluble in aqueous solution.

5. **Types of collagen**
   - About 25 distinct tropocollagen α chains have been identified. Various combinations of α chains in the tropocollagen triple helix give rise to more than **20 biochemically different types of collagen** (Table 5-1).

   a. **Fibrillar (fibrous) collagens** account for 80%–90% of the collagen in the body. Include types I, II, and III, which form typical 67-nm banded fibrils.

   b. **Reticular fibers**, composed of type III collagen with more carbohydrate residues, stain with PAS and silver salts (unlike other collagens).

B. **Elastic fibers** can be **readily deformed or stretched** by a small force, and **reversibly recover** their original dimensions.
   - These fibers are prevalent in extracellular matrix of the **skin, blood vessels**, and **lungs**—tissues that must be strong and elastic in order to function.

   1. **Elastin**, an amorphous protein composed of **tropoelastin subunits**, forms the **core of elastic fibers.**

      a. Elastin has a **high proportion of nonpolar, hydrophobic amino acids**, making it relatively insoluble.

      b. Joining of tropoelastin subunits into elastin is catalyzed by lysyl oxidases, which form covalent **lysine cross-links** and two unusual amino acids, **desmosine** and **isodesmosine.**

   2. **Microfibrils** (11 nm in diameter) form a **scaffold for elastin**, molding it into a fibrous configuration.
      - Several glycoproteins, the predominant one called **fibrillin**, form microfibrils.

TABLE 5-1 Properties of Major Collagen Types

Type	Cells Synthesizing	Major Tissues	Function
I	Fibroblast Odontoblast Osteoblast	Bone and dentin; skin; tendons and ligaments; interstitium of internal organs	• Resists tension
II	Chondroblast	Cartilage (hyaline and elastic); intervertebral disks; vitreous humor	• Resists intermittent pressure
III	Fibroblast	Cardiovascular system; endoneurium; lymph nodes; interstitium of internal organs; lymph nodes	• Forms extensive open network that provides structural support in expandable organs • Is first collagen in wound healing
IV	Epithelial cell Schwann cells Adipocyte Muscle cell	All basal laminae	• Provides support and selective filtration
X	Chondrocyte	Epiphyseal plate	• Provides framework for bone formation

3. **Elastic fiber–producing cells** include **fibroblasts** (generalized connective tissue), **smooth muscle cells** (large arteries), and **chondrocytes** (elastic cartilage).

C. **Diseases involving defective extracellular fibers**

1. **Scurvy** results from a severe impairment of collagen synthesis due to **prolonged deficiency of vitamin C (ascorbate),** which is required for hydroxylation of proline to hydroxyproline during tropocollagen synthesis.
   - Clinical symptoms include **pinpoint hemorrhages** in the skin, **bleeding gums,** and **loosened teeth** as preexisting normal collagen gradually is lost and not replaced.

2. **Ehlers-Danlos syndrome** is caused by a genetic defect that prevents conversion of procollagen to tropocollagen.
   - This disorder is characterized by fragile skin, weakened blood vessels, rupture of the colon, and **hypermobile joints**.

3. **Homocystinuria,** an **autosomal recessive** defect in the enzyme cystathionine synthetase, leads to abnormal tropocollagen cross-linking.
   - This disorder is marked by elevated levels of homocystine and methionine in the blood and urine, as well as musculoskeletal, ocular, and cardiac abnormalities similar to Marfan syndrome.
   - Increased plasma homocystine predisposes individuals to **vessel thrombus.**

4. **Marfan syndrome,** an **autosomal dominant** disorder, is caused by mutation in the fibrillin gene on chromosome 15.
   - Clinical manifestations include abnormally long fingers and toes **(arachnodactyly),** dislocation of the lens, **mitral/tricuspid valve prolapse,** and stretching of the ascending aorta, which may lead to **dissecting aortic aneurysm.**

5. **Lathyrism** is caused by **reduced lysyl oxidase** activity usually due to severe **copper deficiency** or ingestion of excessive amount of **beta-amionopropionitrile** (found in some peas).

V. **Basement Membrane**
   - All epithelia are separated from the subjacent connective tissue by a structurally similar interface, the **basement membrane** (Table 5-2).
   - A basement membrane also surrounds muscle cells, adipose cells, and Schwann cells, and separates epithelial and endothelial cells in kidney glomeruli.

A. **Structural elements of the basement membrane**

1. **Basal lamina,** which ranges in thickness from 40–100 nm, is produced by the **adjacent epithelium.**
   - All basal laminae contain similar components, although their ultrastructural organization may vary in different sites.
   a. **Lamina lucida (rara),** an electron-lucent zone closest to the epithelium, contains two key proteins.

Scurvy and Ehlers-Danlos syndrome (dissecting aortic aneurysm) result from impaired collagen synthesis or surface peptidaic activity.

Homocystinuria: marked by increased plasma homocystine and methionine, vessel thrombus, and marfanoid habitus.

Marfan syndrome: defective formation of elastic fibers; marked by arachnodactyly, lens dislocation, dissecting aortic aneurysm, and mitral/tricuspid valve prolapse.

TABLE 5-2 Terms Referring to Various Epithelia and Subjacent Connective Tissues

Site	Epithelium	Connective Tissue	Epithelium + Connective Tissue
Covering of external body surfaces	Epidermis	Dermis	Skin
Lining of body cavities open to the surface (alimentary, urinary, respiratory tracts)	Epithelium (with or without glands)	Lamina propria	Mucosa
Lining of closed body cavities: Coelomic cavity (peritoneal, pericardial, and pleural)	Mesothelium (no glands)	Submesothelium	Serosa
Cardiovascular cavity	Endothelium	Subendothelium	Intima (vessels) Endocardium (heart)

(1) **Laminin,** which binds type IV collagen, herparan sulfate, and cell-surface integrins
(2) **Perlecan,** a proteoglycan rich in heparan sulfate
b. **Lamina densa** is largely a meshlike network composed of **type IV collagen.**
2. **Lamina reticularis** is produced by the underlying **connective tissue.**
   • It is rich in **collagen** and **reticular fibers** embedded in ground substance.
B. **Functions of the basement membrane**
   1. **Forms selective barrier to movement** of large molecules and cells
   2. **Separates connective tissue** from epithelial cell environment
   3. **Provides elastic support**
   4. **Helps guide migration of cells** during regeneration of injured tissue and development

C. **Alport's syndrome**
   • This **X-linked dominant** or **autosomal dominant** disorder is caused by mutation in the gene encoding one of the α chains of **type IV collagen.**
   • The resulting defects in glomerular basal lamina cause **nephritis** marked by hematuria and progressive **renal failure.** Some patients also manifest **hearing loss** and **ocular disorders.**

6

Nervous Tissue

Target Topics

▷ Ultrastructure and classification of neurons
▷ Functions of neuroglial cells
▷ Changes associated with nerve injury and recovery
▷ Generation of action potentials and impulse transmission at synapses
▷ Myelination and nodes of Ranvier
▷ Blood-brain barrier
▷ Peripheral nerve layers
▷ Meningitis, degenerative diseases of the central nervous system, Guillain-Barré syndrome, Charcot-Marie-Tooth disease, neurofibromatosis

I. Introduction

- **Nervous tissue** is specialized to **receive stimuli** (irritability) and **transmit impulses** (conductibility).

A. Cellular components

1. **Neurons**, which conduct impulses, are the **fundamental structural and functional unit** of the nervous system.
   - They consist of a **cell body (perikaryon)**, which extends into two types of processes, **axons** and **dendrites.**
2. **Neuroglial cells**, which are nonconducting, support and protect neurons.

B. Major divisions

1. **Central nervous system (CNS)** comprises the **brain** and **spinal cord.**
2. **Peripheral nervous system (PNS)**, consisting of neurons located outside the CNS, transmits impulses to and from the CNS.

II. The Neuron

A. Formation of neurons

- Neurons are **nonreplicating, postmitotic cells** derived from precursor cells that are present only during prenatal development.
  1. **Neuroepithelial cells** in the embryonic neuroectoderm give rise to neuroblasts, which differentiate into **neurons of the CNS.**
  2. **Neural crest cells,** derived from a specialized region of the neuroectoderm, migrate throughout the body and give rise to **neurons and neuroglial cells of the PNS.**

B. **Structure of neurons**
  1. **Cell body** contains the **nucleus** and various cytoplasmic organelles, cytoskeletal elements, and inclusions.
     a. **Golgi complex,** located near the nucleus, and **mitochondria** throughout the cytoplasm
     b. **Nissl bodies** (or substance), which are composed of rough endoplasmic reticulum (RER) and free ribosomes
     c. **Lipofuscin granules,** which are the end result of lysosomal activity and increase in number with age
     d. **Neurofilaments** (intermediate filaments) and **neurotu-**

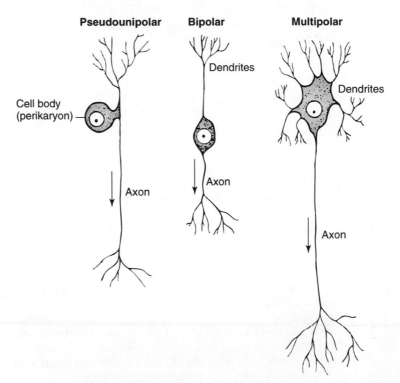

Figure 6-1 Three main morphologic classes of neurons. The single axon extending from pseudounipolar neurons divides into two branches, one functioning as an axon and the other as a dendrite. Bipolar neurons have an axon and a dendrite. Multipolar neurons, which have multiple dendrites and a single axon, are the most abundant. *Arrows* indicate direction of impulse conduction.

bules (microtubules), some of which extend from the cell body into the processes

2. **Neuron processes** vary in number, providing the basis for morphologic classification of neurons (Figure 6-1).

    a. Axons (nerve fibers) conduct impulses away from the cell body.

        (1) Most axons are **long, slender** processes that arise from the **axon hillock** in the cell body and branch at the distal (terminal) end.

        (2) Axonal cytoplasm (**axoplasm**) lacks ribosomes, RER, and Golgi apparatus.

        (3) **Myelin sheath**, composed of many layers of modified plasma membrane, covers some axons.

    b. Dendrites conduct impulses toward the cell body.

        (1) Dendrites usually are relatively **short** and **highly branched.**

        (2) They contain all the cytoplasmic components found in the cell body except Golgi apparatus.

C. Axoplasmic transport

- Because the axon terminus lacks components for synthesizing new proteins or degrading old ones, materials must be transported back and forth between the cell body and terminus.

    1. **Anterograde transport:** cell body → axon terminal

        a. Fast component (50–400 mm per day) transports cytoplasmic proteins and macromolecules required for metabolic and synaptic activity.

        b. Slow component (1–4 mm per day) transports cytoskeletal components down the axon.

    2. **Retrograde transport:** axon terminal → cell body

        - Used membranous components of synaptic vesicles move to the cell body where they are degraded in lysosomes.

D. Functional classification of neurons

    1. **Sensory neurons** transmit impulses from sensory receptors to the CNS.

    2. **Motor neurons** transmit impulses from the CNS to a motor effector organ (muscle or gland).

        a. Somatic motor neurons innervate skeletal muscles.

        b. Autonomic motor neurons innervate some glands, cardiac muscle, and involuntary smooth muscles.

        - Autonomic neurons are classified into two functional types, which generally have opposite effects on target organs (Table 6-1).

        (1) **Parasympathetic neurons:** cell body of first-order (presynaptic) neurons in the cranial and sacral regions of the spinal cord; cell body of second-order (postsynaptic) neurons in or near the organs they innervate

        (2) **Sympathetic neurons:** cell body of first-order neurons in thoracic and lumbar regions of the spinal cord; cell body of second-order neurons in sympathetic ganglia near the spinal cord

Viruses and toxins can be transported from the periphery to the CNS within axons (retrograde transport).

3. Interneurons transmit impulses within the CNS and most commonly connect sensory and motor neurons.

E. Reaction of neurons to injury (Figure 6-2)

   1. Damage to the cell body generally results in the **death of a neuron.**

   • Because neurons cannot undergo cell division and no neural precursor cells are present after birth, **neurons that are destroyed postnatally cannot be replaced.**

TABLE 6-1   Selected Effects of Parasympathetic and Sympathetic Stimulation

Target Tissue/Organ	Parasympathetic Effect	Sympathetic Effect
Adrenal medulla	No effect	Stimulates secretion
Bladder	Promotes voiding	No effect
Bronchi	Constricts	Relaxes
Heart pacemaker cells	Decreases heart rate	Increases heart rate
Pupil of eye	Constricts	Dilates
Salivary glands	Stimulates secretion	Inhibits secretion
Stomach, intestines	Promotes motility and gland secretion	Inhibits motility and gland secretion

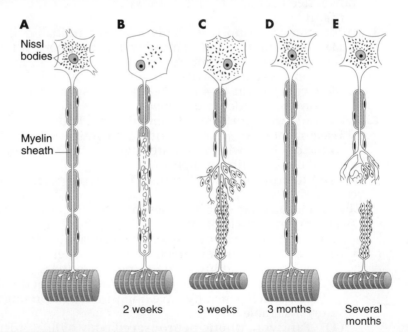

Figure 6-2   Degeneration and regeneration of an axon following injury. **A,** Intact normal nerve cell synapsing on a striated muscle cell. **B,** Following severing of the axon, it undergoes wallerian degeneration distal to the injury. Reactional changes also take place in the cell body. **C,** Axonal sprouts begin to grow in proximal stump. Schwann cells proliferate, forming a tube that the growing axon penetrates. **D,** Successful regeneration occurs when the axon reestablishes contact with muscle cell. Note that the denervation atrophy of the muscle observed soon after nerve injury is reversed once nerve stimulation is restored. **E,** Regeneration is unsuccessful if the axon does not penetrate the tube of Schwann cells. Although the reactional changes in the perikaryon are reversed, further permanent atrophy of the muscle occurs in the absence of stimulation.

2. **Severing or crushing of an axon** leads to characteristic changes (Figure 6-2, *A, B*).
   a. **Wallerian (anterograde) degeneration** occurs in the **distal portion of the axon** (the portion separated from the cell body).
      (1) Axon begins to swell and degenerate; the myelin sheath fragments; and phagocytes remove cellular debris.
      (2) After about 3 weeks, Schwann cells proliferate and form a tube of cells distal to the injury.
   b. **Reactional changes** occur in the **neuron cell body**.
      (1) Cell body swells and the nucleus is displaced peripherally.
      (2) Nissl bodies disperse with a concomitant loss in cytoplasmic basophilia referred to as **chromatolysis.**
   c. **Recovery and regeneration of damaged axons** (Figure 6-2, *C, D*)
      • If the lesion in a peripheral neuron is sufficiently distant from the cell body, the nerve may recover.
      (1) **Axonal sprouts** are produced at the distal end of the axon stump, using materials synthesized in the cell body.
      (2) The axon stump elongates and the sprouts seek the tubes formed by Schwann cells.
      (3) If sprouts penetrate the Schwann-cell tube and reestablish contact with an appropriate effector cell, regeneration is likely.

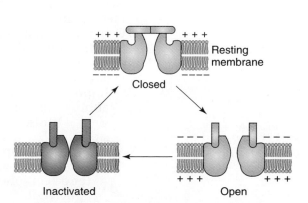

A Kinetics of action potential

B Voltage-gated Na⁺ channel

Figure 6-3 Action potential. **A,** Time course of action potential. Sudden massive influx of Na^+ ions causes a rapid depolarization of the membrane potential from its resting value. Subsequent closing of Na^+ channels and opening of K^+ channels leads to efflux of K^+ ions, briefly hyperpolarizing the membrane potential below its resting value. **B,** Schematic diagrams of changes in conformational states of voltage-gated Na^+ channels during generation of an action potential. In unstimulated neurons, these channels are closed. Their opening, triggered by a small depolarizing stimulus, leads to rapid depolarization of the membrane potential, as shown in **A.**

A Chemical synapse

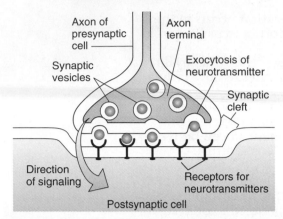

B Electric synapse

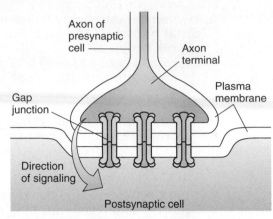

Figure 6-4 Synapses. The two types of synapses, chemical (**A**) and electrical (**B**), differ in structure and the mechanism of impulse transmission. Impulse transmission is faster at electrical synapses than at chemical synapses, although the latter are much more common. See also Figure 1-7, *C*, for structure of gap junctions.

3. **Trophic effects of nerve injury**
    a. **Degeneration of motor neurons** innervating some muscle cells induces **muscle atrophy.**
       • **Motoneuron disease** is any condition in which progressive degeneration of motor neurons at the cervical and lumbosacral levels of the spinal cord leads to **degeneration atrophy of limb muscles** (e.g., amyotrophic lateral sclerosis, polio).
    b. Degeneration of some neurons is transmitted to neurons with which they synapse, causing **transneuronal degeneration.**

III. **Nerve Impulses**
    • Nerve impulses represent **rapid, transient changes in the membrane potential** of neurons, called **action potentials.**
    A. **Generation of action potentials** (Figure 6-3)
       • Action potentials originate at the **axon hillock** and move as a wave of electrical excitation toward the axon terminal.
    B. **Synaptic transmission of nerve impulses**
       • Impulses are transmitted from one neuron (**presynaptic**) to another neuron (**postsynaptic**) or from a neuron to an effector cell (muscle or gland cell) at regions of functional apposition, called **synapses.**
    1. **Chemical synapses** (Figure 6-4, *A*)
       a. **Presynaptic axon terminal:** small knoblike termination (**end-feet**) of transmitting neuron, which contains synaptic vesicles filled with a **neurotransmitter**
       b. **Presynaptic membrane:** thickened region in the plasmalemma of the presynaptic axon terminal containing **voltage-gated Ca^{2+} channels**
          • Arrival of an action potential at axon terminal → opening of Ca^{2+} channels → influx of Ca^{2+} ions →

Action potential: rapid, transient changes in electrical potential across the plasma membrane involving influx of Na^+ ions (depolarization) followed by efflux of K^+ ions (repolarization)

BOX 6-1	**Excitatory and Inhibitory Synapses**

Whether a neurotransmitter promotes or inhibits generation of an action potential in postsynaptic cells depends on the receptor it binds to in the postsynaptic membrane. Acetylcholine produces an excitatory response in some postsynaptic cells but an inhibitory response in other cells. Most neurotransmitters, however, produce either an excitatory or inhibitory response. The effects and sites of action of some common neurotransmitters are listed below:

- **Excitatory:** ACh in skeletal muscle; dopamine, glutamate, and serotonin in CNS
- **Inhibitory:** ACh in heart muscle; GABA, glycine, and met-enkephalin in CNS
- **Excitatory or inhibitory:** ACh in CNS; norepinephrine in CNS and PNS

Important clinical correlations include:

- **Decreased serotonin** is associated with **depression.** Tryptophan is precursor in biosynthesis of serotonin.
- **Increased GABA** in the CNS leads to **hepatic encephalopathy** in patients with chronic liver disease.
- **Decreased ACh** in the CNS is commonly seen in **Alzheimer's disease.**
- **Tetanus toxin** blocks release of inhibitory neurotransmitters (e.g., glycine), leading to continuous stimulation and contraction of muscles.
- Tyrosine is precursor in biosynthesis of dopamine and norepinephrine.

rise in cytosolic Ca^{2+} level promotes exocytosis of neurotransmitter into synaptic cleft.

   c. Synaptic cleft: 20- to 40-nm–wide space separating the presynaptic and postsynaptic membranes across which neurotransmitter diffuses

   d. Postsynaptic membrane: thickened region in plasmalemma of receiving cell containing **neurotransmitter receptors** (Box 6-1)

- At **excitatory** synapse: binding of neurotransmitter to its receptors → **opening of Na^+ channels** in postsynaptic membrane → **depolarization** of the membrane → **action potential** in the postsynaptic cell
- At **inhibitory** synapse: neurotransmitter binding → **opening of K^+ or Cl^- channels** in postsynaptic membrane → **hyperpolarization** of the membrane → **no action potential** in postsynaptic cell

  2. Electrical synapse (Figure 6-4, *B*)

   a. Gap junctions (nexi) directly link the cytoplasm of some presynaptic and postsynaptic cells.

   b. Flow of ions through gap junctions **transmits action potentials** from presynaptic to postsynaptic cell without involvement of neurotransmitters.

   c. Speed of impulse transmission at electric synapses is nearly instantaneous, whereas transmission at chemical synapses involves a delay of about 0.5 ms.

ACh is excitatory neurotransmitter for skeletal muscle (nicotinic ACh receptor) and inhibitory for heart muscle (muscarinic ACh receptor).

IV. Components of the CNS
    A. **Two types of tissue** are distinguishable in the CNS.
        1. **Gray matter** consists of the cell bodies of neurons, neuron processes, and neuroglial cells.
        2. **White matter** contains neuroglial cells and a large number of neuron processes, most of which are myelinated, but lacks neuron cell bodies.
    B. **Neuroglial cells of the CNS** are about 10 times more numerous than neurons (Figure 6-5).
        • Neuroepithelial cells of the **embryonic neuroectoderm** give rise to all CNS neuroglial cells except microglia, which arise from **embryonic mesoderm.**
        • Under appropriate conditions, neuroglial cells are **capable of cell division.**
        1. **Astrocytes,** the largest of the neuroglial cells, have numerous processes with expanded end-feet (**pedicles**) that terminate on capillaries or the pia mater.
            a. **Fibrous astrocytes:** located primarily in the **white matter;** long, spindly processes with few branches
            b. **Protoplasmic astrocytes:** located in the **gray matter;** thick, highly branched process; closely apposed to neuron cell bodies
            c. **Functions of astrocytes**
                (1) Regulate the composition of the intercellular environment or entry of substances into it
                (2) Provide structural support (analogous to fibroblasts)
                (3) Metabolize neurotransmitters
                (4) Mediate the exchange of nutrients and metabolites between the blood and neurons
                (5) Help form noncollagenous scar tissue after injury to the CNS
        2. **Oligodendrocytes**
            a. **In white matter,** oligodendrocytes are the predominate type of neuroglial cell and produce the **myelin sheath** around myelinated fibers.
            b. **In gray matter,** oligodendrocytes are closely associated with neuron cell bodies, functioning as **satellite cells**

Neuroglial tumors, which arise from astrocytes, oligodendrocytes, and ependymal cells, make up about half of all intracranial tumors.

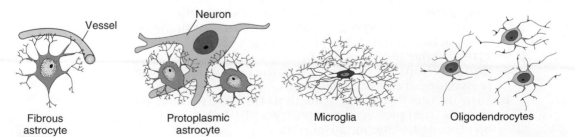

Fibrous astrocyte   Protoplasmic astrocyte   Microglia   Oligodendrocytes

Figure 6-5 Neuroglial cells. Both fibrous and protoplasmic astrocytes have end-feet that terminate on vessel walls. Protoplasmic astrocytes, found mainly in the gray matter, also associate closely with neuron cell bodies. Oligodendrocytes myelinate central nervous system (CNS) neurons. Microglia are phagocytes of the CNS.

along with protoplasmic astrocytes; also surround the axons of unmyelinated fibers.

3. Microglia are small phagocytic cells that enlarge and become mobile following injury to the CNS.

4. Ependymal cells are ciliated cuboidal cells that line the ventricles of the brain and the central canal of the spinal cord.
  • Within the **choroid plexus**, ependymal cells are thought to be the principal cell type that **secretes cerebrospinal fluid** (CSF).

C. Meninges are the three membranous layers that **cover and protect the brain and spinal cord** (Box 6-2).

1. Dura mater (outer meninx) blends with the periosteum of the skull but is separated from the vertebrae by the **epidural space** and from the underlying arachnoid by the **subdural space**.
  • Composed of **dense fibrous connective tissue**
  • Lined by a discontinuous mesothelium on its inner surface in the skull and on both surfaces in the spinal column

2. Arachnoid (middle meninx) is a delicate fibrous layer that extends weblike strands (trabeculae) into the underlying subarachnoid space.
  • Lined on both surfaces by mesothelium
  a. Subarachnoid space lies between the arachnoid and pia mater and contains blood vessels surrounded by CSF.
  b. Arachnoid villi are specialized projections of the arachnoid that terminate in venous spaces and function to **return CSF to the venous system**.
    • **Meningiomas** are derived from arachnoid granulation.

3. Pia mater (inner meninx) is a delicate layer of fibroblasts and collagen fibers directly apposed to the brain and spinal cord.
  a. Perivascular spaces are tunnels covered with pia mater through which blood vessels penetrate the CNS.

Microglial cells, the macrophages of the CNS, are the reservoir cell for HIV in patients with AIDS dementia.

Glioblastoma multiforme, the most malignant type of astrocytoma, is a rapidly growing tumor that usually occurs in the cerebral hemispheres in adults.

BOX 6-2   Meningitis

Infection or inflammation of the meninges usually results from pathogens spreading from other, primary sites of infection via the bloodstream. Meningitis often has a sudden onset and is characterized by severe headache, fever, nausea with vomiting, and stiffness in the neck. Diagnosis of meningitis is confirmed by a lumbar puncture (spinal tap) and analysis of the cerebrospinal fluid.

Bacterial meningitis commonly is caused by *Streptococcus pneumoniae* and *Neisseria meningitidis*. This severe, pus-forming infection requires immediate, high-dose antibiotic therapy.

Viral meningitis, caused by *Coxsackie* viruses and **mumps virus**, generally is self-limiting and resolves within a few weeks.

Fungal meningitis due to *Candida* or *Cryptococcus* can be serious, especially in immunocompromised patients.

• Pia mater disappears as blood vessels are transformed into capillaries.
      b. Choroid plexus consists of infoldings of the pia mater that project into **ventricles of the brain** and are covered by a thin layer of specialized ependymal cells (choroid epithelial cells).
         (1) Blood perfuses through the choroid plexus to form **CSF**, which is an exudate of blood.
         (2) Tight junctions between choroid epithelial cells constitute **blood-CSF barrier.**
   D. Blood-brain barrier prevents passage of certain substances from the blood to nervous tissue in the CNS.
      • Several properties of CNS capillaries **reduce their permeability**, contributing to the functional blood-brain barrier:
      1. Lack of fenestrations and paucity of **pinocytic vesicles** in the endothelial cells
      2. Zonulae occludens (tight junctions) between the endothelial cells
      3. Astrocyte pedicles that completely envelop these capillaries
   E. Degenerative diseases of the CNS (Table 6-2)

V. **Components of the PNS**
   • The PNS is composed of neuron processes and cell bodies located outside the CNS, ganglia that house cell bodies, neuroglial cells, and nerve endings.
   A. Neuroglial cells of the PNS
      1. Satellite cells (amphicytes) form a capsule of cells around neuron cell bodies located in peripheral ganglia.
      2. Schwann cells envelop the axons of unmyelinated fibers and elaborate the **myelin sheath** around myelinated fibers.
   B. Myelin sheath
      • In both the CNS and PNS, **some axons**, but no dendrites, are **surrounded by a myelin sheath.**
      1. Myelin-producing cells
         a. In the CNS, individual **oligodendrocytes** myelinate portions of **several** axons.
         b. In the PNS, individual **Schwann cells** myelinate portions of only a **single** axon.
      2. Composition and formation of myelin sheath (Figure 6-6)
         • Myelin sheath, which is derived from the plasma membrane of a neuroglial cell, is similar in composition to the plasma membrane but has a higher proportion of **lipids.**
      3. Nodes of Ranvier
         a. These interruptions in the myelin sheath around an axon represent **gaps between adjacent myelinating cells.**
         b. Because Na$^+$ channels are concentrated at nodes, impulse conduction along myelinated axons involves "**jumping**" **of action potentials** from one node to the next (**saltatory conduction**).
   C. Ganglia
      • These **encapsulated collections of neuron cell bodies,**

Hydrocephalus results from a decrease in the absorption or outflow of CSF. Typically leads to enlargement of the head and mental retardation.

Alzheimer's disease and Pick's disease are marked by distinct histopathologic changes that cause atrophy of the cerebral cortex, leading to dementia.

Myelin sheath is formed by Schwann cells in PNS and by oligodendrocytes in CNS.

Demyelination can result from viral infection of oligodendrocytes (measles virus), osmotic damage to Schwann cells (in diabetics), or autoantibodies directed against myelin (multiple sclerosis).

TABLE 6-2　Degenerative Diseases of the Central Nervous System

Disease	Pathogenesis	Clinical Features
Alzheimer's disease	Progressive diffuse atrophy throughout cerebral cortex from degeneration of neurons; **senile plaques** (extracellular deposits of beta-amyloid fibrils); **neurofibrillar tangles** within neurons	• Gradual loss of recent memory (decreased ACh), cognition, and judgment, progressing to dementia. • Defects in fine motor skills, restlessness, and fearfulness • Most common cause of dementia after 65 years of age
Amyotrophic lateral sclerosis	Progressive deterioration of upper and lower motor neurons (corticospinal tract), leading to muscle atrophy	• Wasting of muscles beginning in limbs and progressing proximally. • Onset usually in middle age; rapid course leading to severe paralysis, breathing difficulty, and death within 2–5 years
Huntington's chorea	Severe atrophy of the caudate nuclei, cerebral cortex, and extrapyramidal system	• Rapid, jerky movements (chorea) of head, limbs, and tongue; mental deterioration ending in dementia. • Autosomal dominant inheritance with onset at ages 25–45; death within 15 years
Multiple sclerosis	Patchy autoimmune destruction of myelin throughout the CNS and PNS, resulting in slowed impulse conduction along affected fibers	• Numbness in limbs, muscle weakness, incoordination, and visual disturbances. • Onset in young adulthood with recurrent attacks of symptoms and remissions
Parkinson's disease	Loss of neurons within substantia nigra (decreased dopamine) and other portions of extrapyramidal system	• Masklike facies, "pill-rolling" involuntary tremor, shuffling gait, slowing of voluntary movement, muscle rigidity
Pick's disease	Progressive atrophy primarily involving frontal and temporal lobes; globular filamentous inclusions (Pick bodies) within degenerating neurons	• Similar to Alzheimer's disease

located outside the CNS, also contain **satellite cells** (amphicytes) and the usual connective tissue elements.

1. **Craniospinal ganglia** house the cell bodies of **sensory neurons**, which are **pseudounipolar** or **bipolar**.
    - Sensory ganglia are associated with most cranial nerves and the dorsal roots of all the spinal nerves (**dorsal root ganglia**).
2. **Autonomic ganglia** house the cell bodies of multipolar **motor neurons** composing the autonomic nervous system.
    a. **Sympathetic ganglia** are located beside the vertebral column.
    b. **Parasympathetic ganglia** are located within or near the target tissue.

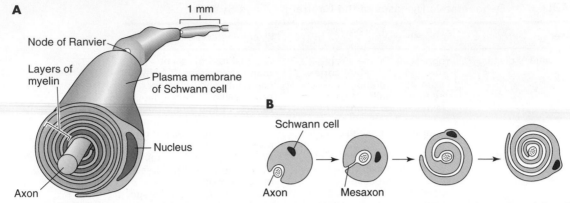

Figure 6-6 Myelination in the peripheral nervous system. **A,** Portion of a myelinated axon with nodes of Ranvier between adjacent Schwann cells. **B,** Mechanism of myelination. After a Schwann cell completely surrounds an axon, the region of edge-to-edge contact of the plasma membrane (mesaxon) elongates and wraps around the axon. As consecutive spirals of infolded plasma membrane are formed, the intervening cytoplasm is squeezed out and the cytosolic surfaces fuse (major dense line). External membrane surfaces are held in close apposition (intraperiod line) by a protein found only in myelinating Schwann cells. In reality, the myelin layers are compacted much more tightly than depicted.

Connective tissue layers of peripheral nerves:
• Endoneurium surrounds a single nerve fiber, including myelin sheath if present.
• Perineurium surrounds a fascicle of nerve fibers, forming permeability barrier.
• Epineurium surrounds entire nerve and carries blood vessels.

D. Peripheral nerves (Figure 6-7)
- A peripheral nerve comprises bundles (**fascicles**) of nerve fibers (axons) that are surrounded by myelin sheaths or Schwann cells and are invested with three connective tissue elements.
1. **Connective tissue elements**
   a. Epineurium: thick fibrous coat that forms the external covering of a nerve
      - Blood and lymphatic vessels supply the epineurium.
   b. Perineurium: layer of dense connective tissue around **each fascicle** of nerve fibers
      - The inner surface is lined with epithelial-like cells joined by **zonulae occludens** (tight junctions), which provide a permeability barrier.
      - This layer must be rejoined in microsurgery for limb reattachment.
   c. Endoneurium: thin **reticular layer** that surrounds each **individual nerve fiber** and contains Schwann cells
      - In myelinated fibers, the endoneurium lies outside and encloses the myelin sheath.
2. **Functional classification of nerves**
   a. Sensory nerves contain axons of sensory neurons (**afferent fibers**), whose cell bodies are located in craniospinal (dorsal root) ganglia.
   b. Motor nerves contain axons of motor neurons (**efferent fibers**), whose cell bodies are located in the spinal cord or autonomic ganglia.
   c. Mixed nerves, the most common type, contain both efferent (motor) and afferent (sensory) fibers.

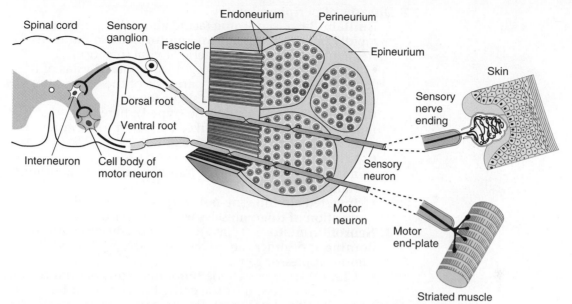

Figure 6-7 Schematic depiction of a typical reflex arc with cross-sectional view of a mixed peripheral nerve. Note the bundles (fascicles) of fibers in the nerve and three types of connective tissue layers. Stimulation of sensory nerve endings in the skin triggers an impulse that is transmitted to the spinal cord via the dorsal root ganglion. The sensory impulse is transmitted to a motor neuron (via an interneuron), triggering a motor impulse that passes to a skeletal muscle. The knee-jerk reflex and heat-induced withdrawal reflex operate in this fashion.

E. **Peripheral nerve endings** (see Figure 6-7)

   1. **Motor endings** are the **axonal** terminations of motor fibers where they synapse with muscles or glands.

      a. Motor end-plate is the chemical synapse between the axon terminal of a motor fiber and a muscle fiber; also called **neuromuscular junction.**

      b. Neurotransmitter released from motor endings **changes permeability of the effector cell** (muscle or gland), causing a wave of depolarization to sweep over the effector cell bringing about contraction or secretion.

   2. **Sensory endings** are specialized **dendritic** terminations that **convert** various internal or external **stimuli into nerve impulses.**

      a. Mechanoreceptors respond to **stretch, touch,** or **pressure;** may be free nerve endings or encapsulated corpuscles (see Figure 8-3).

      b. Chemoreceptors are the free endings of specialized epithelial cells that respond to **taste** sensations and **odors** (see Figure 19-5).

      c. Light receptors are the free endings of **photoreceptor cells in the retina** (see Figure 19-2).

      d. Temperature and pain receptors generally are free nerve endings.

F. Diseases of peripheral nerves
1. **Guillain-Barré syndrome** (acute idiopathic polyneuritis): rapidly progressive **ascending motor neuron paralysis** that frequently is a sequel to enteric or viral infection
   - Clinical manifestations begin with **paresthesias** of the feet, followed by **flaccid paralysis** of the legs that moves upward; accompanied by slight **fever.**
2. **Charcot-Marie-Tooth disease (type I):** hereditary disorder (**autosomal dominant**) marked by loss of innervation to muscles supplied by the **peroneal nerves**
   - Clinical onset in children or young adults leads to **weakness and atrophy of calf muscles** with foot deformities (talipes) common.
   - Inverted **champagne-bottle** appearance results from preservation of thigh muscles with atrophy of calf muscles.
3. **Neurofibromatosis (type 1):** relatively common **autosomal dominant** disorder caused by loss of the *NF-1* or *NF-2* tumor-suppressor gene.
   - Clinical features include **numerous soft, benign tumors** (neurofibromas) over the entire body; **café au lait spots** on the skin; **Lisch nodules** (hamartomas of the iris); and multiple types of **brain tumors** (e.g., acoustic neuromas, meningiomas, optic nerve gliomas).

Muscular Tissue

7

Target Topics

▷ Banding patterns of skeletal muscle in resting, contracted, and stretched state

▷ Key structural/functional differences between skeletal, cardiac, and smooth muscle

▷ Molecular structure of myofibrils and myofilaments

▷ Sliding-filament mechanism of muscle contraction

▷ Role of T tubules and sarcoplasmic reticulum in contraction

▷ Muscular dystrophies, Eaton-Lambert syndrome, myasthenia gravis, botulism, regenerative capacity of muscle

I. **Introduction**
- **Muscular tissue** comprises a population of cells (muscle fibers, **myofibers**) specialized to perform **movement** (locomotion) through the processes of **contraction** and **relaxation**.
- All muscles consist of a **stroma of connective tissue** and **parenchyma of muscle fibers** varying in length and diameter.

Muscle cell = myofiber = fiber.

A. **Classification of muscular tissue**
  - Three types vary in their structure, distribution, and functional properties.
  1. **Skeletal muscle** (muscles of the skeleton)
  2. **Cardiac muscle** (parenchyma of the heart)
  3. **Smooth muscle** (muscles associated with blood vessels, viscera, and internal organs)

B. **Basic properties of muscle fibers**
  1. **Excitability:** ability to respond to a stimulus
  2. **Conductivity:** ability to propagate a limited response
  3. **Contractility:** ability to shorten
  4. **Elasticity and viscosity:** ability to relax (return to original shape) after contraction

II. **Structure of Skeletal Muscle**
- Skeletal muscle fibers are **long cylindrical cells with numerous, peripherally located nuclei.**
  A. **Development of skeletal myofibers**
    1. **Prenatal:** embryonic **mesodermal cells** in somites proliferate, migrate, and fuse into **multinucleated myotubes,** which differentiate into skeletal muscle fibers.
    2. **Postnatal:** growth of muscle before puberty occurs by an increase in the size of muscle fibers (**hypertrophy**) and in their number (**hyperplasia**). Following puberty, growth occurs by hypertrophy only.
  B. **Connective tissue stroma of skeletal muscles** (Figure 7-1)
    1. **Epimysium** envelops an entire muscle.
    2. **Perimysium** separates small bundles (**fascicles**) of muscle fibers.
    3. **Endomysium** envelops each individual muscle fiber.
       a. **External lamina,** which is equivalent to the basal lamina in epithelial tissue, lies between the plasma membrane (**sarcolemma**) and endomysium.
       b. **Satellite cells** (pericytes) located within the external lamina function as stem cells that can **replace damaged muscle** by proliferating, fusing, and differentiating into skeletal muscle fibers.
  C. **Myofibrils**
    - The cytoplasm (**sarcoplasm**) of a muscle fiber is filled with bundles of **myofibrils** composed of long **myofilaments** running parallel to the long axis of the fiber.
    1. **Characteristic striations** evident in each muscle fiber and myofibril arise from the highly organized pattern of myofilaments (see Figure 7-1).
       a. **A band:** darkly staining region (overlapping **thin and thick filaments**)
       b. **I band:** lightly staining region (**thin filaments only**)
       c. **H band:** lightly staining region that bisects each A band (**thick filaments only**)
       d. **Z line (Z disk):** dense region that bisects each I band
       e. **M line:** narrow dark region that bisects each H band
    2. **Sarcomere,** the regularly repeating unit between successive Z lines, is the **smallest unit capable of contraction.**
  D. **Molecular components of myofilaments**
    1. **Thick (myosin) filaments** (≈14 nm thick)
       a. **Myosin** is a dimeric protein with a long **tail** and two **globular heads** at one end.
       b. **Tails** of hundreds of myosin molecules associate to form a **bipolar filament** with the heads located at the distal ends and the tails directed toward the central region (Figure 7-2, *A*).
       c. **Heads** of the myosin molecules, which project from thick filaments, have **actin-binding sites** and **ATPase activity.**
    2. **Thin (actin) filaments** (≈8 nm thick)
       a. **Fibrous F-actin,** a double helical filament, is formed by

Striations in skeletal muscle:
- A band: dark (thick and thin filaments)
- I band: pale (thin filaments)
- H band: pale, center of A band (thick filaments)
- Z line: dark, center of I band
- M line: dark, center of H band

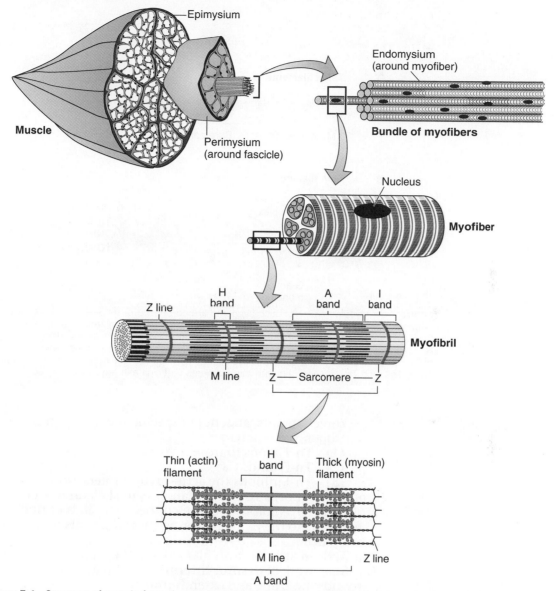

Figure 7-1 Structure of muscle from the gross to the molecular level. Connective tissue layers surround entire muscle, bundles of myofibers (fascicles), and individual myofibers. The regular array of myofilaments within each myofibril and alignment of sarcomeres of adjacent myofibrils produce the characteristic banding pattern. In the region where thick and thin myofilaments overlap, each thick filament is surrounded by six thin filaments in a hexagonal array.

polymerization of 300–400 **G-actin monomers** (Figure 7-2, *B*).
- Each actin monomer possesses a **myosin-binding site.**
b. Tropomyosin, a long polymeric protein, runs in the groove of the F-actin helix.
c. Troponin (Tn), a globular protein complex composed of

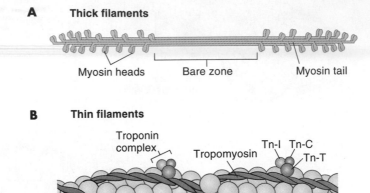

Figure 7-2 Myofilaments. **A,** Thick filaments are composed of myosin molecules, arranged with their long, coiled-coil tails parallel and their heads projecting from the surface. These filaments are bipolar, with each end covered by heads and the central portion devoid of heads. **B,** Thin filaments are composed primarily of F-actin, resulting from polymerization of G-actin monomers. In skeletal and cardiac muscle, tropomyosin and the trimeric troponin complex (Tn-T, Tn-I, and Tn-C) associated with thin filaments participate in regulating contraction.

Elevated troponin level in blood is seen after acute myocardial infarction.

three subunits, attaches to specific sites along the tropomyosin polymer.

(1) Tn-T binds to tropomyosin.

(2) Tn-C binds Ca^{2+}.

(3) Tn-I inhibits the actin-myosin interaction.

E. **Proteins that organize myofilaments in skeletal muscle**

　1. **Titin,** a large fibrous protein, connects the ends of thick filaments to the Z line centering these filaments in the sarcomere.

　2. **α-Actinin** attaches thin filaments to the Z line.

　3. A framework of **desmin intermediate filaments**, which surrounds the Z line and extends into each sarcomere, links myofibrils together laterally and to the sarcolemma.

　　• Desmin is an excellent marker for tumors that are derived from skeletal muscle and smooth muscle and that have a nonvascular origin.

　4. **Dystrophin** is one of the proteins that link α-actinin/desmin complex to cytoplasmic side of the sarcolemma.

　　• Dystrophin gene, located on X chromosome, is mutated in patients with Duchenne and Becker muscular dystrophies.

F. **Sarcoplasmic membrane system in skeletal muscle**
(Figure 7-3)

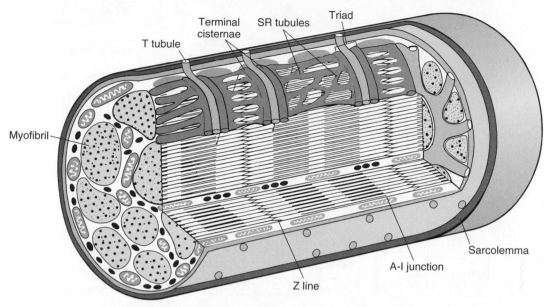

Figure 7-3 Sarcoplasmic reticulum *(SR)* and transverse *(T)* tubules in skeletal muscle fibers. Ca²⁺ ions stored in the SR are released to the cytosol via voltage-gated channels in the terminal cisternae. Opening of channels is triggered by depolarization of the sarcolemma, which is conveyed by the T tubules into the sarcoplasm.

1. **Sarcoplasmic reticulum (SR)**, a modified smooth endoplasmic reticulum, constitutes a meshwork of tubules and cisternae surrounding each myofibril.
   - **Terminal cisternae:** greatly dilated regions of the SR, located at A-I junctions, that **store and release Ca²⁺ ions**
2. **Transverse (T) tubules** are invaginations of the sarcolemma that extend into the sarcoplasm at the level of the A-I junction.
3. **Triads** consist of a central T tubule flanked by two terminal cisternae.

G. Types of skeletal muscle fibers
   - Most skeletal muscles contain a mixture of two or three fiber types.
1. **Red fibers** have large-diameter myofibrils and are capable of sustained activity over long periods of time; also called **slow-twitch** fibers.
   - High myoglobin and low glycogen content; many mitochondria
2. **White fibers** have small-diameter myofibrils and are capable of fast but brief bursts of activity; also called **fast-twitch** fibers.
   - Low myoglobin and high glycogen content; few mitochondria
3. **Intermediate fibers** have characteristics similar to or between those of red and white fibers.

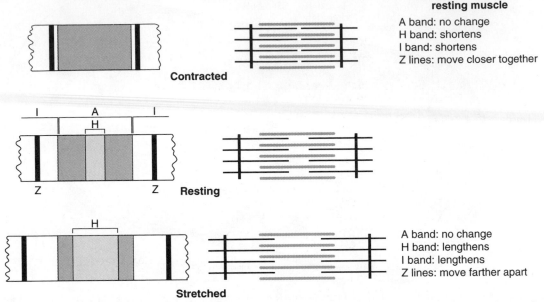

Changes relative to resting muscle

A band: no change
H band: shortens
I band: shortens
Z lines: move closer together

Contracted

I   A   I
    H

Z   Z   **Resting**

H

A band: no change
H band: lengthens
I band: lengthens
Z lines: move farther apart

Stretched

Figure 7-4 Comparison of banding pattern of skeletal muscle in contracted, resting (relaxed), and stretched state. During contraction and stretching, the overlapping of thick and thin filaments changes, but their lengths remain constant.

III. **Mechanism of Skeletal Muscle Contraction**
   A. **Sliding filament model**
     • When a myofibril contracts, thin filaments move past thick filaments, increasing their overlap.
     • Filament sliding during contraction **decreases sarcomere length** but the **lengths of myofilaments remain constant** (Figure 7-4).
   B. **Contraction cycle** (Figure 7-5)
     • Movement of thick and thin filaments past each other requires **adenosine triphosphate** (ATP) and involves **cyclic interactions between myosin and actin.**
     • **In the absence of ATP** (e.g., after death), myosin cannot dissociate from actin filaments and muscles remain in a state of **rigor mortis.**
   C. **Regulation of skeletal muscle contraction**
     1. **Inactive (off) state:** In resting muscle, **tropomyosin** partially covers the myosin-binding sites on thin (actin) filaments, inhibiting the interaction of myosin with actin that occurs during the contraction cycle. In this state, the contraction cycle cannot proceed.
     2. **Active (on) state:** Binding of Ca^{2+} by **troponin C** (Tn-C) leads to a slight shift in the position of tropomyosin on the thin filament, exposing the myosin-binding sites. In this state, the contraction cycle proceeds if ATP is available.
   D. **Initiation and cessation of muscle contraction** (Figure 7-6)
     • Contraction of skeletal muscle is triggered by arrival of a nerve impulse at the **motor end-plate**, or **neuromuscular junction.**

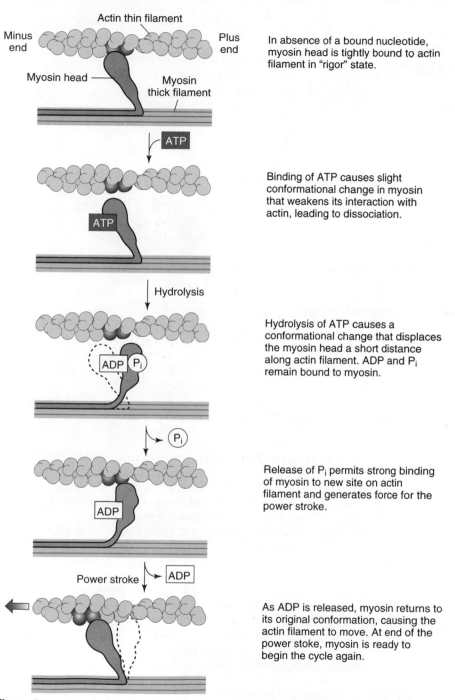

Minus end

Plus end

Actin thin filament

Myosin head

Myosin thick filament

In absence of a bound nucleotide, myosin head is tightly bound to actin filament in "rigor" state.

ATP

ATP

Binding of ATP causes slight conformational change in myosin that weakens its interaction with actin, leading to dissociation.

Hydrolysis

ADP P_i

Hydrolysis of ATP causes a conformational change that displaces the myosin head a short distance along actin filament. ADP and P_i remain bound to myosin.

P_i

ADP

Release of P_i permits strong binding of myosin to new site on actin filament and generates force for the power stroke.

Power stroke

ADP

As ADP is released, myosin returns to its original conformation, causing the actin filament to move. At end of the power stoke, myosin is ready to begin the cycle again.

Figure 7-5 Steps in coupling of adenosine triphosphate *(ATP)* hydrolysis to movement of thick and thin filaments during contraction. *ADP,* Adenosine diphosphate; *P_i,* inorganic phosphate.

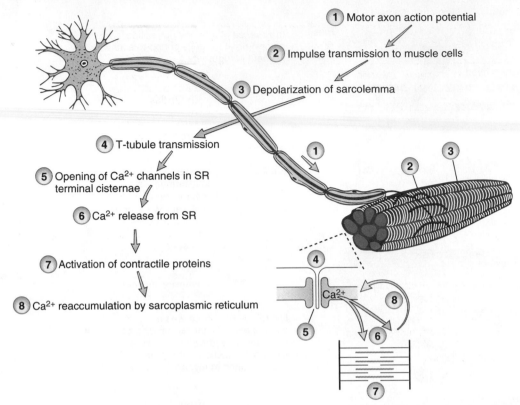

Figure 7-6 Summary of events leading to contraction of skeletal muscle fibers. *SR,* Sarcoplasmic reticulum.

1. **Acetylcholine** (ACh) released from motor nerve endings binds to receptors in the sarcolemma of the muscle fiber.
2. **Wave of depolarization** (action potential) sweeps over the sarcolemma and T tubules and is relayed across the gap between T tubules and terminal cisternae.
3. **Opening of voltage-gated Ca^{2+} channels** in the SR terminal cisternae releases stored Ca^{2+} into the cytosol.
4. **Increase in cytosolic Ca^{2+}** switches actin thin filaments from off to on state, permitting myofibrils to contract. Contraction cycle will continue as long as the cytosolic Ca^{2+} level remains high enough.
5. **Ca^{2+} ATPase** in the SR membrane pumps Ca^{2+} back into the SR, reducing the cytosolic Ca^{2+} level.
   - When cytosolic Ca^{2+} is reduced enough, thin filaments return to their off state and fiber relaxes.

IV. **Disorders of Skeletal Muscle**
   - The two major classes of muscle disorders, **myopathy** and **neuropathy**, generally lead to muscle **atrophy** marked by a decrease in the cross-sectional area of muscle fibers and in the number of myofibrils.

TABLE 7-1 Muscular Dystrophies

Type	Inheritance	Onset/Progression	Signs and Symptoms
Duchenne muscular dystrophy (DMD)	X-linked (dystrophin gene mutated)	Early onset Usually fatal by maturity	• Progressive weakness of pelvic and limb girdles • Early Gowers' sign • Extensive pseudohypertrophy of calf muscles (replacement of lost fibers by connective tissue and fat) • Swaying gait with legs kept wide apart • Cardiac involvement
Becker muscular dystrophy	X-linked (dystrophin gene mutated)	Late onset Slow progression	• Similar to DMD but less severe
Limb-girdle muscular dystrophy	Autosomal recessive	Variable onset (10-30 years) Usually slow progression	• Weakness and wasting of proximal muscles of upper and lower limbs
Myotonic muscular dystrophy	Autosomal dominant	Childhood onset common, but also later Slow progression	• Sustained muscle contraction (myotonia) especially in face and neck followed by muscle atrophy • Distinctive ring fibers • Cataracts, gonadal atrophy, frontal balding, cardiac defects

A. Myopathies: innervation to muscle fibers remains intact.
- **Proximal, symmetrical muscle weakness** commonly occurs in myopathies.
1. **Muscular dystrophies** are hereditary diseases in which muscle fibers exhibit shrinkage and enlargement, **centrally located nuclei**, and eventual necrosis (Table 7-1).
   - **Ring fibers**, formed by wrapping of one dystrophic fiber around another, are a distinctive feature of **myotonic muscular dystrophy**.
2. **Aging, malnutrition,** and **immobilization** can lead to muscle atrophy with retention of innervation.

B. Neuropathies: innervation to muscle fibers is lost.
- **Distal, asymmetrical muscle weakness** commonly occurs in diseases caused by degeneration of motor neurons (e.g., amyotrophic lateral sclerosis, Guillain-Barré syndrome, and Charcot-Marie-Tooth disease; see Chapter 6).

Duchenne muscular dystrophy: X-linked; absence of dystrophin; most severe form of muscular dystrophy with fairly rapid progression.

Becker muscular dystrophy: X-linked; defective dystrophin; similar to Duchenne but with later onset and slow progression.

Eaton-Lambert syndrome: autoantibodies that block release of ACh from motor end-plate; weakening of limb muscles, but ocular muscles usually spared.

Myasthenia gravis: autoantibodies that block ACh receptors in muscle; weakening of muscles, especially those of the eye, face, and throat.

Botulinum toxin inhibits release of ACh at motoneuron ending. Bungarotoxin and other neurotoxins in certain snake venoms bind to and inactivate ACh receptors at neuromuscular junctions.

C. Disorders in which impulse transmission at neuromuscular junction is disrupted
1. **Eaton-Lambert syndrome:** autoimmune disease in which **autoantibodies** to voltage-gated Ca^{2+} channels in motoneuron endings **inhibit release of ACh**
   - **Muscle weakness** affecting the limbs but usually not involving ocular or bulbar muscles. Often associated with **oat cell (small cell) carcinoma of the lung.**
2. **Myasthenia gravis:** autoimmune disease in which **autoantibodies** to ACh receptors in muscle cells **block binding of ACh**
   - Gradual **weakening** (atrophy) of **skeletal muscles,** especially the most active ones. Ptosis, diplopia, dysphagia, and dysarthria are often present.
3. **Botulism:** food poisoning in which **endotoxin** produced by *Clostridium botulinum* **inhibits release of ACh** at motoneuron endings
   - **Visual disorders, muscle weakness, difficulty in swallowing,** sometimes nausea and vomiting. Fatal if untreated, usually due to respiratory failure.
4. **Certain snake venoms** (e.g., bungarotoxin) bind to and inactivate ACh receptors at neuromuscular junctions, leading to **paralysis.**

V. **Cardiac Muscle** (Table 7-2)
   - Cardiac muscle is **striated** because of organization of thick and thin filaments as in skeletal muscle.
   A. **Major structural features that characterize cardiac muscle**
   1. **Cell shape and size:** branched cells shorter than skeletal muscle cells
   2. **Nucleus:** single, centrally located
   3. **Sarcoplasmic membrane system**
      a. **T tubules:** located at the Z line instead of A-I junction because they are in skeletal muscle
      b. **Terminal cisternae:** relatively small and discontinuous
      c. **Diads:** one terminal cisterna associated with T tubule at each Z line
   4. **Intercalated disks**
      - These complex steplike junctions connect adjacent cardiac fibers end-to-end.
      a. **Transverse parts,** which run at right angles to the long axis of cardiac fibers, contain adherens and occludens components.
         - Thin filaments of adjacent cells attach to the transverse parts.
      b. **Lateral part,** which runs parallel with the long axis of cardiac fibers, contains numerous large **gap junctions** (nexi).
         - Action potentials spread rapidly from one fiber to another via these gap junctions, synchronizing contraction of the individual cardiac muscle fibers.

TABLE 7-2 Comparison of Types of Muscular Tissues

Property	Skeletal Muscle	Cardiac Muscle	Smooth Muscle
Structural Properties			
Location	Muscles of skeleton	Heart	Vessels, organs, and viscera
Cell size/shape	Long; cylindrical	Short; branched	Variable size; spindle shape
Nuclei	Many; peripherally located	Single; centrally located	Single; centrally located
Striations	Yes	Yes	No
Z lines	Yes	Yes	Cytoplasmic dense bodies replace Z lines
T tubules and sarcoplasmic reticulum (SR)	Triads at A-I junction	Diads at Z line	Caveolae replace T tubules; sparse SR
Cell junctions	None	Intercalated disk (adherens, occludens, and nexi)	Nexi (gap junctions)
Connective tissue	Epimysium Perimysium Endomysium	Endomysium	Reticular fibers
Association of fibers	Bundles (fascicles)	Sheets	Sheets (primarily)
Functional Properties			
Mode of contraction	Voluntary; all or none	Involuntary; rhythmic all or none	Involuntary; slow, sustained
Stimuli inducing contraction	Neural (somatic efferent)	Intrinsic (pacemaker) modified by autonomic efferent; spread via nexi	Intrinsic (stretching), neural (autonomic efferent), and hormonal; spread via nexi
Mitosis	No	No	Yes
Regeneration	Limited (differentiation of satellite cells)	None	High

B. Contraction of cardiac muscle
- The mechanism of contraction is the same as that in skeletal muscle.
- Certain specialized cardiac myofibers contract through **intrinsically generated impulses,** which are passed to neighboring cells via gap junctions, resulting in the rhythmic heart beat (see Chapter 11).

C. Absence of cardiac muscle regeneration
- Cardiac myofibers are postmitotic cells **incapable of cell division** and are not associated with any stem cells like the pericytes in skeletal muscle.
- Injured cardiac muscle generally is replaced by fibrous connective (scar) tissue.

VI. **Smooth Muscle** (Table 7-2)
- Smooth muscle **lacks striations** because the thin and thick fila-

In adults, smooth muscle cells undergo mitosis, but skeletal and cardiac muscle cells do not.

ments are not organized in the highly ordered arrays found in skeletal and cardiac muscle.

A. **Major structural features that characterize smooth muscle**
1. **Cell shape and size:** fusiform (spindle shaped); considerable variation in size depending on location
2. **Nucleus:** single, centrally located
3. **Sarcoplasmic membrane system:** very sparse and **lacks T tubules**
4. **Caveolae:** depressions in the sarcolemma that may function in regulating cytosolic Ca^{2+} level
5. **Dense bodies:** regions in the sarcoplasm that may be analogous to Z lines
   a. **Thin (actin) filaments** are anchored to sites on the sarcolemma and to dense bodies.
   b. **Intermediate filaments** extend from one dense body to another.
6. **Gap junctions (nexi):** abundant in sarcolemma of smooth muscle fibers, enabling **rapid transmission of action potentials** to adjacent fibers, which are not separately innervated

B. **Contraction of smooth muscle**
1. **Sliding of thin filaments** relative to thick filaments results in shortening and thickening of smooth muscle fibers.
2. **Rise in cytosolic Ca^{2+} level** triggers contraction (as in skeletal muscle), but the mechanism by which it does so differs from that in skeletal muscle.
3. **Rate of ATP hydrolysis** by myosin is slower than in skeletal muscle, so contraction is relatively slow and sustained.
4. **Initiation of smooth muscle contraction** is triggered by various stimuli.
   a. **Nerve impulses** in vascular smooth muscle (usually)
   b. **Stretching of muscle** in visceral smooth muscle
   c. **Oxytocin** in uterus during terminal stages of pregnancy
   d. **Epinephrine** in smooth muscle elsewhere in the body

C. **Regeneration of smooth muscle**
- Because smooth muscle cells **actively divide**, damaged fibers are regenerated.

Regeneration of muscle:
- High in smooth muscle because cells actively divide.
- Limited in skeletal muscle resulting from differentiation of satellite cells.
- None in cardiac muscle, which lacks any stem cells. Injured fibers replaced by scar tissue.

8

Integumentary System

Target Topics

▷ Properties of the epidermis, dermis, and hypodermis
▷ Distinguishing features of the strata of the epidermis
▷ Functions of melanocytes, Langerhans' cells, and Merkel's cells
▷ Differences between thin and thick skin
▷ Hair follicles and skin glands
▷ Innervation of the skin and common encapsulated mechanoreceptors
▷ Epidermal tumors, psoriasis, epidermolysis bullosa, pemphigus vulgaris, keloids, elastosis, acne vulgaris, Kaposi's sarcoma

I. **Introduction**
- The **integumentary system** consists of the skin and its appendages (hair follicles, nails, sweat glands, and sebaceous glands).

A. **Major components of the skin**
1. **Epidermis:** superficial layer of **stratified squamous keratinized epithelium;** primarily of **ectodermal** origin
2. **Dermis (corium):** dense fibrous irregular connective tissue layer beneath the epidermis; **mesodermal** origin
3. **Hypodermis:** layer of loose connective tissue that underlies the dermis and corresponds to **superficial fascia** of gross anatomy
- The hypodermis, which is not actually part of the skin, binds skin to subjacent tissue.
- It may contain **fat cells,** which can form a thick layer (**panniculus adiposus**) in obese individuals or certain regions of the body.

B. **Functions of the skin**
1. **Protective barrier**
a. **Prevents desiccation** (loss of fluids)
b. **Inhibits entry** of foreign substances and microorganisms

> The skin is the largest organ in the body, accounting for 8%–16% of adult body weight.

    c. Disperses light (keratinized layers) and **absorbs ultraviolet (UV)** radiation (melanin)

    d. Undergoes **wound healing**

  2. Thermoregulation

    a. Body temperature is regulated by control of **sweat gland activity** and **blood flow** through dermal capillary network.

    b. Sweat glands are decreased in the elderly, which predisposes them to heat stroke.

  3. Regulation of blood pressure

    a. Opening of dermal capillary network lowers blood pressure.

    b. Closing of dermal capillary network raises blood pressure.

  4. Excretion of metabolic waste products

  5. Sensory reception (touch, pressure, temperature, and pain)

  6. Synthesis of provitamin D

    • Photolysis of 7-dehydrocholesterol in the skin by UV radiation produces cholecalciferol (provitamin D), which is converted to active vitamin D in the liver (25-hydroxylation) and kidneys (1-α-hydroxylation).

II. Epidermis

  A. Epidermal strata (Figure 8-1)

    • **Keratinocytes,** the predominant cell type of the epidermis, form a **stratified squamous keratinized epithelium** containing **five strata** in the following order from deepest to most superficial:

    1. Stratum basale: single layer of **cuboidal to columnar** keratinocytes that are **mitotically active**

      a. Hemidesmosomes attach keratinocytes to adjacent basement membrane.

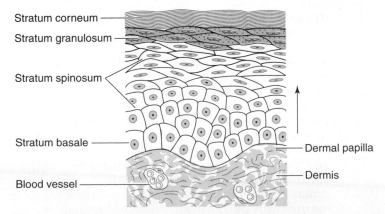

Figure 8-1 Strata of thin skin, which covers most of the body. Keratinocytes arise in the stratum basale and move toward the surface as they differentiate *(arrow),* a process that normally takes 15–30 days. The connective tissue dermis contains blood vessels and nerve endings. The stratum lucidum, a thin layer just below the stratum corneum, is evident only in thick skin (the palms and soles).

    b. Low-molecular-weight keratins are produced by kerati-nocytes in the basal layer.

    c. Basal cells give rise to additional **nondifferentiating stem cells,** which remain in this layer, and to **differenti-ating keratinocytes,** which move into the stratum spinosum.

  2. Stratum spinosum: several layers of **polyhedral-shaped** ke-ratinocytes (**prickle cells**) that **proliferate** and differentiate

    a. High-molecular-weight keratins are produced and as-sembled into intermediate filaments (**tonofibrils**) that terminate in numerous desmosomes.

    b. Lamellar bodies (membrane-coated granules) containing lipid, carbohydrate, and hydrolytic enzymes become evident.

    c. Stratum germinativum = stratum basale + stratum spinosum.

  3. Stratum granulosum: three to five layers of **flattened** kerati-nocytes that **cannot divide**

    a. Disulfide bonds begin to cross-link keratin filaments, which associate with numerous **keratohyalin granules.**

    b. Glycolipid and sterols secreted from lamellar bodies into the intercellular space form an **impermeable, waterproof barrier.**

    c. Lysosomal activity **degrades organelles** as cells move toward next strata.

  4. Stratum lucidum: clear, homogeneous layer composed of flat keratinocytes that **lack nuclei and organelles**

    a. This layer is well-defined only in **thick skin** (palm of hand and sole of foot).

    b. Cytoplasm consists almost entirely of **keratin filaments.**

  5. Stratum corneum: 5–50 layers of flattened, **keratinized** (cornified) **dead cells**

    a. Cells of this superficial layer, called **squames,** are filled with **cross-linked keratin filaments** embedded in a glob-ular amorphous matrix.

    b. Squames are continuously shed from the surface and re-placed by differentiating cells from the basal layer.

      • **Cytomorphosis of keratinocytes** in stratum basale to squames in stratum corneum takes **15–30 days.**

B. Nonkeratinocytes in the epidermis

  1. Melanocytes synthesize a dark brown pigment (**melanin**) that absorbs UV radiation, thereby **protecting DNA** in divid-ing cells of the skin from UV-induced damage.

    • Elevated ACTH increases melanin synthesis.

    a. Location: in **stratum basale, papillary layer** of dermis, and **hair follicles**

    b. Origin: derived from embryonic **neural crest cells** that migrate into skin of a 12- to 24-week embryo

    c. Melanin formation and release

      (1) Synthesis occurs in **melanosomes,** membrane-bounded granules that contain **tyrosinase** and other

Layers of the epider-mis from base to surface: stratum basale, stratum spinosum, stratum granulosum, stratum lucidum (thick skin only), stratum corneum.

Ichthyosis vulgaris: autosomal domi-nant; hyperkeratosis and absence of stratum granulo-sum; most common inherited disease affecting keratinization.

Absence of tyrosi-nase in melanocytes is responsible for albinism.

enzymes involved in conversion of tyrosine to melanin.

Melanocytes synthe-
size melanin, which
is seen in pig-
mented melano-
phores and
chromatophores.

    (2) Processes containing melanin-filled melanosomes are transferred via **cytocrine secretion** from melanocytes to the cytoplasm of keratinocytes (**melanophores**) in the stratum basale and stratum spinosum.

    (3) **Chromatophores** are pigmented cells in the dermis that take up melanin by phagocytosis.

  2. Langerhans' cells have long dendritic processes that radiate throughout the epidermis.

Langerhans' cells
in the epidermis
function as antigen-
presenting cells.

    a. Location: primarily in **stratum spinosum**

    b. Origin: derived from precursor cells in the **bone marrow**

    c. Function: involved in immune response as **antigen-presenting cells** (see Chapter 13)

  3. Merkel's cells contain small, dense-cored **granules filled with catecholamines** (similar to granules in cells of the adrenal medulla).

    a. Location: in **stratum basale** near well-vascularized, highly innervated dermis; present **only in thick skin**

    b. Function: may act as sensory **mechanoreceptors** or as diffuse **neuroendocrine cells**

C. Thickness of epidermis

  • Skin is classified as thin or thick based on relative thickness of the viable epidermis (stratum germinativum) and the stratum corneum.

  1. Thin skin covers most of body (Figure 8-1).

    a. Epidermis: 70–50 µm thick

    b. Viable strata thicker than stratum corneum

    c. Appendages: present

    d. Stratum lucidum: absent

  2. Thick skin lines palms of hands and soles of feet

    a. Epidermis: 400–1500 µm thick

    b. Stratum corneum thicker than viable epidermis

    c. Appendages: not present

    d. Stratum lucidum: present

D. Skin color

  • Skin thickness, vascular supply, and presence of pigments determine the color of skin.

  1. Black/brown color is due to **melanin**.

    • Although blacks and whites have the same number of melanocytes, these cells are larger and transfer more melanin to keratinocytes in blacks.

  2. Yellow color is due to **carotene** in stratum corneum and in adipose cells of the dermis.

  3. Red color is due to **oxyhemoglobin** in blood.

E. Disorders involving the epidermis

  1. Epidermal neoplasms (Box 8-1)

    • Skin tumors arise from cells that are **actively mitotic**, including keratinocytes in the viable epidermis and melanocytes.

BOX 8-1	Epidermal Tumors

Basal cell carcinoma: most common form of malignant skin tumor, arising from keratinocytes in the stratum basale. Usually occurs as small pearly nodule with a central crater that may erode, crust, and bleed. Locally invasive and aggressive, but **rarely metastatic.** Most common on face of adults, especially on sun-exposed areas.

Squamous cell (epidermoid) carcinoma: slow-growing malignant tumor that often originates in sun-damaged areas of the skin and also develops from squamous epithelium in the lung and other sites. **Actinic (solar) keratosis** is a precursor lesion for squamous cell skin cancer. Tumor cells resemble **prickle cells** of the stratum spinosum and are characterized by "**keratin pearls.**" Skin lesions commonly are firm, red, painless small bumps, which initially are localized and superficial, but may later invade and metastasize.

Malignant melanoma: any malignant neoplasm arising from **melanocytes.** Most common type (superficial spreading melanoma) often occurs on lower leg or back and presents as flat, pigmented skin patches that develop over several months or years. Malignant melanomas are deeply invasive and may metastasize throughout the body.

Verruca plana: a generally **benign** epidermal tumor caused by **papillomavirus infection** of keratinocytes. Small, slightly raised, tan or flesh-colored lesions (**warts**) often occur in large numbers on the face, neck, back of the hands, wrists, and knees.

Seborrheic keratosis: a **benign** skin tumor arising from basal cells and usually occurring in middle age. Lesions often develop rapidly in crops, presenting as yellow or brown, raised, soft plaques. Rapid increase in size and number of these lesions, known as **Leser-Trélat sign,** may indicate internal malignancy, especially of the GI tract.

2. **Psoriasis:** chronic skin disease marked by **dry, scaly plaques and papules,** most commonly on the scalp, knees, elbows, and trunk
   - **Psoriatic lesions** result from increased proliferation of keratinocytes in stratum germinativum, faulty keratinization, and reduction in transit time from basal layer to skin surface.

3. **Ichthyosis vulgaris:** most common inherited disorder (**autosomal dominant**) of keratinization with onset in childhood
   - Dry scales present on trunk and extremities; histologically marked by hyperkeratosis and absence of the stratum granulosum.

4. **Pemphigus vulgaris:** chronic, autoimmune disease marked by **flaccid, fragile bullae** that rupture, leaving painful denuded regions
   - **Autoantibodies to adherens junctions** between keratinocytes mediate this disease, the most common form of pemphigus.

III. **Dermis**
- The dermis, composed of **dense, fibrous irregular connective tissue**, varies in density, thickness, and elasticity in different body locations.

A. **Dermal layers**
- Both layers of the dermis contain an **elastic fiber network** continuous throughout the **bundles of collagen** (primarily type I).
  1. **Papillary layer:** moderately dense connective tissue arranged in fine interlacing bands of thin collagenous bundles
     - Has an **irregular contour** that sends projections (**dermal papillae**) into the adjacent basal layer of the epidermis
  2. **Reticular layer:** dense connective tissue arranged in thick interlacing collagenous bands
     - Is continuous with the hypodermis

B. **Cells and other structural components of the dermis**
- Similar elements are also found in the underlying hypodermis.
  1. Fibroblasts
  2. Adipocytes
  3. Smooth muscle fibers
  4. Nerves and nerve endings
  5. Blood vessels
  6. Extensions of epidermal derivatives (hair follicles, sweat glands, and sebaceous glands)

C. **Variation in thickness of the dermis**
  1. On the **back**, the dermis is **very thick**.
  2. On the **abdomen**, the dermis is **very thin**.

D. **Disorders involving the dermis**
  1. **Keloids:** abnormal scar tissue that is elevated, firm, and rounded with irregular margins
     - These lesions result from abnormal wound healing or skin injury involving excessive formation of **type III collagen** in the dermis.
  2. **Elastosis:** loss of skin elasticity (wrinkles) accompanied by increase in stainable elastin in dermis
     - This condition commonly occurs with **aging** and can result from excessive **exposure to sunlight.**

IV. **Appendages of Skin**
- The skin's appendages are **derived from the epidermal layer**, but hair follicles and glands extend into the dermis and sometimes the hypodermis.

A. **Hair and hair follicles** (Figure 8-2)
  1. **Structure**
     a. **Hair shaft** is located in **multi-layered follicle.**
        - Ducts of sebaceous glands and apocrine sweat glands empty into hair follicles.
     b. **Dermal sheath** surrounds each follicle and extends a protrusion (**hair papilla**) through follicular layers into base of the shaft (**hair bulb**).

Basal cell carcinoma: derived from stratum basale; rarely metastatic; small lesions have central crater; common on face.

Squamous cell carcinoma: slow growing with later metastasis possible; firm, painless bumps; keratin pearls in cells.

Malignant melanoma: derived from melanocytes; deeply invasive and metastatic; flat, pigmented skin lesions on lower leg and back.

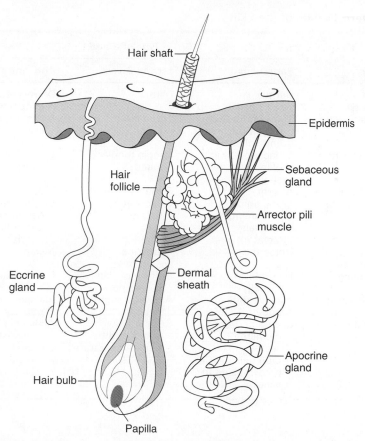

Hair shaft

Epidermis

Hair follicle

Sebaceous gland

Arrector pili muscle

Eccrine gland

Dermal sheath

Apocrine gland

Hair bulb

Papilla

Figure 8-2 General structure of a hair follicle and associated structures. Both the hair shaft and follicle are epidermal derivatives and contain several histologically distinguishable cell layers. Sebaceous glands and apocrine sweat glands empty into hair follicles, whereas eccrine sweat glands empty into pores on the skin surface.

      c. Arrector pili muscle (smooth muscle) originates on the dermal sheath of hair follicle and inserts into papillary layer of the dermis.
        • Contraction elevates the hair (**piloerection**) and depresses the skin where muscle attaches to dermis, causing "goose bumps."
    2. Hair growth
      a. Hair shaft grows from the hair bulb, composed of a **germinal layer** of mitotically active basal cells and a **keratogenous zone** where hair cells become keratinized.
      b. Sex hormones influence hair growth in both males and females.
      c. Usually hair growth is **asynchronous.**
      d. When hair growth is **synchronous** (e.g., postpartum, women on birth control pills), there is massive hair loss.
B. Glands in the skin (see Figure 8-2)
  • Prominent features of **sebaceous, eccrine sweat,** and **apocrine sweat glands** are summarized in Table 8-1.

TABLE 8-1 Glands of the Skin

Property	Type of Gland		
	Sebaceous	**Eccrine Sweat**	**Apocrine Sweat**
Location within skin	Dermis	Dermis	Dermis and hypodermis
Body distribution	Throughout body except for palms and soles	Throughout body	Axilla, mons pubis, areola of nipple, perianal region
General structure	Branched acinar gland with short duct	Simple tubular gland	Large, complex gland
Myoepithelial cells	Absent	Present	Present
Type of secretion	Thick, lipid-containing substance (sebum)	Clear, watery secretion	Viscous substance rich in protein and cellular debris
Secretion mechanism	Holocrine	Merocrine	Mixed
Duct opening	Hair follicle (usually)	Surface of skin (sweat pore)	Hair follicle
Period of activity	Inactive until puberty	Active throughout life	Inactive until puberty
Other features	Excess androgen-mediated secretion can plug hair follicles, predisposing to acne	Secretion stimulated by high temperature and stress	Activity is linked to menstrual cycle in female

1. **Sebum:** oily secretion of sebaceous glands of the skin
   a. Mixture of sebum and sweat is mildly bactericidal and protects skin against drying.
   b. **Androgen receptors** in sebaceous glands function in controlling sebum production.
2. **Seborrhea:** any of several skin diseases marked by very oily skin resulting from **overproduction of sebum**
3. **Acne vulgaris:** chronic inflammatory disease of the pilosebaceous apparatus
   a. Pathogenic features include **abnormal keratinization** of the follicular epithelium, **increased sebum production** (androgen-controlled), and lipase production by *Propionibacterium acnes,* leading to fatty acid release and an inflammatory reaction.
   b. Lesions take various forms including blackheads (comedones), pink papules, and pus-filled cysts, primarily on the face, chest, and upper back.

C. Nails
   • Nails are **hard keratinized plates** resting on a bed of epidermis at the distal end of each digit.
1. **Proximal root** is embedded in deep fold of epidermis.
   a. **Eponychium (cuticle):** stratum corneum of nail fold, which overlies proximal root

Androgen receptors in sebaceous glands function in androgen-mediated control of sebum production.

   b. Nail matrix: region of epidermal cells covered by epo-
      nychium where nail synthesis occurs
   c. Lunula: extension of nail matrix beyond eponychium,
      visible as whitish crescent
2. **Distal (free) edge** is underlain by **hyponychium,** a thickened stratum corneum.
3. **Abnormal nails** are associated with some **diseases.**
   • Nails should appear pinkish, due to blood vessels in un-
      derlying dermis.
   a. Pale or bluish nail bed may indicate **cardiovascular
      problems** or poor oxygenation of circulating blood
      (**cyanosis**).
   b. Split nails are associated **with nutritional deficiencies.**
   c. Clubbing (thickening) at nail base may indicate **lung
      cancer.**
   d. Spoon-shaped nails (koilonychia) are associated with
      iron-deficiency anemia.

V. **Vasculature and Innervation of the Skin**
   A. Blood supply to the skin
      • The **epidermis lacks blood vessels,** however, the dermis,
         hypodermis, and all skin appendages have an extensive
         network of small vessels.
      1. **Arterial plexuses**
         a. Rete cutaneum (reticular plexus) at **dermis/hypodermis
            border**
         b. Rete subpapillare (papillary plexus) at **border of papil-
            lary and reticular layers** of the dermis
            • Arterioles from this plexus give rise to a single capillary
               loop around each dermal papilla.
      2. **Venous plexuses**
         a. Middle of dermis
         b. Between papillary and reticular layers of dermis
         c. Dermis/hypodermis border
      3. **Arteriovenous anastomoses (AV shunts)**
         a. Direct connections between arterioles and venules, which
            occur in deeper parts of the skin, are important in
            thermoregulation.
         b. Blood flow through AV shunts is regulated by autonomic
            nerve fibers and certain hormones.
      4. **Kaposi's sarcoma**
         a. Clinically is characterized by **bluish-red cutaneous
            nodules,** usually first appearing on legs, toes, or feet, that
            slowly enlarge and spread to more proximal sites.
            • In AIDS patients, Kaposi's sarcoma is associated with
               herpes infection (HHV8)
         b. Histologically, lesions exhibit vascular proliferation with
            slitlike channels composed of malignant **spindle-
            shaped cells,** probably of endothelial origin.
   B. Nerves of the skin
      1. **Motor nerves:** postganglionic fibers from **sympathetic**
         ganglia of paravertebral chain

Sympathetic inner-
vation of the skin
functions largely in
thermoregulation by
controlling blood
flow, secretion of
sweat glands, and
piloerection.

Kaposi's sarcoma:
spindle cell carci-
noma of vascular
origin that com-
monly arises in the
skin and presents as
bluish-red nodules.
Most common
cancer found in
AIDS patients, in
whom it is associ-
ated with HHV8
infection; lesions are
aggressive and
often metastasize.

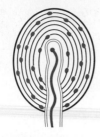
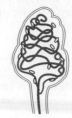
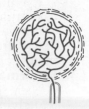
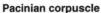

	Pacinian corpuscle	Meissner corpuscle	Krause end bulb
Location:	Ligaments, joint capsules, serous membranes	Palms, soles, digits	Skin, mucous membranes, conjunctiva
Detects:	Pressure, coarse touch, vibration, tension	Light touch on hairless skin	Cold, mechanical stimulation

Figure 8-3 Encapsulated mechanoreceptors. Their relative size is Pacinian corpuscle > Meissner corpuscle > Krause end bulb (not to scale).

- Autonomic nerve supply functions primarily in **thermo-regulation** by regulating blood flow to the skin, secretion by sweat glands, and piloerection.
2. **Sensory nerve endings:** most dense on the hands and feet, on the face (especially around the mouth), and in anogenital region.
    a. **Free nerve endings,** located at epidermal opening and root sheath of hair follicles, function as **mechanoreceptors.**
    b. **Encapsulated sensory receptors,** located in the skin and associated mucous membranes, are summarized in Figure 8-3.

Cartilage, Bone, and Joints

Target Topics

▷ Features distinguishing cartilage and bone
▷ Functions and locations of hyaline, elastic, and fibrous cartilage
▷ Interstitial vs appositional growth of cartilage
▷ Stages in intramembranous and endochondral ossification
▷ Hormonal and vitamin influences on bone formation and resorption
▷ Bone repair
▷ Different types of joints
▷ Osteogenesis imperfecta, osteopetrosis, osteoporosis, Paget's disease of bone, osteosarcoma, rickets, osteomalacia, arthritis, ankylosing spondylitis

I. Cartilage
   • A specialized **avascular connective tissue**, cartilage functions primarily to support soft tissues and in development and growth of long bones.
   A. Structure of cartilage
      1. **Cartilage cells**, which arise from **stellate mesenchymal cells**, synthesize and secrete **extracellular matrix components.**
         • Eventually these cells become roundish and completely surrounded by matrix except for the small spaces, or **lacunae**, in which they reside.
         a. **Chondroblasts:** less mature form that actively produces matrix
         b. **Chondrocytes:** more mature form that is less active in matrix synthesis

101

   2. Matrix of cartilage consists of fibers, ground substance, and water.

   a. Fibrous component contains collagen types I and II, elastic fibers, and reticular fibers depending on cartilage type.

   b. Ground substance contains **hyaluronic acid** and **chondroitin sulfate** and **keratan sulfate proteoglycans**, primarily in the form of aggregates (see Figure 5-3).

   c. Bound water provides avenue for diffusion of nutrients and oxygen to chondrocytes and confers gel-like property to cartilage matrix.

   3. Perichondrium, the vascularized connective tissue investment surrounding cartilage, comprises two layers.

   a. Outer fibrous layer of fibroblasts

   b. Inner chondrogenic layer

B. Types of cartilage (Table 9-1)

C. Growth of cartilage

   1. Interstitial growth results from mitosis of preexisting chondrocytes and chondroblasts in lacunae.

   a. Isogenous (isogenic) groups of two or four daughter cells trapped in lacunae are formed by interstitial growth.

   b. Cartilaginous fetal bones **elongate** by interstitial growth.

   2. Appositional growth results from differentiation of mesenchymal cells in the **chondrogenic layer** of the perichondrium.

   a. This growth process involves formation of new chondrocytes and additional matrix at the periphery.

   b. Cartilaginous fetal bones **increase in width** by appositional growth.

TABLE 9-1   Properties of Cartilage Types

Cartilage Type	Primary Fibers	Major Body Locations	Other Properties
Hyaline (most abundant)	Type II collagen	Articular surfaces at diarthrotic joints Ventral ends of ribs (costal cartilages) Tracheal rings Larynx	Functions as temporary skeleton during fetal growth Matrix has smooth, glassy appearance in light microscope
Elastic	Type II collagen Elastic fibers	Pinna of external ear Wall of external auditory canal Epiglottis Larynx (cuneiform and corniculate cartilages)	Found in flexible, semirigid structures Has yellowish color when unstained Matrix shows elastic fibers in light microscope
Fibrocartilage (least abundant)	Type I collagen	Pubic symphysis Intervertebral discs	Located where support and tensile strength needed Lacks perichondrium

D. Calcification of cartilage
1. When **chondrocytes hypertrophy,** they release alkaline phosphatase, which leads to **precipitation of calcium phosphate** in the matrix.
2. The calcified matrix compromises the nutrient supply so that cartilage **cells die.**
3. During **endochondral ossification,** large spicules of calcified cartilage function as scaffolding for bone formation.

II. **Bone** (Table 9-2)
* A specialized **vascular connective tissue,** bone contains several cell types embedded in or on a **mineralized matrix.**
A. **Bone matrix** is a roughly 1:1 mixture of inorganic and organic components.
1. **Hydroxyapatite crystals,** $Ca_{10}(PO_4)_6(OH)_3$, constitute the bulk of the inorganic part of bone matrix.
2. **Osteoid,** the organic part of the matrix, is composed of **type I collagen fibers; proteoglycans; osteonectin,** which anchors mineral salts to collagen; and **osteocalcin,** a calcium-binding protein.
a. **Eosinophilic** if unmineralized
b. **Basophilic** after mineralization
B. **Covering tissues**
1. **Periosteum:** a vascularized connective tissue that covers most external surfaces of bone
a. An outer fibrous layer and inner osteogenic layer compose the periosteum.
b. **Sharpey's fibers,** which are collagen fibers present in the periosteum, sweep into bone, anchoring the periosteum to it.

TABLE 9-2   Comparison of Cartilage and Bone

Property	Cartilage	Bone
Ground substance	Proteoglycan aggregates Hyaluronic acid No mineral component	Proteoglycans Osteonectin and osteocalcin Hydroxyapatite crystals and small amounts of other minerals
Collagen fibers	Type I (fibrocartilage) Type II (hyaline and elastic cartilage)	Type I
Blood supply	Lacking (nutrients diffuse through ground substance)	Present
Nerve supply	Lacking	Present
Mitotic activity	Chondroblasts: Yes Chondrocytes: Yes	Osteoprogenitor cells: Yes Osteoblasts: Maybe Osteocytes: No
Regenerative ability	Low	High
Communicating gap junctions	None	Between osteocytes

Four major cell
types in bone:
• Osteoblasts =
bone-forming cells
• Osteocytes =
relatively inactive os-
teoblasts in lacunae
• Osteoclasts =
bone-resorbing cells
• Osteoprogenitor
cells = undifferenti-
ated mesenchy-
mal cells that give
rise to osteoblasts

  2. **Endosteum:** a thin cell layer that lines internal surfaces of bone and has osteogenic capability
C. **Bone cells**
  1. **Osteoblasts** are **bone-forming** cells that arise from stellate **mesenchymal cells** and retain their stellate morphology.
    a. These cells produce **osteoid** (unmineralized bone matrix) and have a basophilic cytoplasm containing well-developed rough endoplasmic reticulum (RER) and Golgi apparatus typical of protein-synthesizing cells.
    b. Separate **receptors for vitamin D and parathyroid hormone** (PTH) are present on surface of osteoblasts.
  2. **Osteocytes** (mature bone cells) are osteoblasts that have been trapped within the matrix they produce.
    a. Cells retain stellate shape and are housed within matrix-bounded lacunae.
    b. Tunnels (**canaliculi**) form around cytoplasmic processes as matrix is deposited.
      • Tissue fluid in the small space between matrix of canaliculi and osteocyte plasmalemma supplies nutrients and metabolites to osteocytes.
    c. Adjacent osteocytes communicate with each other via **gap junctions** between their cytoplasmic processes.
    d. Osteocytes are relatively **inactive in osteoid production** but are capable of **osteocytic osteolysis**, the removal of some calcium from newly mineralized matrix.
    e. Because osteocytes do not undergo cell division, there is **no interstitial growth of bone** (in contrast to cartilage).
  3. **Osteoclasts** are **bone-resorbing** cells located at sites of active bone resorption.
    • They often are located in depressions, called **Howship's lacunae,** in the bone being resorbed.
    a. Morphology of osteoclasts
      (1) **Multinucleated giant cells** formed by fusion of several monocytes
      (2) **Ruffled border** on the resorptive surface adjacent to the eroding bone
      (3) Many mitochondria, vesicles, and lysosomes; well-developed RER and Golgi apparatus
    b. Resorptive activity of osteoclasts
      (1) **Collagenase** and other enzymes (e.g., **lysosomal hydrolases**) secreted by osteoclasts digest the osteoid, releasing previously stored minerals in the bone matrix.
      (2) **PTH increases** osteoclastic activity by inducing release of **osteoclast activating factor** (interleukin-1) from osteoblasts, leading to rise in blood Ca^{2+}.
      (3) **Calcitonin** and **estrogen decrease** osteoclastic activity, the latter by inhibiting osteoclast activating factor.

Vitamin D and
PTH promote bone
growth by stimu-
lating the pro-
liferation and
differentiation of os-
teoprogenitor cells
into osteoblasts.

Osteoporosis is
caused by increased
osteoclastic activity
(postmenopausal
form) or decreased
osteoblastic activ-
ity (senile form),
leading to a
decrease in
bone mass.

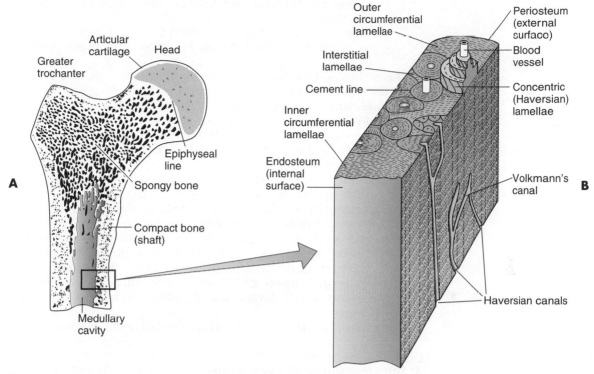

Figure 9-1 Two views of bone structure. **A,** Spicules of spongy bone adjacent to the marrow-filled shaft of a long bone are surrounded by compact bone containing numerous Haversian systems (osteons). **B,** Enlarged section through shaft of a long bone reveals lamellar organization of compact bone.

4. **Osteoprogenitor (osteogenic) cells** are undifferentiated mesenchymal cells located in the inner layer of the periosteum (osteogenic layer) and in the endosteum.
   a. Proliferation and differentiation of these cells generates osteoblasts.
   b. Although relatively inactive in adults, osteoprogenitor cells begin to proliferate under certain conditions (e.g., following a fracture).
D. **Types of bone** (Figure 9-1, *A*)
   1. **Cancellous (spongy) bone** consists of **endosteum-covered spicules of bone** and has a honeycomb appearance.
      • After birth, cancellous bone is found adjacent to epiphyseal plates and cavities filled with bone marrow.
   2. **Compact bone**, which has no spicules, forms the **shaft of typical long bones** surrounding the medullary cavity.
      • **Matrix** of compact bone **is deposited in lamellae** (rows), leaving cells trapped in lacunae.
      a. **Outer circumferential lamellae** are produced by periosteum.
      b. **Inner circumferential lamellae** are produced by endosteum.

Metastases to bone are much more common than primary tumors arising in bone. Osteolytic metastases cause increased bone resorption; osteoblastic metastases cause increased bone density.

         c. Haversian lamellae are circular lamellae located between the inner and outer circumferential lamellae.

         d. Interstitial lamellae are derived from incompletely resorbed Haversian lamellae produced during remodeling of bone.

    E. Haversian system (osteon) in compact bone

        1. Osteon structure (Figure 9-1, *B*)

            a. Group of concentric (Haversian) lamellae surround a central vascular channel, forming a **long cylindrical structure** that runs **parallel to the long axis.**

            b. Cement line, a thin zone that lacks canaliculi, defines the periphery of an osteon.

        2. Formation of osteons occurs continually as a consequence of bone remodeling.

            a. Resorption tunnels created by osteoclasts are "filled in" by osteoblasts, forming new osteons.

            b. Osteon formation proceeds from **the outside toward the center**, with the oldest lamellae at the outer edge and youngest lamellae adjacent to the Haversian canal.

        3. Volkmann's canals are vascular canals that branch from Haversian canals at various angles and **interconnect osteons.**

    F. Bone disorders unrelated to vitamin deficiencies (Box 9-1)

  III.   Histogenesis of Bone

    A. Intramembranous ossification

      • This process of bone formation involves **differentiation of mesenchyme directly into bone** without formation of an intervening cartilaginous model.

      • **Flat bones of the skull** and **subperiosteal lamellar bone** are formed by intramembranous ossification.

      1. Steps in intramembranous ossification

         a. Stellate mesenchymal cells differentiate into osteoblasts, forming **spicules of aggregated cells.**

         b. Osteoblasts begin producing osteoid, which eventually traps some osteoblasts as osteocytes in the interior of spicules.

         c. Mineralization of the developing spicule occurs gradually.

            (1) Basophilic core = mineralized, older osteoid

            (2) Thin, eosinophilic peripheral zone = nonmineralized, younger osteoid

         d. Spicules anastomose with each other, producing **immature (woven) bone**, which has the following characteristics:

            (1) Absence of lamellae

            (2) Loosely packed, randomly arranged collagen fibers, which impart a woven appearance

            (3) High cell density (greater than that for mature bone)

         e. Anastomosing spicules eventually enclose mesenchymal areas, which contain blood vessels and nerves.

BOX 9-1 Bone Disorders

Osteogenesis imperfecta: group of diseases caused by mutation in a gene encoding one of the α chains of **type I collagen**, leading to disturbance in the amount and quality of bone collagen. Marked by fragile bones prone to fracture, lax joints, and discolored teeth. Characteristic **blue sclerae** result from thinning of the sclerae and increased visibility of the underlying choroidal veins. The most common and mildest form (type I) exhibits **autosomal dominant** transmission.

Osteopetrosis: hereditary disease characterized by abnormally dense bone usually due to **decreased resorption** by dysfunctional osteoclasts. Most severe form (**autosomal recessive**), occurring in infancy and childhood, leads to obliteration of marrow cavity and lack of bone remodeling. Bone fractures, anemia, and cranial nerve palsies (bone entrapment) are common complications. Bone marrow transplants have been helpful.

Osteoporosis: a metabolic disorder characterized by **decreased bone mass** caused by an imbalance between bone formation (decreased) and bone resorption (increased). All forms are associated with increased risk of **fracture** after minor trauma and may cause pain (especially in the lower back), loss of body height (compression vertebral fractures), and deformities.

- **Postmenopausal osteoporosis**, occurring in women 3–20 years after menopause, results from **excessive bone resorption** by osteoclasts. Lowered estrogen level in postmenopausal women is a risk factor because estrogen inhibits osteoclast activating factor.
- **Senile osteoporosis**, occurring in both men and women over age 70, results from **decreased bone formation** by osteoblasts.
- **Immobilization**, endocrine disorders (e.g., **hyperparathyroidism**), and other diseases also can cause osteoporosis.

Paget's disease of bone (osteitis deformans): chronic, often asymptomatic bone disorder that occurs primarily in individuals over age 40. Repeated episodes of increased osteoclastic activity followed by excessive attempts at repair (osteoblastic activity) results in weakened, thickened bones, called *mosaic bone*. Bowing of long bones, spinal curvature (kyphosis), bone pain, and multiple fractures are common manifestations.

Osteosarcoma (osteogenic sarcoma): second most common malignant tumor of bone origin, mainly affecting young males. It generally involves the metaphysis of distal femur or proximal tibia and often spreads to the lungs. Tumors are highly variable and are classified based on the major histologic component.

    f. Appositional deposition of osteoid is greatest on the side of the spicule nearest the vessels and nerves, thereby forming an immature osteon.

  2. Remodeling of immature bone yields mature (compact) bone.

B. Endochondral ossification

- This process of bone formation begins with **differentiation of mesenchyme into a hyaline cartilage model**, which is reworked into adult (compact) bone.

- **Long bones of the limbs**, as well as the vertebral column, shoulder and pelvic girdles, and ribs, are formed by endochondral ossification.
  1. **Formation of diaphyseal (primary) center of ossification** (Figure 9-2, steps 1–4)
     a. **Hyaline cartilage model**, formed from fetal mesenchyme, contains chondroblasts and chondrocytes and is surrounded by perichondrium except at the ends.
     b. **Interstitial growth** increases length of model, and **appositional growth** from perichondrium increases its width.
     c. **Vascularization of the perichondrium** induces differentiation of osteoblasts from regional mesenchyme, thereby transforming the outer layer into **periosteum.**
     d. **Periosteal collar of bone** is produced by **intramembranous ossification of periosteum** around center of model.
     e. **Hypertrophy and death of chondrocytes** at the center of the cartilage model leaves **spicules of calcified cartilage** and empty lacunae that form **primitive marrow cavity.**
     f. **Enlargement of marrow cavity** occurs by addition of bone on the outside of the diaphyseal collar and removal of bone from its endosteal surface.
     g. **Periosteal bud**, containing blood vessels, osteoprogenitor cells, and mesenchymal cells, extends from the diaphyseal periosteum into center of the degenerating cartilage model.
     h. **Osteoprogenitor cells** of the periosteal bud attach to "naked" spicules of calcified (basophilic) cartilage and become osteoblasts, establishing the **primary center of ossification.**
     i. **Osteoblasts begin elaborating matrix,** the oldest of which soon becomes mineralized, forming a spicule.
        - Spicules have calcified cartilage in the center surrounded by mineralized bone matrix, which is surfaced by a thin zone of unmineralized (eosinophilic) matrix directly underneath the layer of osteoblasts.
     j. **Bone formation proceeds toward both epiphyseal ends** by repetition of steps b–i (above).
     k. **Marrow cavity is enlarged** by osteoclastic removal of oldest spicules of endochondral ossification.
  2. **Formation of epiphyseal (secondary) centers of ossification** (see Figure 9-2, steps 5–7)
     a. After birth, a center of ossification develops in **each epiphysis** by the same endochondral process used in formation of the diaphyseal center.
     b. Epiphyseal and diaphyseal centers of ossification are separated by **epiphyseal plates** composed of **hyaline cartilage.**
     c. Continual addition of new hyaline cartilage at the epiphyseal ends of long bones and its replacement by bone at the diaphyseal ends "moves" the epiphyseal plates outward, leading to lengthening of long bones.

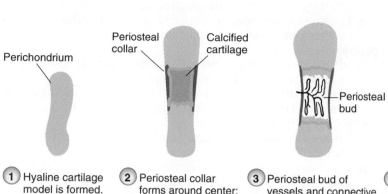
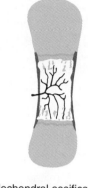
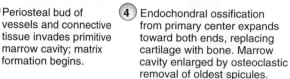

① Hyaline cartilage model is formed.

② Periosteal collar forms around center; cartilage calcification begins.

③ Periosteal bud of vessels and connective tissue invades primitive marrow cavity; matrix formation begins.

④ Endochondral ossification from primary center expands toward both ends, replacing cartilage with bone. Marrow cavity enlarged by osteoclastic removal of oldest spicules.

Perichondrium

Periosteal collar

Calcified cartilage

Periosteal bud

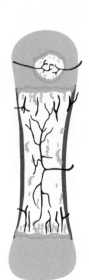
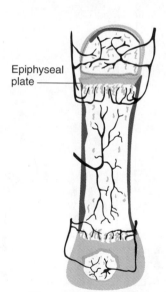
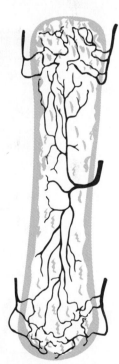

Epiphyseal plate

⑤ First epiphyseal (secondary) center of ossification forms in upper epiphysis.

⑥ Upper epiphyseal plate develops; formation of other epiphyseal center of ossification begins in lower epiphysis. Continued ossification at both plates lengthens the bone.

⑦ Disappearance (closure) of the epiphyseal plates marks end of growth of long bones, establishing adult height.

Figure 9-2 Overview of development of a long bone. Steps 1–4 establish the primary (diaphyseal) center of ossification, which forms during fetal development. Centers of ossification in the epiphyses develop after birth (steps 5 and 6). Subsequent increase in length of a long bone occurs by endochondral ossification at the two epiphyseal plates, which remain the same thickness but "move" outward.

     d. Epiphysis is enlarged by interstitial growth of hyaline cartilage in the articular region and its ossification.

     e. Epiphyseal surface remains covered by hyaline (articular) cartilage and has no periosteum.

C. Epiphyseal plates

- **Pituitary growth hormone** stimulates overall growth, especially bone formation at epiphyseal plates.

   1. Zones in epiphyseal plates can be distinguished histologically and occur as follows from the epiphyseal to diaphyseal side (Figure 9-3):

     a. Zone of resting cartilage: small, randomly arranged chondrocytes

     b. Zone of proliferation: interstitial growth of chondrocytes giving rise to rows of isogenous cell groups

     c. Zone of hypertrophy: enlarged chondrocytes that release **alkaline phosphatase**

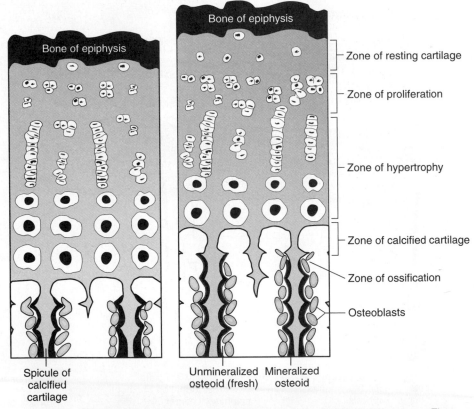

Figure 9-3 Endochondral ossification at an epiphyseal plate of a growing long bone. The two diagrams are of the same regions but the one on the left is earlier in time than that on the right. Formation of new cartilage at the epiphyseal end of the plate and its ossification at the diaphyseal end leads to lengthening of the bone shaft. In the zone of ossification, osteoblasts attached to spicules of calcified cartilage secrete osteoid onto the spicule surface. In time, the osteoid is mineralized (dark band), starting with the oldest, which is closest to the cartilage spicule. At the diaphyseal end of the mineralized spicules (not shown), osteoclasts remove the calcified cartilage-mineralized matrix complex, thereby enlarging the diaphyseal marrow cavity.

   d. Zone of calcified cartilage: dying or dead chondrocytes
      and calcified cartilage spicules (intensely basophilic)
   e. Zone of ossification: continuous secretion of osteoid
      (eosinophilic) by osteoblasts attached to spicules of calci-
      fied cartilage and subsequent mineralization of older
      osteoid (basophilic), producing tricolored appearance of
      spicules
  2. Closure of epiphyses refers to the change within epiphyseal
     plates that makes them nonfunctional.
   a. Depending on the bone, closure occurs in young adults at
      20–30 years of age.
   b. Epiphyseal closure marks the **end of growth in length of
      long bones.**
   c. Epiphyseal line in "older" long bones marks site of
      former epiphyseal plate.
**D. Effect of vitamin and hormonal abnormalities on bone
   formation**
  1. Vitamin C deficiency impairs collagen synthesis by osteo-
     blasts, although the osteoid that is produced is mineralized.
   • Results in thin spicules of mineralized bone, as seen in
      scurvy (see Chapter 5)
  2. Vitamin D deficiency causes poor intestinal absorption of
     calcium and phosphorus, leading to poor mineralization
     of osteoid (**soft bone**).
   • Results in thick spicules of bone containing excessive
      amounts of eosinophilic, unmineralized osteoid
   a. Rickets in children is due to poor mineralization before
      closure of epiphyseal plates.
    • Clinical features include short stature, flaring of ribs,
       bowlegs, knock-knees, **craniotabes** (soft skull), and
       rachitic rosary (nodular swellings where ribs join their
       cartilages).
   b. Osteomalacia in adults is due to poor mineralization
      after closure of epiphyseal plates.
    • Clinical features include thickened osteoid seams,
       bone pain, muscle weakness, and fatigue.
  3. Excess of vitamin A causes premature epiphyseal closure,
     resulting in short stature.
  4. Excess of growth hormone stimulates liver-derived
     somatomedin, leading to excessive bone formation.
   a. Before epiphyseal closure → **pituitary gigantism** (elon-
      gated long bones)
   b. After epiphyseal closure → **acromegaly** (thickened
      long bones)
  5. Deficiency of growth hormone before epiphyseal closure
     causes **pituitary dwarfism.**
E. Remodeling of bone
  1. Continual bone remodeling results from combined activ-
     ity of osteoclasts (bone resorption) by osteoclasts (bone
     formation).
  2. Immature bone is remodeled more rapidly than
     mature bone.

Bone formation by osteoblasts requires vitamin C for synthesis of collagen fibers and vitamin D for intestinal absorption of the Ca^{2+} and phosphorus used in mineralization of osteoid.

Serum alkaline phosphatase (released by enlarged chondrocytes) is three to five times higher in children than in adults because of the rapid bone growth in children.

Growth hormone deficiency before epiphyseal closure causes pituitary dwarfism.

Growth hormone excess before epiphyseal closure causes pituitary gigantism marked by elongated long bones. Excess after epiphyseal closure causes acromegaly marked by thickened long bones.

   3. Typical adult bone turns over completely in about **7–10 years**, so that roughly each decade a new skeleton is formed.
   4. Bone density is promoted by weight lifting and walking, and reduced by lack of gravity in space.
F. Broken bones and their repair
   1. Initial events following a fracture
      a. Thrombus formation
      b. Arrival of neutrophils (PMNs) and macrophages, which remove debris
      c. Hypoxia of the bone matrix distal to fracture caused by blood vessel damage
      d. Death of osteocytes in osteons
   2. Development of bony callus on internal and external surfaces at a fracture site
      a. Differentiation of osteoprogenitor cells in endosteum and periosteum into chondroblasts and chondrocytes
      b. Formation of cartilaginous bridge, or **callus**, across break on the periosteal side (external callus) and endosteal side (internal callus)
      c. Endochondral ossification of callus to produce cancellous bone
   3. Remodeling of bony callus into mature compact bone across the fracture site
      a. Forces of stress (**weight bearing**) cause remodeling to original architecture.
      b. Bone develops structure most suited to resist the forces acting on it (**Wolff's law**).

IV.   **Joints**
   A. Synarthroses
      • These **immovable joints** are classified based on the type of tissue connecting the bones.
      1. Syndesmoses: bone joined to bone by **dense fibrous connective tissue** (e.g., sutures of the skull during childhood)
      2. Synchondroses: bone joined to bone by **cartilage** (e.g., epiphyseal plate, which is temporary, and union between ribs and sternum)
      3. Synostoses: bone joined to bone by **bone** (e.g., sutures of skull in adult)
   B. Amphiarthroses
      • These **slightly movable joints** are composed of **fibrocartilage** (e.g., pubic symphysis and intervertebral disks).
   C. Diarthroses
      • These **freely movable joints**, which generally unite long bones, are also known as **synovial joints**.
      1. Synovial fluid-filled cavity separates two bones.
      2. Hyaline (articular) cartilage covers the opposing bone surfaces, which lack perichondrium.
         • Parallel collagen fibers lie close to the joint cavity (deeper fibers run in arches or arcades)
         • Small pieces of cartilage ("**joint mice**") may be present in the synovial fluid.

3. **Joint capsule** connects the ends of adjacent bones.
   a. **Inner capsular layer** contains nonepithelial cells that secrete **hyaluronic acid**, the joint lubricant.
      • This layer, also called the **synovial membrane**, functions in formation of a blood dialysate that enters the joint cavity and together with hyaluronic acid forms **synovial fluid**.
   b. **Outer capsular layer** supports the synovial membrane.
      • Fibrous type withstands pressure.
      • Areolar type allows sliding.
      • Adipose type provides cushion.
4. **Menisci** are cushions of fibrocartilage present in some synovial joints (e.g., knee joint).

D. **Joint disorders**
   1. **Osteoarthritis:** noninflammatory, degenerative disease that commonly affects joints of the hand, cervical and lumbar spine, hip, and knee
      • Pathologic changes include **degeneration of articular cartilage**, thickening and polishing of subchondral bone (**eburnation**), and formation of bony spurs (osteophytes) that often extend into the joint.
   2. **Rheumatoid arthritis:** chronic **inflammatory** arthritis caused by **autoimmune** mechanisms and involving systemic effects
      • Inflammation and proliferation of synovial membrane leads to formation of rheumatoid **pannus**, the characteristic joint lesion. Muscle atrophy and ankylosis occur in later stages.
   3. **Ankylosing spondylitis:** chronic degenerative inflammatory disease that primarily affects males under age 30 and initially involves the spine.
      • Marked by **synovitis without pannus formation** and inflammation of ligaments at their insertion into bone; may progress to ankylosis of the spinal column
      • Often associated with **inflammatory intestinal diseases**

Osteoarthritis: most common noninflammatory joint disease; degeneration of articular cartilages with osteophyte formation at the joint margins.

Rheumatoid arthritis: autoimmune origin; synovitis with pannus formation, muscle atrophy and ankylosis (late).

Majority of patients with ankylosing spondylitis are HLA-B27 positive.

10

Respiratory System

Target Topics

▷ Histologic features characterizing different portions of respiratory tract
▷ Cell types composing respiratory epithelium
▷ Pathway of gaseous exchange (air–blood barrier)
▷ Cell types in alveoli
▷ Lung cancer, chronic bronchitis, asthma, respiratory distress syndrome, emphysema, pneumoconiosis (coal miner's lung, silicosis, asbestosis), heart-failure cells

I.   **Introduction**
   - The structures throughout the **respiratory system** possess characteristic lining epithelia, supporting tissues, and glands (Table 10-1).
   A. **Conducting portion** comprises a series of progressively smaller passageways that convey inspired air to small conducting bronchioles within the lungs.
      - No gaseous exchange occurs in these airways, which constitute the **dead-air space** of pulmonary physiology.
   B. **Respiratory portion**, located entirely within the lungs, comprises structures where **gaseous exchange** occurs.

II. **Respiratory Epithelium**
   - **Pseudostratified ciliated columnar epithelium**, commonly known as **respiratory epithelium**, lines all or part of the larger conducting structures.
   A. **Cell types composing respiratory epithelium**
      1. **Goblet cells** secrete mucus, which traps inhaled particles (bacteria, pollen, dust).
      2. **Ciliated columnar cells** beat their cilia toward the oropharynx, thereby moving mucus upward so it can be swallowed or expectorated.

TABLE 10-1   Histology of Respiratory System Components

Structure	Epithelium*	Cilia	Goblet Cells	Supporting Tissue	Other Features
Conducting Portion					
Nasal cavity:					
Respiratory	Respiratory	Yes	Yes	Bone, hyaline cartilage	Nasal sinuses; glands
Olfactory	Olfactory	No	No	Bone	Olfactory bipolar neurons; Bowman's glands
Nasopharynx	Respiratory, oral	Yes	Yes	Muscle	Pharyngeal tonsil; glands
Larynx	Respiratory, oral	Yes	Yes	Hyaline and elastic cartilages	Epiglottis and vocal cords; glands
Trachea and primary bronchi	Respiratory	Yes	Yes	C-rings (hyaline cartilages); smooth muscle (trachealis)	Glands
Intrapulmonary bronchi	Respiratory	Yes	Yes	Hyaline cartilage blocks; smooth muscle	Glands
Conducting bronchioles	Respiratory to simple cuboidal	Some	In larger ones	Smooth muscle	Clara cells
Respiratory Portion					
Respiratory bronchioles	Simple cuboidal	Some	None	Smooth muscle	Clara cells; some alveoli
Alveoli and alveolar ducts	Pneumocytes (type I and II)	None	None	Elastic and reticular fibers in interalveolar septa	Surfactant covering surface; alveolar macrophages

*Respiratory epithelium, pseudostratified ciliated columnar epithelium containing five cell types; oral epithelium, nonkeratinized stratified squamous epithelium.

3. **Nonciliated columnar cells** have microvilli on their apical surface but no cilia.
4. **Basal cells** are undifferentiated **stem cells** whose progeny can differentiate into goblet cells or columnar cells (ciliated and nonciliated).
5. **Small granule cells** are neuroendocrine cells that synthesize and release **catecholamines**.

B. **Lamina propria beneath respiratory epithelium**
   - Formed of **loose areolar connective tissue** that contains **glands** (seromucous, mucous) and **diffuse lymphatic**

tissue including plasma cells, lymphocytes, and macrophages

III. **Conducting Portion**
- During its passage through the conducting portion, inspired air is **warmed, moistened,** and **cleaned.**
- The structures of the conducting portion are arranged in the following order: **nasal cavity → nasopharynx and oropharynx → larynx → trachea → bronchi → bronchioles → terminal bronchioles.**

A. **Nasal cavity and nasopharynx**
1. **Portions of the nasopharynx** that experience "wear and tear" (e.g., uvula) are covered by **nonkeratinized stratified squamous epithelium,** or **oral epithelium,** rather than respiratory epithelium.
2. **Watery secretion** of glands in the lamina propria moistens inspired air.
3. **Large number of blood vessels** in the lamina propria help to warm inspired air.
4. **Olfactory mucosa** is present on the superior aspect of each nasal cavity (see Chapter 19).

B. **Larynx**
- Several **hyaline** and **elastic cartilages** help support thin walls of the larynx and function in phonation.
1. **Epiglottis,** the anterior superior extension of the larynx, is shared by respiratory and digestive systems.
   - During swallowing, the epiglottis folds on itself, closing the airway.
   a. **Elastic cartilage** forms the core of the epiglottis and is surrounded by a lamina propria.
   b. **Digestive part,** which constitutes the anterior aspect, tip, and upper part of the posterior aspect, is covered by **oral epithelium.**
   c. **Respiratory part,** which constitutes lower part of the posterior aspect, is covered by **respiratory epithelium.**
2. **Vocal apparatus,** distal to the epiglottis, consists of two pairs of **folds of the laryngeal mucosa** spanning the laryngeal space.
   a. **False vocal cords (vestibular folds)** are the **superior pair** of folds, which play no role in phonation.
      - Covered by respiratory epithelium and contain seromucous glands in the lamina propria
   b. **True vocal cords (folds)** are the **inferior pair** of folds, which **produce sound** as air passes over them.
      - Covered by oral epithelium and lack seromucous glands in the lamina propria
      (1) **Vocal ligament:** mass of elastic tissue forming core of each vocal cord
      (2) **Vocalis muscle:** small skeletal muscle deep to the vocal ligament

C. Trachea
   1. **Mucosa** is surfaced by **respiratory epithelium** with an underlying lamina propria.
   2. **Submucosa,** containing **many seromucous glands,** is separated from the mucosa by a layer of elastic fibers.
   3. **C-shaped hyaline cartilages (C-rings)** lie deep to the submucosa.
      * These supporting cartilages are covered by a perichondrium, which is surrounded by an adventitia of loose connective tissue shared with the esophagus.
      a. Open end of each C-ring faces posteriorly, toward the esophagus.
      b. Smooth muscle (**trachealis**) bridges the open end of each cartilage.
   4. **Extrapulmonary (primary) bronchi,** which arise by division of the trachea outside the lungs, are histologically similar to the trachea.
D. Intrapulmonary bronchi
   * Within the lungs, the bronchi divide many times.
   1. **Hyaline cartilages** are variably shaped and eventually break up into **small blocks** in the walls of the intrapulmonary bronchi.
   2. **Respiratory epithelium** and other histologic layers of the wall progressively **diminish in thickness.**
E. Conducting bronchioles
   1. **Characteristic features**
      a. Absence of cartilages (i.e., loss of rigid support)
      b. Abundant **smooth muscle** in walls
         * Contraction and relaxation of smooth muscle **determines the diameter of bronchioles.**
         * **Epinephrine relaxes** this muscle.
      c. Transition of the inner layer as bronchioles become smaller:
         * Respiratory epithelium → ciliated columnar → ciliated cuboidal → nonciliated cuboidal
      d. Absence of seromucous glands
      e. Mucus-producing goblet cells only in larger bronchioles
   2. **Terminal bronchioles**
      * Constitute smallest (diameter <0.5 mm), most distal part of the conducting tree and terminate in the first component of the respiratory branch
      a. Some ciliated cuboidal cells but no goblet cells are present, assuring that **all mucus production occurs upstream of cilia.**
      b. Parallel branching converts turbulent airflow to laminar airflow.
   3. **Clara cells**
      a. Prevalence: as number of ciliated cells decreases in conducting bronchioles, the number of Clara cells increases.

Terminal bronchioles are the primary site for "small airway" diseases such as asthma.

    b. Morphology: rounded, dome-shaped apical surface (with short, blunt microvilli but no cilia); cytoplasmic ultrastructure is typical of secretory cells.

    c. Function

        (1) Secretion of a **surface-active lipoprotein** that prevents collapse of terminal bronchioles, especially during exhalation

        (2) Metabolism of airborne toxins by cytochrome P450 enzymes

F. Diseases involving bronchi and bronchioles

  1. Bronchogenic carcinoma (a squamous cell carcinoma) is the most common type of cancer of the lung.

    • **Cigarette smoke,** which is ciliotoxic and stimulates excess production of mucus, is the most common causative agent.

    a. Carcinogenesis involves progressive changes in the respiratory epithelium of bronchi, as illustrated in Figure 10-1.

    b. Cessation of smoking can lead to reversal of mild dysplastic changes but not anaplastic changes.

        (1) Reversal results from differentiation of remaining basal cells into goblet cells and ciliated and nonciliated columnar cells, thereby restoring the normal respiratory epithelium.

        (2) Risk for carcinoma slowly returns to almost normal after about a decade of no exposure to smoke.

  2. Chronic bronchitis results from irritation of the bronchi, commonly by cigarette smoke, leading to **excess mucus production** and narrowing of the airway, primarily the terminal bronchioles.

    • Is defined clinically as a **sputum-producing cough** for at least 3 months per year for 2 successive years

  3. Asthma is marked by recurrent **bronchospasms** in which widespread **constriction of smooth muscle** in the bronchi

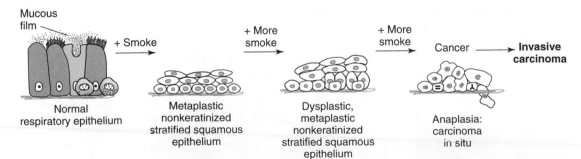

Figure 10-1 Changes in respiratory epithelium caused by smoking. Normal respiratory epithelium first undergoes metaplasia (replacement of one adult cell type by another adult cell type) to normal-appearing nonkeratinized stratified squamous epithelium. These metaplastic cells then undergo atypical changes in their size, shape, and organization (dysplasia). Further dysplastic changes lead to complete cytological disorganization of the epithelium (anaplasia), initially producing a carcinoma in situ (confined to epithelium above basement membrane) and then an invasive carcinoma (extending through the basement membrane into adjacent tissues).

and bronchioles decreases their diameter, leading to expiratory wheezing.

   a. Asthma attacks often are associated with **immediate (type I) hypersensitivity reactions** during which vasoconstrictive mediators are released (see Figure 13-5).

   b. Common treatment for mild asthma is **β$_2$-agonists** (e.g., albuterol), which relax the bronchiolar smooth muscle and decrease its tonus, thus enlarging the air passages.

IV. **Respiratory Portion**

   A. Pulmonary lobules

   • Distal to terminal bronchioles, the lung is composed of lobules, each containing a central **respiratory bronchiole** that gives way to **alveolar ducts** whose distal end terminates in one or more **alveolar sacs.**

   1. Deoxygenated blood is carried into each lobule by a branch of the pulmonary artery that accompanies the respiratory bronchiole and terminates in dense capillary networks in the walls of alveoli.

   2. Oxygenated blood is drained from the periphery of each lobule by pulmonary veins contained in delicate connective tissue septa arising from the visceral pleura.

   B. Alveoli

   • These saclike evaginations in the walls of respiratory bronchioles, alveolar ducts, and alveolar sacs are the **sites of gaseous exchange.**

   • Alveoli are the smallest (200–300 µm in diameter) and most abundant (300 million per lung) air-containing structures in the respiratory tract.

   1. Interalveolar septa: connective tissue partitions separating adjacent alveoli and containing **pulmonary capillaries**

   2. Pores of Kohn: holes in interalveolar septa through which adjacent alveoli normally share air (thus equalizing the pressure)

   3. Alveolar walls: lined by an epithelium composed of two types of pneumocytes

   a. Type I pneumocytes have an extremely thin cytoplasm and cover about 95% of the alveolar surface.

   • Tight junctions connect adjacent type I cells.

   • Basal lamina of these cells may be fused with the basal lamina of nearby capillary endothelial cells.

   b. Type II pneumocytes (great alveolar cells) are somewhat rounded cells that bulge into the alveolar lumen, covering about 5% of the alveolar surface.

   • These cells, the primary repair cells of alveoli, can divide and replace damaged type I pneumocytes, which normally do not divide.

   4. Pulmonary surfactant: phospholipid–protein mixture secreted by **type II pneumocytes** that spreads over alveolar walls

β$_2$-Agonists used to treat asthma (e.g., albuterol) reduce bronchospasm and enlarge airways by relaxing bronchiolar smooth muscle.

Lobar pneumonia results from spread of microorganisms throughout a lung via the pores of Kohn connecting adjacent alveoli.

Atelectasis: proximal plugging of the terminal bronchioles with mucus. In this condition, air in the alveoli is resorbed through the pores of Kohn.

Type II pneumocytes secrete pulmonary surfactant, which reduces surface tension of pulmonary fluids, thereby contributing to the elasticity of alveoli and patency of the small airways on expiration.

a. **Reduction in surface tension** due to surfactant permits alveoli to expand easily during inspiration without collapsing during expiration.

b. **Respiratory distress syndrome (RDS) of the newborn** is caused by a **deficiency** in the amount and quality of **pulmonary surfactant.**

- This disorder is most common in **premature infants** (surfactant production normally begins late in gestation) and in infants with diabetic mothers (insulin inhibits surfactant production).

- **Labored breathing** is evident shortly after birth, followed by **cyanosis** of the skin and mucous membranes. If newborn survives for 3–5 days, disease usually resolves.

5. **Pulmonary emphysema:** abnormal increase in the residual volume of the lungs (hyperinflation) accompanied by a decrease in vital capacity and increase in total lung capacity

a. **Decrease in normal elasticity** of the alveolar walls eventually causes distention of the alveoli, rupture of their walls, and obliteration of alveolar capillaries.

- Decreased elasticity can result from cigarette smoke or a hereditary condition that reduces activity of α_1-**antitrypsin**, which normally protects the lungs' elastic fibers from degradation by elastase released from neutrophils.

b. In advanced cases, **chronic hypoxemia** (low arterial Po_2) causes pulmonary artery hypertension, which makes the right side of the heart work excessively, resulting in **cor pulmonale** associated with right ventricular hypertrophy.

C. **Gaseous exchange**

1. **Mechanism:** oxygen diffuses from the alveolar airspace across the air–blood barrier into red blood cells where it binds to heme groups in hemoglobin, releasing bound carbon dioxide, which diffuses back to the alveolar airspace.

2. **Respiratory membrane (air–blood barrier):** about 0.2 μm thick at its thinnest points, the "barrier" to gas diffusion comprises the following components in the air-to-blood direction (Figure 10-2):

- Surfactant → type I pneumocyte → basal lamina of type I pneumocyte → basal lamina of capillary endothelial cell → endothelial cell → blood plasma → plasmalemma of red blood cell

D. **Alveolar macrophages (dust cells)**

- These phagocytic cells, derived from monocytes that migrate out of capillaries in the interalveolar septa, wander over the alveolar surface **ingesting bacteria** and other **inhaled particles.**

1. **Pneumoconiosis:** accumulation of nondegradable particulate matter in phagocytic cells in the lungs.

a. **Anthracosis (coal miner's lung, black lung)** caused by deposition of inert carbon particles

---

Deficiency of pulmonary surfactant causes RDS, which is most common in premature infants or those with diabetic mothers.

Pneumoconiosis: any disease caused by accumulation of airborne, nondegradable particles in the lungs: anthracosis (coal miner's lung, black lung), asbestosis, and silicosis.

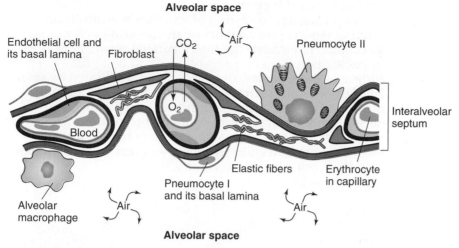

Figure 10-2   Respiratory membrane (air–blood barrier). Thin cytoplasm and underlying basal lamina of type I pneumocytes extend over most of the alveolar surface, which is covered with a layer of surfactant secreted by type II pneumocytes. Gas exchange is most efficient where the membrane is thinnest.

BOX 10-1   **Formation of Heart-Failure Cells**

Left-sided heart failure causes sluggish blood flow in the lungs resulting from a backup of blood from the failed left side of the heart into the pulmonary veins and capillaries. As the pulmonary capillary pressure increases, blood, plasma, and RBCs escape into the interalveolar septa. Excess tissue fluid and extravascular RBCs eventually move into the alveolar airspaces, causing **pulmonary edema.** As alveolar macrophages ingest and digest the RBCs, the macrophages become filled with **hemosiderin,** a brownish breakdown product derived from hemoglobin. Accumulation of these heart-failure cells leads to a **brown induration** of the lung and a **rusty-colored sputum.**

- Pulmonary fibrosis and emphysema eventually develop.
  b. Silicosis resulting from deposition of silica dust
    - Acute exposure can lead to **pulmonary edema** and **alveolar damage.**
    - Prolonged exposure is marked by development of fibrous nodules that may enlarge, causing **massive fibrosis** of the lungs.
  c. Asbestosis resulting from deposition of asbestos fibers
    - Interstitial fibrosis of the lungs occurs to varying degrees. Often associated with benign pleural plaques, pleural **mesothelioma,** and **bronchogenic carcinoma** (most common cancer).
  2. Heart-failure cells: hemosiderin-containing macrophages found in the pulmonary alveoli and sputum in left heart failure (Box 10-1).

Emphysema, caused by decreased elasticity of alveolar walls, can lead to cor pulmonale (right-sided ventricular hypertrophy) with pulmonary hypertension.

V. **Visceral and Parietal Pleurae**
  A. **Serous membranes**, consisting of a surface **mesothelium** and underlying lamina propria, enclose the **pleural cavity**.
  - Visceral pleura invests the lungs; parietal pleura lines the thoracic cavity.
  - Sliding of these pleurae over each other, facilitated by small amount of serous secretion lying between them, permits **movement of the lungs** within the thoracic cavity.
  B. **Mesothelioma**, resulting from malignant transformation of the mesothelium, can be triggered by exposure to **asbestos**.
  - Most commonly seen in **shipyard workers** and individuals who have worked as **roofers** for >20 years.

11

Cardiovascular System

Target Topics

▷ Histologic features distinguishing different types of arteries, veins, and lymphatic vessels
▷ Properties of continuous, fenestrated, and sinusoidal capillaries
▷ Formation of tissue fluid and lymph
▷ Cardiac tunics and their relation to pericardium
▷ Pathway of impulse conduction in the heart
▷ Arterioscleroses, edema, tumor angiogenesis, ischemic heart disease, valvular stenosis

I. **Blood Vessels**
   A. **Vascular tunics**
   - The walls of all blood vessels, except capillaries, consist of three layers (Figure 11-1).
   - The composition and thickness of vascular tunics vary in different types of vessels.
   1. **Tunica intima** (inner layer)
      a. Endothelium and its basal lamina
         - **von Willebrand's factor VIII**, a platelet adhesion factor produced in endothelial cells, is an immuno-chemical marker for endothelium.
      b. Subendothelial connective tissue
      c. Internal elastic membrane
   2. **Tunica media** (middle layer)
      a. Circular smooth muscle and some fibroblasts
      b. Collagen and elastic fibers
   3. **Tunica adventitia** (outer layer)
      a. Loose areolar connective tissue
      b. Irregular fibroelastic connective tissue containing adipocytes (outer aspect)
      c. Small vessels (**vasa vasorum**) and nerves

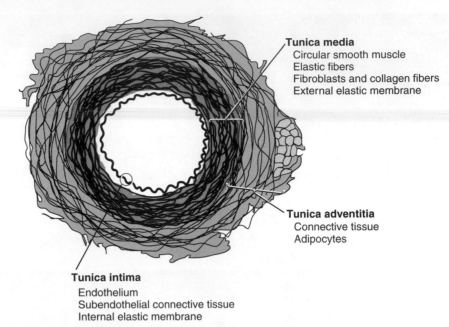

Tunica media
Circular smooth muscle
Elastic fibers
Fibroblasts and collagen fibers
External elastic membrane

Tunica adventitia
Connective tissue
Adipocytes

Tunica intima
Endothelium
Subendothelial connective tissue
Internal elastic membrane

Figure 11-1 Structure of a generalized blood vessel. Except for capillaries, blood vessels contain three well-defined tunics. Some arteries possess an external elastic membrane between the media and adventitia. See Table 11-1 for variations among different-sized arteries.

B. Arterial vessels
- As arteries extend out from the heart, they become progressively smaller and the composition of their tunics changes (Table 11-1).
  1. Elastic (conducting) arteries include the aorta, pulmonary trunk, and their large branches.
  a. During systole, elastic arteries **stretch** as they receive blood.
  b. During diastole, their **passive elastic recoil** plays a major role in maintaining diastolic blood pressure.
  2. Muscular (distributing) arteries include all other named arteries of gross anatomy.
  a. Transition from elastic to muscular type of artery occurs gradually.
  b. Smooth muscle in tunica media contracts and relaxes in response to **hormones** and **autonomic stimulation** (e.g., facial blush).
  c. The lumen diameter and thickness of tunica media decrease as muscular arteries get farther from the heart.
  3. Arterioles are small arteries that have only **one to three smooth muscle layers** in their tunica media.
  a. They give rise to **metarterioles,** the smallest arteries, which possess a discontinuous layer of smooth muscle cells.
  b. Maintenance of **mean arterial pressure** depends primarily on proper **tonus of smooth muscle** in arterioles (peripheral resistance arterioles).

TABLE 11-1   Selected Characteristics of Arterial Tunics

Tunica Components	Elastic Arteries	Muscular Arteries	Arterioles
Intima			
Endothelium	Yes	Yes	Yes
Basal lamina	Yes	Yes	Yes
Subendothelial layer	Yes	Yes	In some
Internal elastic membrane	Incomplete	Thick, complete	Few elastic fibers
Media			
Smooth muscle (circular)	Interspersed between elastic membranes	Many layers	1–3 layers
Fenestrated elastic laminae	Many	None	None
Fibroblasts and collagen	Yes	Yes	Yes
External elastic membrane	No	Yes	No
Adventitia			
Loose connective tissue	Yes	Yes	No
Adipose connective tissue	Abundant	Some	Little
Vasa vasorum	Yes	In some	No
Nerve fibers	Yes	Yes	Yes

(1)   **Vasodilation:** below-normal tonus that leads to **decreased** diastolic blood pressure, which can result in **shock.**

(2)   **Vasoconstriction:** above-normal tonus that leads to **increased** diastolic blood pressure

4. **Arteriosclerosis** refers to any condition marked by **thickening and hardening of arterial walls.**

   a. Atherosclerosis: deposition of fibrous fatty plaques (**atheromas**) in **tunica intima** of arteries, weakening the wall of elastic arteries and reducing the luminal diameter of muscular arteries

   • Subsequent exposure of subendothelial collagen fibers to blood may cause platelet aggregation and **thrombus formation** (see Chapter 12).

   b. Medial calcific sclerosis (Mönckeberg's arteriosclerosis): calcium deposition in tunica media of large and medium-sized arteries (e.g., uterine arteries)

   c. Hyperplastic arteriolosclerosis: hyperplasia of smooth muscle cells in arterioles, leading to **onionskin appearance;** occurs in **malignant hypertension**

   d. Hyaline arteriolosclerosis: deposition of hyaline material in the wall of arterioles with consequent narrowing of the lumina; occurs in **diabetes mellitus** and **hypertension**

C. **Capillaries**

   • Capillaries, which branch from metarterioles, consist of a **single endothelial layer** rolled into a tube that is surrounded by a **basement membrane** and occasional **pericytes.**

In atherosclerosis of muscular arteries, luminal diameter of arteries is reduced by deposition of fibrous fatty plaques in tunica intima.

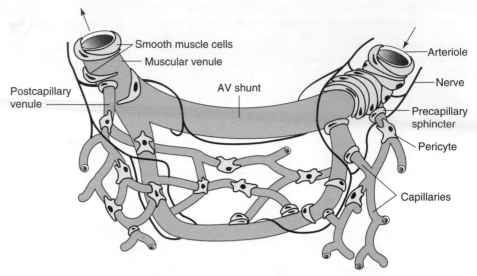

Figure 11-2 Simplified view of a capillary bed. *Arrows* indicate direction of blood flow. Capillary walls are designed for transport of gases, nutrients, and waste products between the blood and tissue spaces.

1. **Capillary bed** is an intricate network of capillaries interposed between arterioles and venules (Figure 11-2).
   a. **Precapillary sphincters** control blood flow into capillaries.
   b. **Lumen of capillaries** (7–9 μm in diameter) is just sufficient to permit passage of RBCs one at a time.
   c. **Arteriovenous anastomoses (AV shunts)** provide direct connections between arterioles and venules. Numerous in the lips, ears, toes, nose, and fingertips.
      (1) **Closed** AV shunt directs blood into capillary bed.
      (2) **Open** AV shunt permits blood to by-pass capillary bed.
2. **Pericytes** are undifferentiated mesenchymal cells that wrap around capillaries encased within the basal lamina (see Figure 11-2).
   a. **Presence of actin and myosin** in pericytes suggests that they may be contractile and help move blood through capillaries.
   b. Normally pericytes are quiescent but can be activated (e.g., during wound healing) to differentiate into fibroblasts and other cell types.
3. **Classification of capillaries** is based on differences in the structure of their endothelial cells (Figure 11-3).
   a. **Continuous capillaries**
      • Transendothelial transport of larger molecules is mediated by **pinocytic vesicles.** Maculae occludens between adjacent cells permit passage of water and small hydrophilic molecules.
   b. **Fenestrated capillaries** (e.g., glomerular capillaries)

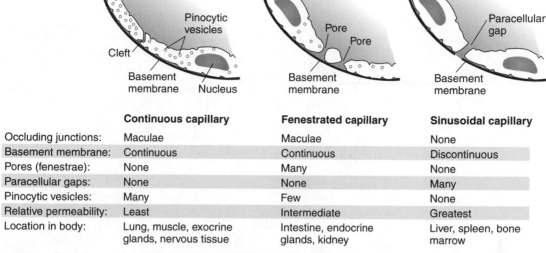

	Continuous capillary	**Fenestrated capillary**	**Sinusoidal capillary**
Occluding junctions:	Maculae	Maculae	None
Basement membrane:	Continuous	Continuous	Discontinuous
Pores (fenestrae):	None	Many	None
Paracellular gaps:	None	None	Many
Pinocytic vesicles:	Many	Few	None
Relative permeability:	Least	Intermediate	Greatest
Location in body:	Lung, muscle, exocrine glands, nervous tissue	Intestine, endocrine glands, kidney	Liver, spleen, bone marrow

Figure 11-3 Comparison of endothelial cells in three types of capillaries. In contrast to continuous capillaries in most tissues (shown here), those in nervous tissue have few pinocytic vesicles, zonulae occludens (tight junctions), and a thick basement membrane, all of which reduce their permeability (blood–brain barrier). Except in renal glomeruli, a thin diaphragm bridges the pores in fenestrated capillaries.

- Transendothelial transport occurs primarily through **pores** (fenestrae) in endothelial cells.

    c. Sinusoidal capillaries (e.g., splenic sinusoids)
- Transendothelial transport occurs primarily through large **paracellular gaps**.

4. Portal system constitutes two capillary beds connected by one or more veins.

    a. Liver portal system: intestinal capillary beds → portal vein → liver sinusoids → central vein

    b. Hypophyseal portal system: capillary beds in median eminence → hypophyseal portal veins → capillary beds in pars distalis

D. Venous vessels
- Veins have larger lumens, thinner walls, and a lower hydrostatic pressure than comparable arteries.

1. Valves, paired folds of the tunica intima, are present in many veins that work against gravity.
- These valves prevent backward blood flow and pooling of blood in the extremities, especially the lower ones.

2. Layer of longitudinal smooth muscle is found in walls of the largest veins (e.g., inferior vena cava)
- This extra muscle layer, located in the inner aspect of the tunica adventitia (not in the tunica media), makes the adventitia the thickest of the three tunics in these veins.

E. Interstitial fluid
- The formation and recovery of interstitial (tissue) fluid occurs primarily in capillary beds (Figure 11-4).

1. Forces driving fluid movement in and out of vessels

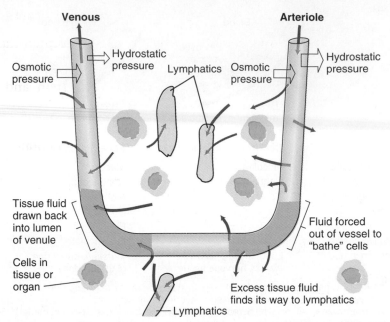

Figure 11-4 Movement of fluid between capillaries and the interstitium. Direction of fluid movement *(black arrows)* at any point within a capillary loop depends on the difference between the hydrostatic pressure, which decreases from arterial to venous side, and the osmotic pressure, which is constant. Fluid forced out at the arterial end of a capillary loop forms the interstitial, or tissue, fluid. This is returned at the venous end or enters blind-ended lymphatic vessels, forming the lymph.

Transudate, a protein- and cell-poor fluid, is produced in edema resulting from increased hydrostatic pressure or decreased osmotic pressure.

    a. Osmotic pressure, created by high concentration of albumin in the blood, **draws fluid into capillaries** from surrounding interstitium.

    b. Hydrostatic pressure, created by blood flow against capillary walls, **forces fluid out of capillaries** into the surrounding interstitium.

  2. Arterial side: hydrostatic pressure > osmotic pressure
- **Net effect:** fluid but not formed elements (a **transudate**) is forced out of blood, forming **interstitial fluid.**

  3. Venous side: osmotic pressure > hydrostatic pressure
- **Net effect:** most, but not all, interstitial fluid returns to the blood.
- Blind-ending lymphatic capillaries take up interstitial fluid not returned to venous blood, forming the **lymph.**

F. Causes of edema (excess interstitial fluid in a body region)

  1. Increased venous hydrostatic pressure
- Left-sided heart failure → **pulmonary edema**
- Pregnant uterus pressing on common iliac veins → **pitting edema** of lower extremities
- Right-sided heart failure → **pitting edema** of lower extremities

  2. Obstruction of lymphatic drainage

- **Axillary node removal/radiation** → lymphedema of ipsilateral superior extremity
- Parasitic infection of lymphatic vessels → **elephantiasis**

   3. Increased permeability of endothelium
- Acute inflammation with histamine-enhanced increase in venule permeability → accumulation of protein- and cell-rich fluid (**exudate**) in the interstitial space

   4. Reduction in osmotic pressure of blood due to decreased concentration of macromolecules in blood
- **Hepatic cirrhosis, nephrotic syndrome**, and **malnutrition** → increased loss of fluid on arterial side of capillary bed and decreased return on venous side → **abdominal ascites** and **pitting edema** of lower extremities

G. Tumor angiogenesis (neoangiogenesis)

   1. Tumor angiogenesis factor (TAF), produced by tumor cells, stimulates nearby endothelial cells to proliferate, migrate into the neoplasm, and form new blood vessels supplying it.
- Growth of a tumor to a large size requires direct blood supply to provide nutrients to cells throughout the mass.

   2. Inhibitors of neoangiogenesis may be useful in treating tumors.
- Monoclonal antibody to TAF and two natural proteins, **endostatin** and **angiostatin**, prevent neoangiogenesis, so that neoplasms must rely on diffusion of local nutrients only and thus remain small.

II. Lymphatic Vessels
- The system of lymphatic vessels drains most tissues except the nervous system and bone marrow.

A. Lymphatic capillaries begin as blind-ending endothelial tubes near blood capillaries.

   1. Unique structural features of lymphatic capillaries
   a. Single layer of **highly attenuated endothelial cells**
   b. Absent or intermittent basal lamina
   c. Anchoring filaments that extend from exterior surface of endothelium into surrounding connective tissue
- These filaments prevent the very thin-walled lymphatic capillaries from collapsing.

   2. Absorption by lymphatic capillaries
   a. Excess tissue fluid and macromolecules in the interstitium are absorbed relatively easily by lymphatic capillaries.
   b. Lipids from fatty meal are taken up by lymphatic vessels, called **lacteals**, in intestinal villi (see Figure 14-4).

B. Larger lymphatic vessels possess valves and are generally similar in structure to small veins but have larger lumens and thinner walls.
- Lymph is filtered in lymph nodes, which are interspersed along the lymphatic tree (see Figure 13-7).

Exudate, a protein- and cell-rich fluid, is produced in edema resulting from increased endothelial permeability (e.g., pus formed in acute inflammation).

In cirrhosis of the liver and nephrotic syndrome, blood albumin levels decrease, reducing osmotic pressure of the blood and promoting edema.

Because of their thin weak walls, lymphatic capillaries are easily invaded by cancer cells, leading to lymphatic spread of cancer.

Cardiac tunics
(inside → outside):
• Endocardium
(endothelium +
subendothelial
connective tissue)
• Myocardium
(cardiac muscle)
• Epicardium
(fibroelastic con-
nective tissue +
mesothelium)

Damaged cardiac
muscle does not re-
generate because
these cells cannot
divide. Lost cells
are replaced by scar
tissue with adjacent
cardiomyocytes
hypertrophying.

C. Right lymphatic duct and thoracic duct, the large trunks resulting from convergence of lymphatic vessels, have three tunics similar to blood vessels.

III. **Heart**

A. Cardiac tunics: three layers composing wall of heart; homologous to those of blood vessels (Figure 11-5)

1. **Endocardium** (inner layer), comprising an endothelium and thin subendothelial connective tissue layer, is continuous with the tunica intima of major blood vessels entering and leaving the heart.

   • Between the endocardium and myocardium is a thin connective tissue layer, the **subendocardium**, that contains nerves and components of the **impulse-conducting system.**

2. **Myocardium**, the parenchyma of the heart, consists of cardiac muscle cells and is **thickest in the ventricles.**

   a. Cardiac myocytes are **incapable of cell division.**

      (1) Cardiac muscle cells that are lost, as in myocardial infarction (MI), are replaced by scar tissue (healed MI), which stains blue with trichrome stain.

      (2) Adjacent parenchymal cells assume extra work load, leading to their **hypertrophy.**

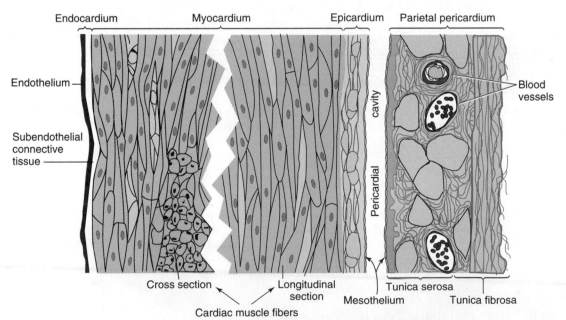

Figure 11-5 Cardiac tunics and their relation to the pericardium. The three tunics are homologous to those of blood vessels: endocardium = tunica intima; myocardium = tunica media; and epicardium = tunica adventitia. The pericardium is composed of two layers: the outer parietal pericardium and the epicardium, or visceral pericardium, which is in contact with the heart and roots of the great vessels. The parietal pericardium has two regions: a serosa facing the pericardial cavity and, peripheral to that, a fibrosa.

    b. **Atrial natriuretic peptide (ANP)** is produced by myofibers in the left and right atria and stored in neuroendocrine granules.

        (1) **Above-normal blood volume** in atria stretches the myofibers, causing **release of ANP**.

        (2) **ANP increases secretion of sodium and water** by distal convoluted tubules in the kidney, leading to **decrease of blood volume**.

  3. **Epicardium** (outer layer) is equivalent to the **visceral layer of the pericardial sac.**

    a. Simple squamous epithelium (**mesothelium**) covers the external surface facing the pericardial cavity.

    b. Underlying fibroelastic connective tissue contains adipocytes, nerves, and coronary vessels.

B. **Cardiac skeleton:** dense collagenous connective tissue from and into which myocardial fibers originate and insert

C. **Heart valves:** endocardial folds with a core of dense connective tissue (dermatan sulfate) that is continuous with the cardiac skeleton

D. **Impulse-conducting system**

  • The heartbeat is initiated and regulated by several structures composed of **cells specialized for conduction** rather than contraction.

  1. **Sinoatrial (SA) node,** located in the wall of the superior vena cava at its junction with the right atrium, normally functions as the heart's **pacemaker.**

    • Small **cardiomyocytes** in the SA node **spontaneously generate impulses** that are transmitted to ordinary atrial myofibers, causing **atrial contraction.**

  2. **Atrioventricular (AV) node,** located in wall of the right atrium near the tricuspid valve, receives impulses from the SA node.

    • The AV node is histologically similar to the SA node and can act as the pacemaker if the SA node becomes nonfunctional.

  3. **AV bundle (bundle of His)** is a band of small special myocytes that radiate from the AV node into the interventricular septum.

    • After dividing into two branches, the bundles enter the subendocardium and continue as Purkinje fibers on either side of the septum.

  4. **Purkinje fibers** are large specialized cardiac muscle cells that carry impulses to ordinary cardiac myocytes in the papillary muscle of each ventricle and at the apex of the heart, causing **ventricular contraction.**

    • These cells contain a few peripherally displaced myofibrils and possess perinuclear masses of glycogen.

E. **Cardiovascular disorders**

  • Numerous acquired or congenital defects in the **heart muscle, heart valves,** and/or the **impulse-conducting system** can compromise heart function.

> Cardiac impulse conduction: SA node (pacemaker) → AV node → bundle of His → Purkinje fibers → papillary muscles

1. **Ischemic heart disease** results from interruption in the coronary artery blood supply to the heart muscle.
   a. **Angina pectoris:** myocardial pain, often radiating to the arms, in the absence of ischemic necrosis of cardiac muscle
   b. **Acute myocardial infarction:** severe pain often with pallor, perspiration, nausea, and shortness of breath associated with ischemic necrosis of cardiac muscle
2. **Arrhythmias** include any changes in normal pattern of the heartbeat.
   - **Heart block** commonly involves impairment of impulse conduction in the AV node or bundle of His.
3. **Valvular stenosis** involves narrowing of any of the heart valves.
   a. The most important long-term sequel of untreated **rheumatic fever** in childhood is scarring and reduced elasticity of the **mitral valve** (most common) and **aortic valve.**
   b. Elderly individuals often have **isolated aortic stenosis** resulting from **calcific degeneration.** Severe left ventricular hypertrophy develops; **dizziness** and **syncope on exertion** are common symptoms.

Rheumatic fever is the most common cause of mitral valve stenosis, which may be accompanied by aortic valve stenosis.

12

Blood Cells and Their Formation

Target Topics

▷ Hematocrit, blood count, differential count, and band/stab count
▷ Major histologic features and functions of different blood cells
▷ Stages and clinical signs of inflammation
▷ Prenatal and postnatal sites of blood formation
▷ Hematopoietic stages and precursors in different lineages
▷ Anemias, von Willebrand's disease, lazy leukocyte syndrome, leukocyte-adhesion deficiency, polycythemia, leukemias

I. **Introduction**
   • **Blood** is a **specialized connective tissue** of mesodermal origin.
   A. **Constituents of blood**
      1. **Formed elements**, the erythrocytes, leukocytes, and platelets, constitute about **45% of blood volume.**
      2. **Plasma**, the fluid matrix in which the formed elements are suspended, constitutes about **55% of blood volume.**
         a. **Major plasma proteins** include albumin, fibrinogen, and the globulins. Gamma globulins function as **antibodies** (see Chapter 13).
         b. **Serum** is the supernatant remaining after blood has clotted.
   B. **Turnover of blood cells**
      1. **Life span** of almost all blood cells is **relatively short**, and millions are formed each day to replenish the supply.
      2. **Hematopoiesis**, the formation of new blood cells, occurs primarily in the **red bone marrow.**

TABLE 12-1   Number, Size, and Life Span of Peripheral Blood Cells

Cell Type	No./mm³	Differential Count (%)	Diameter in Smear (μm)	Life Span
Erythrocyte	$4.5–5.5 \times 10^6$		7–8	120 days
Platelet	$1.5–4 \times 10^5$		2–5	7–12 days
Leukocytes:	$5–9 \times 10^3$			
Neutrophil		50–70	10–12	Hours to days
Eosinophil		1–3	10–12	8–12 days
Basophil		0.5–1	10–12	? (quite long)
Lymphocyte		20–40	7–12	Months to years
Monocyte		1–6	9–12	Months

Normal hematocrit (volume of formed elements in centrifuged blood) is 45. Lower values indicate disorders such as anemia or chronic hemorrhage.

Deviations from normal blood counts are indicated by suffixes. Above-normal counts: cytosis or philia (e.g., monocytosis, eosinophilia). Below-normal counts: penia (e.g., neutropenia).

HbA: major normal hemoglobin in adult (two α-globin and two β-globin chains). HbA$_2$: minor normal hemoglobin in adult (two α-globin and two δ-globin chains). HbF: normal hemoglobin in fetus: two α-globin and two γ-globin chains. HbS: abnormal hemoglobin associated with sickle-cell anemia.

II. Blood Cells

A. Numerical measures of blood cells

- Table 12-1 summarizes the size, number, and life span of the blood's formed elements.

1. **Hematocrit:** volume of formed elements determined by centrifugation of whole blood
   - Because red blood cells (RBCs) are much more numerous than other formed elements, the hematocrit is determined largely by the number of RBCs.
2. **Blood count:** number of each type of blood cell per cubic millimeter of blood
3. **Differential count:** number of each type of white blood cell (WBC) expressed as a percentage of the total WBC count

B. Erythrocytes (RBCs)

1. **Morphology:** small, highly deformable **biconcave disks** that lack a nucleus (**anucleate**) and most cytoplasmic organelles
2. **Hemoglobin:** iron-containing protein in RBCs that carries oxygen and carbon dioxide
3. **Effect of tonicity on RBCs**
   - The interior of RBCs has a tonicity equivalent to 0.9% saline.
   a. **In isotonic medium** (0.9% saline), RBCs retain their normal size and shape.
   b. **In hypertonic medium** (>0.9% saline), water leaves the cells, so RBCs **shrink and become wrinkled** (crenation).
   c. **In hypotonic medium** (<0.9% saline), water enters the cells, so RBCs **swell and burst** (hemolysis).
4. **Erythrocyte cytoskeleton**
   - Extensive **cortical microfilament network** maintains the shape of RBCs. This network is linked to the plasma membrane by **spectrin** and other proteins (see Chapter 2).
5. **Anemia:** any condition characterized by a low count of normal RBCs or decreased amount of hemoglobin in peripheral blood (Table 12-2)

TABLE 12-2   Selected Anemias

Disease	Cause	RBC Morphology	Other Clinical Features
Iron-deficiency anemia	Impaired Hb production resulting from low iron intake, chronic blood loss, or increased demand for iron (e.g., in pregnancy)	Small RBCs with large area of central pallor (microcytic-hypochromic anemia)	• Pallor • Brittle nails, oral lesions • GI complaints
Pernicious anemia	Impaired production of RBCs resulting from vitamin B_{12} deficiency resulting from inadequate synthesis of intrinsic factor	Large, abnormal RBC precursors in bone marrow and blood (megaloblastic anemia)	• Weakness, bilateral tingling and numbness in hands and feet • Red, painful tongue • Subacute degeneration of posterior and lateral spinal column
Sickle cell anemia	Production of abnormal HbS resulting from mutation in β chain; autosomal recessive (heterozygotes usually asymptomatic)	Fragile, misshapen RBCs (sickle cells) with decreased survival time (hemolytic anemia)	• Joint pain, attacks of abdominal pain • Increased bilirubin levels • Ulcerations of lower extremities • Increased risk of *Salmonella* osteomyelitis
Hereditary spherocytosis	Mutation in spectrin causing defect in RBC membrane; usually autosomal dominant	Fragile, round, hyperchromic RBCs sensitive to lysis	• Jaundice • Splenomegaly
β-thalassemia	Various mutations in Hb β chain; autosomal recessive (heterozygotes asymptomatic or show mild disease)	Small, pale, short-lived RBCs (microcytic, hypochromic, hemolytic anemia)	• Splenomegaly • Bone deformities

C. Platelets (thrombocytes)

   1. Morphology: anucleate disk-shaped fragments of **megakaryocyte cytoplasm**

      a. Granulomere: central, densely staining region marked by granules of various sizes

         (1)   Alpha (α) granules (largest) contain platelet-derived growth factor, thromboplastin, von Willebrand's factor VIII, fibrinogen, and factor V.

         (2)   Delta (δ) granules (mid-size) contain serotonin, histamine, and ADP.

         (3)   Lambda (λ) granules (smallest) contain lysosomal enzymes.

b. **Hyalomere:** peripheral, light-staining region filled with microtubules and microfilaments
  - A system of canaliculi that open to the surface aids in delivering granule contents to the outside.

2. **Role of platelets in hemostasis and disease**
  a. **Injury of small vessels** (e.g., capillaries, venules) is followed by **adherence of platelets** to the injured endothelium and their **aggregation** to form platelet plugs bound together by fibrin strands (thrombi).
    (1) **von Willebrand's factor VIII,** which is produced by both megakaryocytes and endothelial cells, mediates platelet adhesion.
    (2) **ADP,** which promotes platelet aggregation, is released from platelet delta (δ) granules after adhesion occurs.
    (3) **Thromboxane A_2,** a potent aggregating and vasoconstricting agent, is synthesized by platelets after the initial release reaction.
  b. **Arterial thrombi** usually develop over areas of turbulence (e.g., atherosclerotic plaques) in both muscular and elastic arteries.
    - Arterial thrombi are primarily composed of platelets held together by fibrin strands.
    (1) In **muscular arteries** (e.g., coronary arteries), thrombi may lead to vessel occlusion and **infarction** (e.g., coronary thrombosis → acute myocardial infarction).
    (2) In **elastic arteries** (e.g., aorta, bifurcation of the carotid arteries), thrombi contribute to formation of **fibrofatty plaques,** the primary lesion of atherosclerosis, and also may occlude the vessel, leading to **infarction** (e.g., thrombus overlying an atheromatous plaque at the bifurcation of the carotid arteries → brain infarction, or **stroke**).
  c. **Venous thrombi** most commonly develop in the **deep veins of the calf.**
    (1) **Stasis of blood** causes activation of the clotting system, leading to formation of **fibrin clots** on top of the platelet thrombus.
    (2) Red blood cells and platelets are trapped in the clots, and vessel lumen eventually is occluded.

3. **von Willebrand's disease (vascular hemophilia)** is caused by a genetic defect that results in reduced synthesis of von Willebrand's factor (vWF) by endothelial cells and platelets.
  - Sudden nosebleeds and bleeding from gums occur in severe cases.

D. **Leukocytes (WBCs)**
  - All WBCs are **nucleated** and contain the usual **cytoplasmic organelles,** as well as nonspecific **azurophilic granules.**

Iron-deficiency anemia: microcytic-hypochromic; decreased hemoglobin synthesis.

Pernicious anemia: megaloblastic; decreased production of RBCs; impaired absorption of vitamin B_{12} usually due to reduced synthesis of intrinsic factor.

Aspirin and other NSAIDs reduce synthesis of thromboxane A_2 in platelets by inhibiting cyclooxygenase. As a result, formation of platelet thrombi is curtailed.

When individuals who are taking aspirin cut themselves shaving, cessation of bleeding takes much longer than normal due to absence of platelet thrombi to stop blood flow.

Anticoagulants (e.g., warfarin, heparin), which inhibit the coagulation system, block formation of venous thrombi.

Aspirin in low doses reduces the incidence of acute MI and stroke by decreasing development of platelet thrombi in arteries.

TABLE 12-3 Selected Properties of Granulocytes

Property	Neutrophil	Eosinophil	Basophil
Nuclear shape	3 to 5 lobes	Bilobed	Irregular
Azurophilic granules	Many	Few	Few
Color of specific granules (Giemsa or Wright's stain)	Dusty rose	Red/orange	Dark blue to black
Size of specific granules	Small	Large	Large
Phagocytic activity	High (bacteria)	Moderate (antigen-antibody complexes)	None
Other	H_2O_2 formed during phagocytosis	Specific granules are lysosomes with a crystalline core of major basic protein (MBP)	Degranulation induced by allergens releases histamine

- They commonly **migrate from the blood** through spaces between capillary endothelial cells, entering connective tissue areas.

1. **Granulocytes**
   - Three types of WBCs, the granulocytes, possess **characteristic nuclear shapes** and **cell type–specific granules** containing degradative enzymes and/or inflammatory mediators (Table 12-3).
   a. **Neutrophils**, the premier cells for **phagocytosing and killing bacteria,** commonly are found at sites of **acute inflammation.**
      (1) Mature neutrophils are also called **polymorphonuclear leukocytes (PMNs).**
      (2) **Bands (stabs)** are **immature neutrophils** with a nonlobed, bean-shaped nucleus; normally constitute 1%–3% of peripheral WBCs.
   b. **Eosinophils** participate in **allergic reactions** and in the response to invasive **parasitic infections.**
   c. **Basophils** contribute to **immediate hypersensitivity reactions** (see Figure 13-5).

2. **Lymphocytes (B and T cells)**
   a. Have a **large, round nucleus** surrounded by a thin rim of cytoplasm containing few organelles and azurophilic granules
   b. Possess **antigen-binding receptors** in their plasma membrane and are responsible for **specific immune responses** (see Chapter 13)

3. **Monocytes**
   a. Have a characteristic **kidney-shaped nucleus** with a clumpy, stringy chromatin pattern.
   b. Migrate into tissues and give rise to **macrophages,** which are phagocytic and present antigens to T cells.

4. Leukocytic disorders
  a. Lazy leukocyte syndrome is due to a genetic defect in the contractile actin microfilaments of PMNs, which severely impairs their mobility.
  - Clinically, this disorder is marked by a severe decrease in the number of circulating PMNs and recurrent **low-grade infections** (e.g., sinusitis, stomatitis, and otitis media).
  b. Leukocyte-adhesion deficiency (LAD) results from a defect in several integrins normally expressed on the surface of leukocytes.
  - Defective leukocytes have reduced ability to migrate into tissues and adhere to target cells.
  - Affected individuals show recurrent **bacterial infections** and **impaired wound healing.** In newborns, the umbilical cord fails to separate.

III. **Inflammation**
  - A localized protective response to tissue infection or injury, inflammation is **aseptic** if no bacteria are involved and **septic** if bacteria are involved.
  - Various **inflammatory mediators** are released from leukocytes in connective tissue near the site of infection or injury.

  A. **Classic signs of acute inflammation**

Four cardinal signs of inflammation: rubor (redness); calor (heat); tumor (edema); and dolor (pain).

  - **Histamine** released from mast cells causes vasodilation and increased permeability.
  1. **Dilation of vessels** and subsequent increased blood flow to the affected area causes **rubor** (redness) and **calor** (heat).
  2. **Increased vessel permeability** leads to **tumor** (swelling, or **edema**) resulting from excess tissue fluid and to **dolor** (pain) resulting from pressure on nerve endings and presence of bradykinin and prostaglandin E_2.

  B. **Stages in inflammatory response**
  1. **Acute phase: PMNs** migrate from bloodstream into damaged area.
    a. Adherence of circulating PMNs to endothelium (margination) is mediated by **cell-adhesion molecules (CAMs)** in the plasma membranes of the interacting cells.
    b. Diapedesis involves movement of adhered PMNs between endothelial cells into surrounding connective tissue.
    c. Chemotactic factors that "attract" neutrophils also play a role in neutrophil adherence and transendothelial migration.
  2. **Subacute phase: lymphocytes, monocytes,** and **plasma cells** enter affected tissue, mixing with PMNs.
  3. **Chronic phase: macrophages** predominate, with lymphocytes and plasma cells also present; few PMNs present.

  C. **Changes in band count during acute infection**

Higher band/stab count (left shift) indicates infection.

  1. **Shift to the left:** severe infection results in the release of **immature** PMNs (bands or stabs) from bone marrow, leading to an **increase in the band/stab count.**

2. **Shift to the right:** as inflammation subsides, the band/stab count **decreases** toward normal.

IV. **Hematopoietic Sites**
   A. **Prenatal sites of blood formation**
      1. **Yolk-sac of embryo**
         a. **Blood islands**, or **angiogenic cell clusters**, in the wall of the yolk sac give rise to **nucleated erythrocytes** from about **2 to 8 weeks' gestation.**
         b. No leukocytes form during this stage.
      2. **Liver and spleen**
         a. Formation of erythrocytes and leukocytes occurs primarily in the fetal liver and spleen from **8 to 28 weeks' gestation.**
         b. Hematopoiesis in liver and spleen normally ceases about time of birth.
      3. **Red bone marrow**
         • Starting at 6 months' gestation, the red bone marrow exhibits hematopoietic activity and soon becomes the major site of hematopoiesis.
   B. **Postnatal sites of blood formation**
      1. **Prior to puberty:** hematopoiesis occurs in the skull, ribs, sternum, vertebrae, clavicles, pelvis, and long bones.
      2. **After puberty:** hematopoiesis occurs in the same sites, except for long bones.
      3. **Extramedullary hematopoiesis:** formation of blood cells occurs in liver and spleen following birth in certain disease states.
   C. **Histology of red bone marrow**
      1. **Stroma** contains fibroblasts (produce collagen and reticular fibers), reticular cells, fat cells, and endothelial cells.
         • **Hematopoietic growth factors** are synthesized and secreted by stromal cells.
      2. **Parenchyma** contains hematopoietic cells of different lineages in various stages of differentiation.
      3. **Hematopoietic cords** are bands of parenchyma and stroma lying **between sinusoids** that connect arterial and venous vessels within red bone marrow.
         • Mature blood cells produced in parenchyma of the cords gain access to the circulation by passing through sinusoid walls.
   D. **Distribution of hematopoietic cells within bone marrow parenchyma**
      1. **Total number of cells**
         a. **60% in granulocytopoiesis** (formation of neutrophils, basophils, and eosinophils)
         b. **30% in erythrocytopoiesis** (formation of erythrocytes)
         c. **10% in thrombocytopoiesis, monocytopoiesis, and lymphocytopoiesis** (formation of platelets, monocytes, and lymphocytes, respectively)
      2. **Myeloid/erythroid ratio:** ratio of **total volume** (or number) of cells undergoing granulocytopoiesis to total volume (or

Iliac crest is primary site for bone marrow biopsy; secondary site is sternum.

number) of cells undergoing erythrocytopoiesis in the red bone marrow

   a. Normal M/E ratio is 3:1 (2:1 to 4:1).

   b. High M/E ratio (e.g., 8:1) indicates decreased erythrocytopoiesis and/or increased granulocytopoiesis (as in **chronic myelogenous leukemia**).

   c. Low M/E ratio (e.g., 1:5) indicates increased erythrocytopoiesis (as in **polycythemia**) and/or decreased granulocytopoiesis.

  V. **Stages in Hematopoiesis**

- Formation of each type of blood cell progresses through distinct cell kinetic "compartments" during which the degree of **potentiality decreases** and the extent of **differentiation increases.**

  A. Stem cell compartment

- This compartment comprises vegetative intermitotics (VIMs), which are **self-sustaining** and **self-renewing** cells. The various stem cell populations are **cytologically indistinguishable.**
- Hematopoietic stem cells are referred to as **colony-forming units (CFUs)** because they give rise to self-renewing colonies in the spleen, of irradiated mice injected with bone marrow.

  1. Totipotent stem cells (CFUs) are capable of giving rise to **all** types of blood cells.

  2. Pluripotent stem cells arise from daughter cells of totipotent stem cells that become committed to either the myeloid or lymphoid pathways.

   a. Lymphoid stem cells (CFU-Ly) give rise to lymphocytes.

   b. Myeloid stem cells (CFU-GEMMeg, or CFU-S) give rise to all the other blood cell lines.

  3. Unipotent and multipotent stem cells arising from myeloid stem cells are committed to one of three lineages (Figure 12-1):

   a. Erythrocyte line (CFU-E)

   b. Megakaryocyte/platelet line (CFU-Meg)

   c. Granulocyte/monocyte line (CFU-GM)

- CFU-GM subsequently gives rise to CFU-G, committed to the granulocyte line, and CFU-M, committed to the monocyte line.

  B. Differentiating/multiplicative compartment

- Each lineage of committed stem cells gives rise to differentiating intermitotics (DIMs), or **precursor cells,** which undergo continuous **cell division** and **cytodifferentiation** in this compartment.
- The first **histologically distinct precursors** of mature blood cells arise at this stage.
- All the daughter cells eventually differentiate into highly specialized, postmitotic cells; thus this compartment must be replenished by influx from the stem cell compartment.

  C. Functional compartment

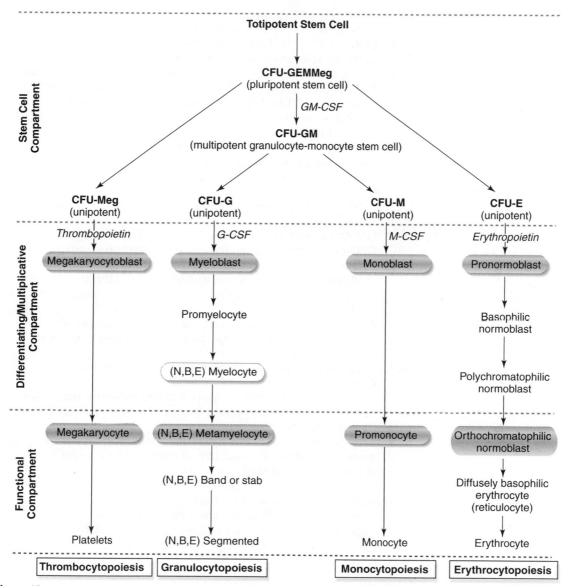

Figure 12-1 Flow chart of hematopoiesis showing named stages of cytodifferentiation, key stimulating factors *(in italics)*, and cell kinetic compartments. The first histologically distinct cells in the two, non–stem cell compartments are indicated by *shading*. The three granulocyte lineages—neutrophilic *(N)*, basophilic *(B)*, and eosinophilic *(E)*—become distinguishable from each other at the myelocyte stage. Totipotent stem cells also give rise to lymphoid stem cells, whose differentiation into lymphocytes is not illustrated. *CFU,* Colony-forming unit (stem cell); *CSF,* colony-stimulating factor; *E,* erythrocyte; *G,* granulocyte; *M,* monocyte; *Meg,* megakaryocyte.

- Mature blood cells in each lineage and their immediate precursors compose this compartment. The mature cells enter the bloodstream or are held in reserve until they are needed.
- These **fixed postmitotic cells** (FPMs) function, age, and in time die (see Table 12-1). They are replaced by cell influx from the differentiating compartment.

D. Time course of hematopoiesis
   1. Stem cell → granulocytes: about 12 days
   2. Stem cell → erythrocytes: about 7 days
E. Hematopoietic growth factors (see Figure 12-1)
   - Three general classes of growth factors—**colony-stimulating factors (CSFs), interleukins,** and **erythropoietin**—are responsible for directing cells into different hematopoietic pathways and promoting proliferation/cytodifferentiation within lineages.
   1. Granulocyte/monocyte colony-stimulating factor (GM-CSF) stimulates granulocytopoiesis and monocytopoiesis
      - Treatment with GM-CSF **ameliorates neutropenia** associated with myelosuppressive chemotherapy or radiation therapy.
   2. Granulocyte colony-stimulating factor (G-CSF) directs CFU-G to differentiate along the neutrophilic pathway.
      - Treatment with G-CSF, which produces a **dose-dependent neutrophilia,** shortens the duration of neutropenia following myelosuppressive chemotherapy or radiation therapy.
   3. Monocyte colony-stimulating factor (M-CSF) commits CFU-GM to the monocytic pathway, thereby increasing monocytopoiesis.
F. Clinical uses of hematopoietic stem cells
   - Cancer patients who receive aggressive chemotherapy and/or radiation often require a **bone marrow transplant** to restore their hematopoietic stem cells, which are destroyed by such treatments.
   - Separation of stem cells from harvested bone marrow **greatly reduces the volume of marrow** that must be infused into a patient.

VI. Histology of Blood Cell Precursors
   - Each of the hematopoietic stem cells committed to a particular lineage proceeds through a series of histologically distinct precursors as it undergoes cytodifferentiation.
A. Granulocytopoiesis: CFU-G → neutrophil, basophil, and eosinophil

Granulocytopoiesis: CFU-G → myeloblast → promyelocyte → myelocyte → metamyelocyte → band → mature stages.

   1. Granulocyte precursors (see Figure 12-1)
      a. G-CSF stimulates CFU-G to proliferate and differentiate into the first histologically recognizable granulocyte precursor, the **myeloblast,** a relatively large cell that is **similar in all three granulocyte lineages.**
      b. The **three lineages**—neutrophilic (N), basophilic (B), and eosinophilic (E)—are **first distinguishable** with the appearance of lineage-specific cytoplasmic granules **at myelocyte stage (N, B, E).**
      c. Maturation of each lineage, yielding segmented neutrophils (PMNs), basophils, and eosinophils, is **completed within the bone marrow.**

    2. **Common cytological changes during granulocytopoiesis**
      a. Number of nonspecific and then specific granules **increases.**
      b. Size of entire cell and of nucleoli **decreases.**
      c. Lobation of nucleus **increases.**
      d. Cell deformability increases.
      e. Cell motility increases.
      f. Adhesiveness increases.
      g. Phagocytic capability increases.

B. Erythrocytopoiesis: CFU-E → erythrocyte
    1. **Erythropoietin** (EPO), produced in the kidney, **stimulates CFU-E** to proliferate and differentiate into the first histologically recognizable erythrocyte precursor, the **pronormoblast** (proerythroblast).
      • **Decrease in O_2 saturation** of blood **stimulates erythropoietin production.**
    2. **Diffusely basophilic erythrocyte**, or **reticulocyte**, the final stage of erythrocytopoiesis within the bone marrow, represents an immature anucleated RBC.
      a. After entering the bloodstream, reticulocytes lose their remaining ribosomes and mitochondria, becoming mature RBCs.
      b. Reticulocytes normally constitute 1%–3% of circulating RBCs.
      c. Excessive loss of mature RBCs (e.g., during hemorrhage) causes release of more reticulocytes from the bone marrow and their percentage in the blood increases.
    3. **Secondary polycythemia:** any **abnormal increase in total RBC mass** resulting from tissue **hypoxia**, which stimulates release of erythropoietin from the kidney.
      a. Tetralogy of Fallot, a congenital heart defect, is accompanied by **hypoxia** because not enough blood is routed to the lungs to be oxygenated. Children with this defect commonly are polycythemic.
      b. Cigarette smoke contains carbon monoxide, which binds to hemoglobin much more tightly than oxygen, producing hypoxia. Thus smokers tend to be polycythemic.
    4. **Polycythemia vera:** a neoplastic disease involving stem cells (myeloproliferative disease) marked by **increased RBC mass** with **low EPO** levels
      • Clinical manifestations include, headache, dizziness, ruddy face, thrombotic episodes, and **hepatosplenomegaly.**

C. Thrombocytopoiesis: CFU-Meg → platelets
    1. **Megakarycytoblast**, the first differentiating precursor in this pathway, undergoes DNA replication but not cytokinesis, a process called **endoreduplication.**
    2. **Megakaryocyte**, a giant, **polyploid** cell with a huge, multilobed nucleus, is generated by repeated endoreduplication.

Thrombocytopoiesis: CFU-Meg → megakaryoblast → megakaryocyte → filopodia → platelets.

a. Ploidy level varies among postmitotic megakaryocytes with most cells being $8n$, $16n$, or $32n$ (lower n = younger cell).

b. Filopods (thin pseudopodia) are extended through the walls of marrow sinusoids into the lumen.
- Also known as proplatelets, filopods "shatter," releasing **platelets** directly into the circulation.

D. Monocytopoiesis: CFU-M → monocyte

1. **Monoblast**, the first differentiating precursor, gives rise to a **promonocyte**, which matures into a monocyte.
2. **Monocytes** enter the bloodstream, circulate for 1 or 2 days, and then migrate into connective tissue areas and body cavities where they function as **tissue macrophages**.

E. Lymphocytopoiesis: CFU-Ly → pre-B and pre-T cells → mature B and T cells

1. **Pre-B cells** develop into mature antigen-recognizing B cells in the **bone marrow**.
2. **Pre-T cells** migrate from the bone marrow to the **thymus** where they develop into mature antigen-recognizing T cells.
3. **Proliferation and differentiation of mature B and T cells**
   a. Unlike the other types of blood cells, lymphocytes released from the bone marrow and thymus are **not** fixed postmitotics incapable of cell division.
   b. After encountering a specific antigen, appropriate B and T cells proliferate (**clonal expansion**) and differentiate into **effector cells** and **memory cells** that function in specific immune responses (see Chapter 13).

F. Leukemias: abnormal proliferation and development of leukocytes and their precursors in the bone marrow
- Common symptoms include **fatigue**, **pallor**, **dyspnea** on exertion, and **hepatosplenomegaly**, and generalized **lymphadenopathy**.

1. **Acute myelogenous leukemia (AML)** marked by accumulation of blast cells containing **Auer rods** (red refractile bodies) in bone marrow.
   - Most commonly occurs in individuals 15–59 years of age develop AML. Poor prognosis.
2. **Chronic myelogenous leukemia (CML)** is associated with **Philadelphia chromosome** resulting from translocation between chromosomes 9 and 22.
   - Clinical features include **leukocytosis** and **massive splenomegaly** with progression to acute leukemia typical.
   - Adults **35–55 years** of age are most commonly affected.
3. **Acute lymphoblastic leukemia (ALL)** is characterized by proliferation of **blast cells with lymphocyte differentiation markers**. Classified into three types (L1–L3) based on morphology of blast cells.
   - ALL primarily affects **children** and is responsive to chemotherapy.

All forms of leukemia are characterized by abnormal proliferation of one or more types of immature blood cells within the bone marrow.

AML: most common leukemia between the ages of 15–59 years.

Leukemic cells in CML have short chromosome 22 (Philadelphia chromosome) and long chromosome 9 with *bcr-abl* oncogene.

ALL: most common cancer of any type affecting children.

4. Chronic lymphocytic leukemia (CLL) usually involves B cells with many broken cells (**smudge cells**) seen in peripheral blood smear.

- Complications include hypogammaglobulinemia and autoimmune hemolytic anemia.
- Adults >**60 years** of age are most commonly affected.

CLL: most common of all the leukemias; found most commonly in patients >60 years of age.

Immune System

13

Target Topics

▷ Properties and functions of immune system cells
▷ Antigen presentation and MHC molecules
▷ Antibody structure and immunoglobulin isotypes
▷ Immediate hypersensitivity reaction
▷ Activation and clonal expansion of lymphocytes in lymph nodes and spleen
▷ Splenic filtration of blood
▷ Autoimmune diseases, graft rejection, graft-versus-host disease, X-linked agammaglobulinemia, selective IgA deficiency, DiGeorge syndrome, lymphomas

Immune system has two major cellular components:
• B cells involved in antibody-mediated immunity
• T cells involved in cell-mediated immunity

I. Introduction
   A. **General components of the immune system**
      1. Lymphoid tissues and organs
      2. B and T lymphocytes (B and T cells), which have **specific antigen-binding** receptors in the plasma membrane
      3. Phagocytic cells and **antigen-presenting cells** (Table 13-1)
   B. **General functions of the immune system**
      1. Recognition and destruction of non-self substances (antigens)
         • Antigens may be soluble or present on the surface of microorganisms and cells.
      2. Removal of defective, worn-out self-cells and cell products
      3. Functional branches
         a. Antibody-mediated (humoral) response primarily involves **B cells** (B lymphocytes).
         b. Cell-mediated response involves **T cells** (T lymphocytes).

TABLE 13-1 **Cells of the Immune System**

Cell Type	Primary Functions in Host Defense
Lymphocytes:	
T cells	• Destruction of cells bearing intracellular (endogenous) antigens (cytotoxic T cells)
	• Secretion of cytokines that regulate the intensity and duration of immune responses (T_H cells)
B cells	• Clearance of extracellular (exogenous) antigens by secreted antibodies
	• Processing and presentation of exogenous antigens to T_H cells
Natural killer cells	• Antigen-specific and nonspecific cytotoxicity for tumor cells and virus-infected cells
Granulocytes:	
Neutrophils	• Release of inflammatory mediators
	• Nonspecific phagocytosis and killing of bacteria
Eosinophils	• Defense against parasitic organisms
Basophils	• Release of mediators in certain allergic reactions
Other:	
Mast cells	• Release of mediators in certain allergic reactions
Macrophages	• Nonspecific phagocytosis of exogenous antigens, dead host cells, cellular debris, and bacteria
	• Processing and presentation of antigens to T_H cells
Dendritic cells (various types)	• Processing and presentation of exogenous antigen to T_H cells

C. Clonal expansion of B and T lymphocytes (Figure 13-1)
   1. "Virgin," immunocompetent lymphocytes are activated by exposure of appropriate antigen to blastlike cells.
   2. Proliferation and differentiation of blastlike cells generates large numbers of two types of cells:
      a. Effector cells, which have various functions in clearing antigen from the host
      b. Memory cells, which have no effector function but can react faster than virgin lymphocytes to a second exposure to the same antigen
D. Immunologic tolerance
   1. Self-tolerance: during fetal and early neonatal period, a host normally develops tolerance to its own self-antigens but not to the foreign antigens of others.
   2. Tolerance to foreign antigens: introduction of a foreign antigen before the end of the tolerance-generating period will induce tolerance to that antigen.
E. Autoimmune diseases
   • A breakdown in the mechanisms ensuring natural tolerance to self-antigens leads to numerous clinical manifestations depending on the self-antigens recognized and nature of the response; for example:
   1. Hashimoto's disease: autoantibodies to thyroid proteins block iodine uptake and cause inflammatory response against thyroid tissue.
      • Hypothyroidism eventually develops.

An individual is naturally tolerant of own self-antigens but not of foreign antigens.

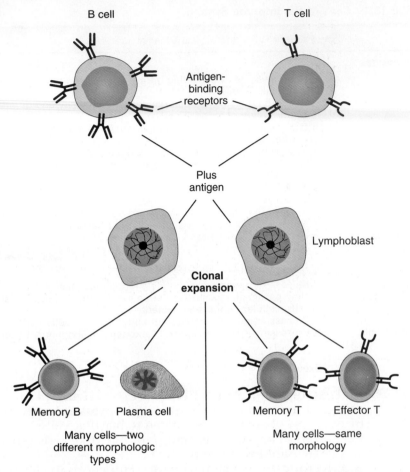

B cell

T cell

Antigen-binding receptors

Plus antigen

Lymphoblast

Clonal expansion

Memory B   Plasma cell

Memory T   Effector T

Many cells—two different morphologic types

Many cells—same morphology

Figure 13-1 T-cell and B-cell clonal expansion in response to exposure to an appropriate antigen. Binding of appropriate antigen to cell-surface receptors on virgin T and B cells activates them to lymphoblasts. These divide mitotically (clonal expansion), producing many daughter cells, which differentiate into effector cells or memory cells with the same antigen specificity as the activated lymphocyte from which they arose.

2. **Insulin-dependent diabetes mellitus (type 1):** delayed hypersensitivity reaction causes destruction of insulin-producing (beta) cells in the pancreas.
   - Insulitis with a subsequent decrease in insulin production results.
3. **Systemic lupus erythematosus (SLE):** autoantibodies against RBCs, platelets, and other self-antigens (e.g., **anti-dsDNA, anti-Sm**) trigger tissue-destroying inflammatory reactions.
   - Vasculitis, erythematous rash, arthritis, neutropenia, and hemolytic anemia are common manifestations.
4. **Goodpasture's syndrome:** autoantibodies to capillary **basement membranes** in kidneys and lungs mediate tissue destruction.

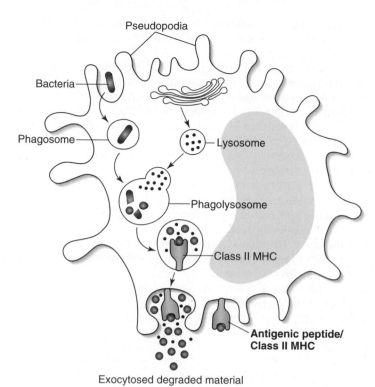

Pseudopodia

Bacteria

Phagosome

Lysosome

Phagolysosome

Class II MHC

**Antigenic peptide/
Class II MHC**

Exocytosed degraded material

Figure 13-2 Phagocytosis, processing, and presentation of antigen by macrophages. Phago-cytosed material is degraded by lysosomal enzymes and most of the products are exocytosed. However, antigenic peptides that interact with class II MHC molecules form complexes that move to the cell surface for presentation to T_H cells.

- Lung hemorrhages, nephritis with proteinuria, and renal failure may result.
5. **Other autoimmune diseases** include **Graves' disease** (see Chapter 1), **myasthenia gravis** (see Chapter 7), and **pemphigus vulgaris** (see Chapter 8).

II. Cell-Mediated Immunologic Response

- **Intracellular pathogens, virus-infected cells, foreign grafts,** and **autologous neoplasms** bearing tumor-specific antigens trigger cell-mediated responses.
A. **Antigen recognition by T cells** occurs only when antigen is present on the membrane of a cell in association with a **major histocompatibility complex (MHC) molecule.**
  1. **MHC molecules** are membrane proteins that have **binding sites for antigenic peptides** in their extracellular domain.
    a. **Class I MHC** molecules: on the surface of **most somatic cells**
    b. **Class II MHC** molecules: on the surface of **antigen-presenting cells** only
  2. **Antigen-presenting cells (APCs)** internalize **exogenous antigens** (produced outside the cell) and degrade them into smaller peptides, which associate with **class II MHC molecules** on the cell surface (Figure 13-2).

An immune response is triggered by antigen exposure followed by clonal expansion of activated antigen-specific B or T cells.

B cells and T cells express antigen-binding receptors on their surface; NK cells, a third type of lymphocyte, do not.

- **Dendritic cells, macrophages, Langerhans' cells** (in dermis), and **B cells**, as well as glial cells and vascular endothelial cells, function as APCs.
3. **Target cells** degrade **endogenous antigens** (produced within the cell) into smaller peptides, which associate with **class I MHC molecules** on the cell surface.
   - Common target cells are virus-infected cells, defective self-cells, tumor cells, and foreign graft cells.
B. **Effector T cells** are divided into two major types, which have different functions and express different **CD (cluster of differentiation) antigens** on their surface.
   1. **Activated T helper (T_H) cells**
      - Arise by clonal expansion and differentiation of T_H cells, which express **CD4** and **recognize antigen–class II MHC complexes** (Figure 13-3, *A*)
      - Produce and release **cytokines**, which are small, soluble protein factors that **regulate the intensity and duration** of immune responses (Table 13-2)

T_H cells are CD4+ and class II MHC restricted. T_C cells are CD8+ and class I MHC restricted.

   a. **T_H1 cells** promote formation of cytotoxic T lymphocytes (CTLs) and activation of macrophages.
   b. **T_H2 cells** help B cells respond to antigenic stimulation.
   2. **Cytotoxic T lymphocytes (CTLs)**
      - Arise by clonal expansion and differentiation of T cytotoxic (T_C) cells, which express **CD8** and **recognize antigen–class I MHC** complexes (Figure 13-3, *B*)
      - **Cause lysis of target cells** by a perforin-mediated process
C. **Natural killer (NK) cells** belong to the population of peripheral lymphocytes (**null cells**) that do not express antigen-specific receptors and other surface markers characteristic of B and T cells.
   - Exhibit both **nonspecific (antigen-independent) cytotoxicity** and **specific cytotoxicity**, which depends on the presence of antibody on target cells (e.g., tumor cells and virus-infected cells)
   - Perform a **surveillance function** by attacking tumor cells that arise regularly

TABLE 13-2 **Properties of Selected Cytokines**

Cytokine	Secreted by	Major Biological Functions
IL-1	Macrophages, other antigen-presenting cells	• Promotes T_H-cell activation
IL-2	T_H1 cells	• Promotes proliferation of T_H and T_C cells • Enhances activity of NK cells
IL-4	T_H2 cells, mast cells	• Promotes clonal expansion of B cells • Enhances IgG and IgE synthesis by plasma cells
IL-6	T_H2 cells, macrophages	• Promotes terminal differentiation into plasma cells
IFN-γ	T_H1 cells, NK cells	• Enhances macrophage activity • Inhibits T_H2 response

D. Macrophages, which express **class II MHC molecules** but no antigen-specific receptors on their membrane, are derived from **monocytes in the blood** that migrate into tissues and differentiate.

  1. **Types of macrophages**
     - **Fixed** macrophages are attached to reticular fibers, whereas **free** macrophages are motile and wander throughout the stroma of different organs.

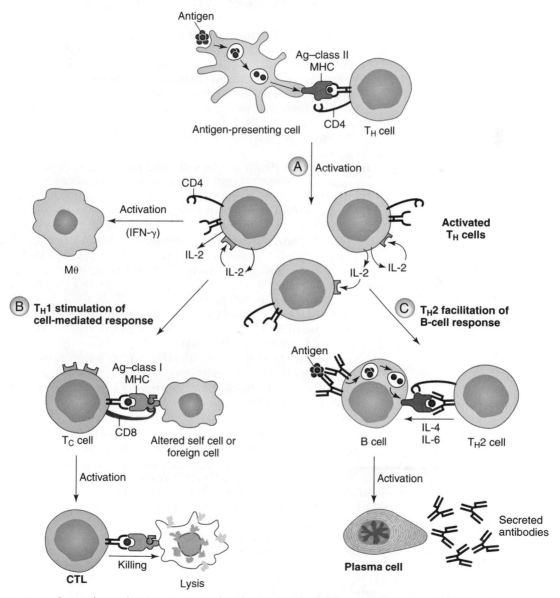

Figure 13-3 Generation and action of effector lymphocytes (activated T_H cells, CTLs, plasma cells). Antigen-presenting cell activates T_H cells *(A)*. Cytokines secreted by the T_H1 and T_H2 subsets of activated T_H cells preferentially promote cell-mediated responses *(B)* and antibody-mediated responses *(C)*. *CTL*, Cytotoxic T lymphocytes; *IFN*, interferon; *IL*, interleukin; *Mθ*, macrophage.

          a. Kupffer cells in liver
          b. Alveolar macrophages in lung
          c. Histiocytes in connective tissue
          d. Microglial cells in brain
       2. **Functions of macrophages**
          a. Phagocytosis and degradation of aged, defective, and dead self-cells
          b. Nonspecific processing and presentation of nonself antigens in context of class II MHC molecules (see Figure 13-2)
          c. Secretion of complement proteins and various cytokines that promote inflammation, elimination of pathogens and tumor cells, and hematopoiesis

   E. **Transplantation-associated immune responses**
      1. **Graft rejection** is caused primarily by the host's cell-mediated response to antigens expressed on cells of a grafted tissue or organ.
        • Intensity of rejection reactions depends on the type of graft:
          a. Autografts (from self to self) and **isografts** (between genetically identical individuals) usually are **accepted.**
          b. Allografts (between individuals of the same species) and **xenografts** (between individuals of different species) are **rejected** unless immune response is suppressed.
            (1) Immunosuppressive drugs (e.g., **cyclosporine**) that selectively suppress the function of T_H cells and NK cells reduce graft rejection but significantly increase the risk of developing cancer (e.g., squamous cell cancer of the skin).
            (2) Natural suppression of maternal cell-mediated immunity during pregnancy helps prevent rejection of allogeneic fetal tissue.
      2. **Graft-versus-host disease (GVHD)** occurs when donor T_C cells in a graft recognize the recipient's cells as nonself and mount a cell-mediated response leading to destruction of the recipient's tissue.
        • GVHD is most likely to occur when a graft containing immunocompetent donor T_C cells is transplanted into a **recipient with a compromised immune system.**

Donor T_C cells in transplanted tissue may mediate an immune response against the recipient's cells, causing GVHD.

Plasma cells, which secrete circulating antibody, arise by differentiation of antigen-stimulated B cells.

III. **Antibody-Mediated (Humoral) Immunologic Response**
    • **Soluble antigens** (e.g., foreign proteins) and antigenic substances on the surface of **extracellular pathogens** trigger humoral responses.
    • Clonal expansion and differentiation of B cells requires direct **B cell/T_H cell interaction** and **cytokines** released from activated T_H cells (see Figure 13-3, *A, C*).
   A. **Plasma cells** are the only type of **effector B lymphocyte.**
    • Plasma cells, which arise from antigen-stimulated B cells (primarily within **lymph nodules**), are terminally differenti-

ated cells and **cannot divide.** They have the following characteristic properties:

1. **Production and secretion of immunoglobulins,** the active agents of humoral immunity
2. **Absence of antigen-binding receptors** on their surface (unlike effector T cells)
3. **Short life span** (about 2–3 weeks)
4. **Abundant rough endoplasmic reticulum (RER) and well-developed Golgi apparatus,** typical of protein-secreting cells
5. **Eccentric nucleus** with clockface chromatin pattern

B. **Immunoglobulins** function as **antibodies** (i.e., they interact specifically with antigens).
1. **Secreted (soluble) and membrane-bound antibodies**
   a. Immunoglobulins **secreted by plasma cells** bind to antigens, forming **antigen-antibody complexes** that are cleared from the body by various mechanisms that may involve **complement proteins.**
   b. Immunoglobulins expressed on the **surface of mature virgin B cells** function as antigen-binding receptors.
2. **Antibody structure and specificity**
   a. Monomeric immunoglobulins have a Y-shaped structure consisting of **two identical heavy (H) chains** and **two identical light (L) chains** (Figure 13-4, *A*).
   b. **Antigen-binding sites,** located at the outer ends of the "arms" of the molecule, exhibit variable amino acid sequences.
      (1) The **variable regions** are responsible for the **antigen specificity** of an antibody molecule.
      (2) Total number of possible different antigen-binding specificities that can be produced in each person is estimated at 10^9–10^{11}.
   c. **Complement-binding** sites are located on heavy chains in CH_2 domains just below the hinge region.
3. **Immunoglobulin classes** (Figure 13-4, *B*)
   • Sequence differences in the Fc region of heavy chains define five immunoglobulin classes, or **isotypes,** which exhibit class-specific functional properties.
   a. **IgM:** predominant secreted antibody produced during **primary immune response**
      • Exists as **pentamer** that **strongly activates complement** system
   b. **IgG:** predominant secreted antibody produced during **secondary immune response**
      • **Promotes phagocytosis** by macrophages
      • **Crosses placenta**
   c. **IgA:** present in external secretions (e.g., tears, saliva, colostrum, mucous secretions of the GI and respiratory tracts) as **dimeric secretory IgA**

Immunoglobulin isotypes:
• IgG: most abundant antibody in blood; promotes phagocytosis; secondary response
• IgA: dimer; in external secretions
• IgM: pentamer; complement activation; primary response
• IgE: type I hypersensitivity reactions (allergy and systemic anaphylaxis)
• IgD: membrane form predominant

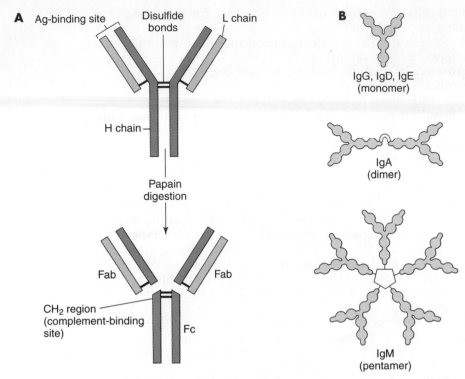

Figure 13-4 Schematic diagrams of immunoglobulin structure. **A,** Y-shaped monomers have a binding site for antigen (Ag) at the end of each arm. Papain digestion yields two Fab fragments, which bind antigen, and an Fc fragment, which binds to receptors on macrophages, mast cells, and basophils. **B,** Dimeric IgA and pentameric IgM have a higher antigen-binding valency than monomeric IgG, IgD, and IgE.

IgE-induced release of histamine, prostaglandins, and other mediators may cause localized allergic reactions (e.g., runny nose, itchy eyes, skin rash) or systemic anaphylaxis, a shock-like, potentially fatal state.

Selective IgA deficiency is the most common immunodeficiency disorder.

    d. IgD: mostly membrane-bound antibody on unstimulated B cells
- Functions primarily in B-cell activation

    e. IgE: only Ig that triggers **immediate (type I) hypersensitivity reactions** (Figure 13-5)

C. Monoclonal antibody is secreted by all the plasma cells derived from a single B cell (i.e., a **clone** of plasma cells).
- Each molecule of a monoclonal antibody has the **same antigen-binding specificity.**

D. Humoral immunodeficiency diseases

    1. X-linked agammaglobulinemia: complete absence of mature B cells, plasma cells, and antibodies
- Marked by recurrent **pyogenic infections** beginning after 6 months of age

    2. Selective IgA deficiency: normal levels of all isotypes except IgA
- Marked by recurrent **sinopulmonary infections** and increased incidence of allergy, GI diseases (e.g., celiac disease), and certain autoimmune diseases

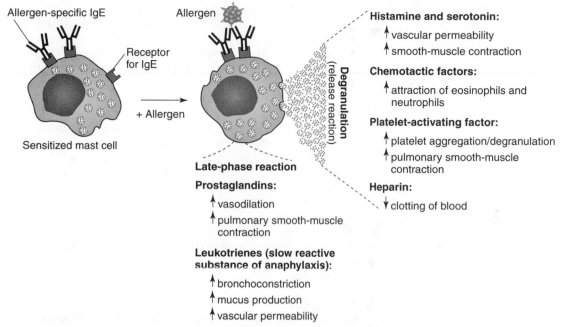

Allergen-specific IgE

Receptor for IgE

Sensitized mast cell

Allergen

+ Allergen

Degranulation (release reaction)

Histamine and serotonin:

↑vascular permeability

↑smooth-muscle contraction

Chemotactic factors:

↑attraction of eosinophils and neutrophils

Platelet-activating factor:

↑platelet aggregation/degranulation

↑pulmonary smooth-muscle contraction

Heparin:

↓clotting of blood

Late-phase reaction

Prostaglandins:

↑vasodilation

↑pulmonary smooth-muscle contraction

Leukotrienes (slow reactive substance of anaphylaxis):

↑bronchoconstriction

↑mucus production

↑vascular permeability

Figure 13-5 Mechanism of immediate (type I) hypersensitivity reactions. Secreted IgE produced following first exposure to an allergen binds to mast cells and basophils, which have receptors for the Fc portion of IgE antibodies. On subsequent exposure to the same allergen, cross-linking of receptor-bound IgE molecules by allergen induces degranulation, releasing preformed mediators. These act to increase (↑) or decrease (↓) various parameters, leading to localized allergic symptoms (e.g., runny nose, itchy eyes, skin rash) or systemic anaphylaxis. Following the release reaction, mast cells synthesize and release prostaglandins and leukotrienes, which mediate the late phase reaction.

E. Multiple myeloma
- This neoplastic disease results from bone marrow–based clonal proliferation of B cells that mature into abnormal but recognizable plasma cells.
- Clinical manifestations include widespread **osteolytic lesions, bone pain**, pathologic fractures, hypercalcemia, and **Bence Jones (light chains) proteinuria**.

IV. Lymphoid Tissues
- **A. Diffuse lymphatic tissue** comprises scattered clusters of plasma cells, macrophages, and lymphocytes in connective tissue (stromal) areas and other sites.
  1. **Cutaneous-associated lymphoid tissue:** in papillary layer of the dermis
  2. **Lamina propria–associated lymphoid tissue**
     - **a. MALT** = mucosal-associated lymphoid tissue
     - **b. BALT** = bronchial-associated lymphoid tissue
     - **c. GALT** = gut-associated lymphoid tissue
- **B. Lymph follicles (nodules),** which are not enclosed by a capsule, occur singly or in aggregates and are sites of **B-cell localization and proliferation.**

Bence Jones protein: monoclonal antibody light chains produced by multiple myeloma cells and excreted in urine.

MALT, BALT, and GALT: diffuse lymphoid tissue associated with the lamina propria in general mucosae, bronchi, and gut, respectively.

1. Structure of follicles

a. Primary (1°) follicles are round tightly packed accumulations of virgin B cells and dendritic reticular cells that **have not been exposed to antigen.**

b. Secondary (2°) follicles arise from 1° lymph follicles that have been **exposed to nonself antigen.**

- Secondary follicles are not present before birth or after birth in individuals kept in a germ-free environment.

(1) Corona: dark peripheral region composed largely of **densely packed B lymphocytes**

(2) Germinal center: central, lighter-staining region composed largely of **B lymphoblasts, memory B cells, plasma cells,** and **dendritic reticular cells,** which trap antigen on their surface

2. Aggregated lymph follicles are located beneath but in contact with the epithelium at several sites.

a. Palatine, pharyngeal, and lingual tonsils

b. Peyer's patches in the submucosa of the ileum (see Chapter 14)

- These are major sites of antibody production in children.

c. Appendix

V. Lymphoid Organs

- In **primary** lymphoid organs (**thymus** and **bone marrow**), lymphocyte **precursors mature** into immunocompetent cells, each programmed to recognize a specific antigen.

- In **secondary** lymphoid organs (**lymph nodes** and **spleen**), trapped antigen stimulates **clonal expansion** of mature B and T cells (and memory cells).

A. Bone marrow: maturation of B cells (see Chapter 12)

B. Thymus: maturation of T cells (Figure 13-6)

- Connective tissue **capsule** of the thymus extends trabeculae into the parenchyma, dividing the organ into **incomplete lobules,** each composed of a distinguishable outer, darker region (**cortex**) and inner, lighter region (**medulla**).

- **Efferent lymphatic vessels** but no afferent lymphatics serve the thymus; thus lymph does not circulate through the organ.

1. Thymic cortex

- Basic dyes such as H&E **densely stain** the thymic cortex, which is filled with epithelial reticular cells and T cells in various stages of differentiation.

a. Epithelial reticular cells secrete **thymosin** and other protein factors that promote maturation of T cells.

- These cells, of endodermal origin (pharyngeal pouch), have **long processes** that surround capillaries and form a meshwork in which T cells are closely packed.

b. T-cell maturation occurs as lymphoblasts (**thymocytes**) in the outer cortex proliferate and become **programmed to recognize a specific antigen** as they migrate toward the inner cortex.

Adenoids: hypertrophy of pharyngeal tonsils in posterior wall of the nasopharynx.

Primary lymphoid organs: thymus (T-cell maturation) and bone marrow (B-cell maturation).

Maturing T cells are programmed to recognize specific antigens as they move from the outer thymic cortex to the deeper cortex. Cells that recognize self-antigens are destroyed, so that the individual exhibits tolerance to these antigens.

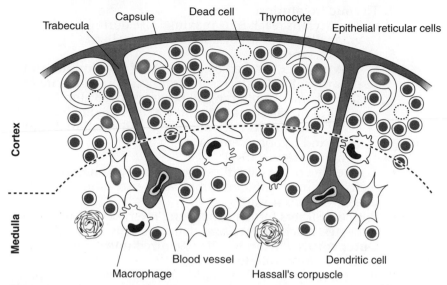

Figure 13-6 Schematic cross-section of a portion of the thymus. The cortex is densely populated with immature T cells (thymocytes) and epithelial reticular cells. Some of these wrap around many thymocytes, forming large multicellular complexes. As they mature, thymocytes move towards the medulla. Only about 5% of thymocyte progeny survive and reach the medulla.

- T cells programmed against self-antigens or unable to recognize self-MHC molecules undergo programmed cell death, called **apoptosis** (>95% of thymocyte progeny do not survive).
- Mature, immunocompetent T cells that remain **recognize nonself antigen in the context of MHC molecules.**

2. **Thymic medulla**
   - Medulla is **lighter staining** than cortex because cells are relatively loosely packed.
   a. **Mature T cells** exit the medulla, via postcapillary venules and efferent lymphatic vessels, and circulate to secondary lymphoid organs.
   b. **Hassall's corpuscles**, found predominantly in the thymic medulla, are concentric arrays of squamous epithelial cells containing **keratohyaline granules.**
      - Probably derived from nearby third branchial/pharyngeal cleft ectoderm during embryogenesis.
3. **Blood–thymus barrier in the thymic cortex**
   a. **Function:** prevents antigens in the bloodstream from reaching developing T cells in the thymic cortex
      - **Barrier is leaky during fetal life**, allowing for development of immunologic tolerance to self-antigen.
   b. **Components:** endothelium → endothelial basal lamina (may house pericytes) → perivascular space → basal lamina of reticular cell → reticular cell → thymic parenchymal cells

4. **Thymic involution**
   - The thymus reaches its maximal size during puberty and gradually atrophies by apoptosis thereafter.
5. **DiGeorge syndrome**
   - This disorder, marked by **agenesis of the thymus and parathyroid glands**, results from congenital failure of the 3rd and 4th pharyngeal pouches to develop.
   - Clinical manifestations include a severe reduction in T-cell count, **markedly depressed cell-mediated immunity**, and **hypocalcemia**.

C. **Lymph nodes** (Figure 13-7)

Secondary lymphoid organs: lymph nodes and spleen. Sites of antigen-stimulated activation and clonal expansion of T and B cells.

- Connective tissue **capsule** surrounding lymph nodes is pierced by many afferent lymphatic vessels and sends trabecular extensions inward.
- **Reticular fibers** form a supporting meshwork in which lymphocytes, macrophages, and dendritic cells can be found.

1. **Outer cortex:** rich in **B cells** organized into primary and secondary **lymph follicles**
2. **Paracortex:** high concentration of **T cells** but no lymph follicles
   a. **Postcapillary venules,** which are lined by cuboidal to low columnar epithelium, are present in paracortex.
   b. **Circulating B and T cells** in the blood can **pass through**

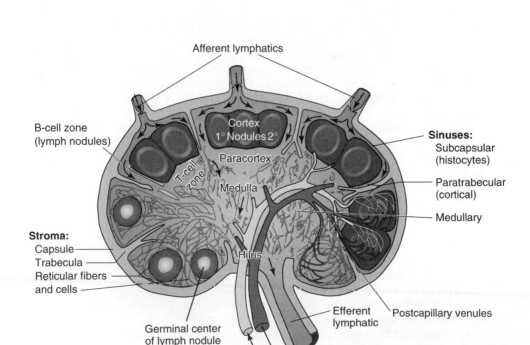

Figure 13-7 Histophysiologic sketch of a lymph node as a filter of lymph. Lymph enters afferent lymphatics, which pierce the capsule and drain into the subcapsular sinus → paratrabecular sinus → medullary sinus → efferent lymph vessels. Clonal expansion of B cells occurs in the outer cortex and of T cells in the paracortex.

these "**high-endothelial**" **venules** to enter the parenchyma of a node.

3. **Medulla:** central, lighter area containing some B and T cells and plasma cells
4. **Hilum:** region where arteries enter a node, and veins and efferent lymphatic vessel exit from it
5. **Sinuses:** endothelium-lined spaces lying just below the capsule, along trabeculae, and in the medulla
   - These spaces are bridged by reticular cells stretched out on reticular fibers (cobweb appearance); they also contain macrophages and lymphocytes.
6. **Filtration of lymph** as it passes through a node largely **removes antigens** and **cellular debris** carried in the lymph.
   - Malignant cells metastasizing to and through a node follow the same pathway as lymph (see Figure 13-7).

D. **Spleen**
   - **Mesothelium-lined** connective tissue **capsule** contains some smooth muscle fibers and sends trabeculae into the splenic parenchyma.
   - During **fetal life**, the spleen functions as a **hematopoietic organ.**
1. **White pulp of the spleen** is the site of **clonal expansion** of antigen-stimulated lymphocytes.
   a. **B-cell area** contains 2° lymph follicles in which the central arteriole of the germinal centers is "off center."
   b. **T-cell area** consists of numerous T lymphocytes located around central arteries of the white pulp, forming the **periarterial lymphatic sheath (PALS).**
2. **Marginal zone of the spleen** forms a **sinusoidal interface** between the red and white pulp.
   a. **Antigen-presenting cells** are abundant in the marginal zone.
   b. **Lymphocytes first encounter antigen** here, and activated T_H cells help in activation of B cells.
3. **Red pulp of the spleen**, which constitutes 80% of the organ, functions to **filter the blood.**
   a. **Cords of Billroth** (Figure 13-8)
      (1) These cords, forming the **red pulp parenchyma,** contain fixed and free **macrophages**, reticular cells and fibers, and various types of blood cells.
      (2) **Terminal capillaries** open into the substance of the cords, delivering blood directly to them (i.e., **open circulation** = not contained by endothelium).
      (3) **Aged, defective RBCs are destroyed by macrophages** in the cords of Billroth.
   b. **Venous sinusoids**
      (1) Splenic sinusoids are lined by endothelial cells that are separated by paracellular gaps and have a discontinuous basement membrane (see Figure 11-3).
      (2) Healthy RBCs pass from cords of Billroth into the sinusoids, which serve as **storage sites for RBCs.**

Splenic red pulp is involved in filtration of blood. Splenic white pulp has both T-cell and B-cell areas plus a marginal zone in which interaction between B and T cells occurs frequently.

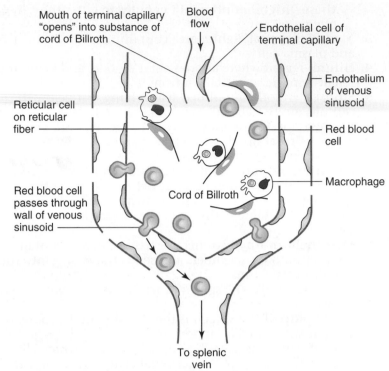

Mouth of terminal capillary
"opens" into substance of
cord of Billroth

Blood
flow

Endothelial cell of
terminal capillary

Endothelium
of venous
sinusoid

Reticular cell
on reticular
fiber

Red blood
cell

Macrophage

Cord of Billroth

Red blood cell
passes through
wall of venous
sinusoid

To splenic
vein

Figure 13-8 Schematic depiction of blood filtration in red pulp of the spleen. Terminal capillaries open directly into the red pulp parenchyma, which is divided into the cords of Billroth by venous sinusoids. As the blood and its formed elements pass through a cord, defective and aged red blood cells (RBCs) are phagocytosed and degraded by macrophages in the cord. RBCs and other elements in the "filtered" blood pass from a cord through the highly permeable endothelial wall of venous sinusoids, thereby regaining access to the bloodstream.

Reed-Sternberg cells: large, generally binucleated neoplastic cells (owl's eye appearance) that are seen in Hodgkin's disease.

E. Lymphomas: tumors of the lymphoid system, which all present with enlarged, painless, firm lymph nodes

1. **Hodgkin's disease:** type of malignant lymphoma characterized by the presence of **Reed-Sternberg cells**, which are giant neoplastic cells that typically have two large, vacuolated nuclei each with prominent nucleoli
   - Neoplastic lymph nodes develop in localized areas either above and/or below the diaphragm.
   - Other clinical manifestations include fever, **night sweats, weight loss, leukocytosis,** and pruritis.

2. **Non-Hodgkin's disease:** large group of malignant lymphomas characterized by neoplastic transformation of B cells (most common), T cells, or histiocytes.
   - **Painless enlargement of one or more lymph nodes** is most common initial feature; generally more disseminated than Hodgkin's disease.
   - Incidence increases with age.

14

Digestive System

Target Topics

▷ Common histologic plan of GI tract and characteristic regional specializations

▷ Myenteric (Auerbach's) and submucosal (Meissner's) plexuses

▷ Gut-associated lymphoid tissue (GALT) and secretory IgA

▷ Secretions from gastric and intestinal glands

▷ Hormones produced by enteroendocrine cells and their functions in GI tract

▷ Histophysiologic organization and ultrastructure of the liver

▷ Pancreatic exocrine secretions

▷ Oral lesions, Plummer-Vinson syndrome, gastroesophageal reflux disease (GERD), peptic ulcer disease, Hirschsprung's disease, cirrhosis of the liver, gallstones, pancreatitis, GI tract neoplasms

I. Introduction

- The **digestive system** consists of a **continuous hollow tube** extending from the lips to the anus, plus several **extramural glands** whose secretions are delivered to the lumen.

A. Basic histologic plan of the alimentary canal (Figure 14-1)

- The wall of the alimentary canal (esophagus → anus) consists of four major layers throughout its length.

  1. Mucosa: three distinct sublayers

  a. Epithelium lining the lumen may have **secretory, absorptive,** and/or **protective functions.**

  b. Lamina propria of loose areolar connective tissue lies below luminal epithelium.
  - Various **glands** and **gut-associated lymphatic tissue (GALT)** are present in the lamina propria.

  c. Muscularis mucosae comprises one to three layers of **smooth muscle.**

General plan of gut wall:
- Mucosa (epithelium, lamina propria, muscularis mucosae)
- Submucosa (connective tissue)
- Muscularis externa (2 or 3 smooth muscle layers)
- Adventitia (retroperitoneal portions) or serosa (intraperitoneal portions)

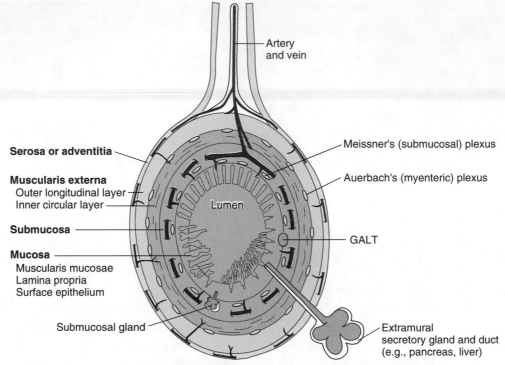

Figure 14-1 Schematic diagram of the general histologic plan of the alimentary canal. The mucosa consists of the surface epithelium, lamina propria, and usually a thin layer of smooth muscle (muscularis mucosa) adjacent to the submucosa, which is inside the muscularis externa. Serosa covers intraperitoneal regions; adventitia covers retroperitoneal regions. The extent of mucosal folding varies in different regions. It is relatively simple in the colon, as depicted here, and more complex in the stomach and small intestine. *GALT,* Gut-associated lymphatic tissue.

Submucosal (Meissner's) autonomic plexuses control local secretion from gut wall.

Myenteric (Auerbach's) autonomic plexuses control gut motility.

2. **Submucosa:** dense irregular connective tissue
   - **Submucosal autonomic plexuses/ganglia (Meissner's)** are located here.
3. **Muscularis externa:** inner circular and outer longitudinal layer of **smooth muscle**
   - **Myenteric autonomic plexuses/ganglia (Auerbach's)** lie between muscle layers.
4. **Outermost layer:** either a serosa *or* an adventitia (fibrosa)
   a. **Serosa** consists of a mesothelial lining and a layer of submesothelial connective tissue.
      - Forms the **visceral peritoneum**, which is a reflection of the serosal lining of the abdominal wall (**parietal peritoneum**)
      - Covers **intraperitoneal** portions of the alimentary canal, surface of the gallbladder exposed to peritoneal cavity, and surface of the colon facing peritoneal cavity
   b. **Adventitia (fibrosa)** consists of dense irregular connective tissue containing adipose tissue.
      - Blends with connective tissue around adjacent organs
      - Covers **retroperitoneal** portions of alimentary canal, surface of gallbladder embedded in the liver, and surface of colon facing the posterior body wall

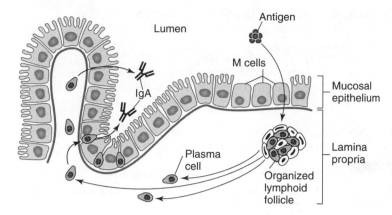

Figure 14-2 Formation of secretory IgA in response to antigens in the GI tract. M cells are specialized epithelial cells that transport antigens from the lumen to the underlying lamina propria. B lymphocytes, present within isolated or aggregated lymphoid follicles (e.g., Peyer's patches), interact with the antigen and differentiate into plasma cells that secrete IgA. As IgA is transported across the mucosa into the lumen, it acquires a protective secretory piece.

B. Turnover of luminal epithelium
  1. High rates of cell loss and cell birth characterize mucosa.
  2. Pap smear cytology can be performed on desquamated cells captured by swabs or lavages (e.g., gastric lavage).
  3. Gastrointestinal (GI) toxicity of radiation and chemotherapy agents results from high rate of cell division.
    • Common clinical signs of toxicity are **bloody diarrhea** and **ulcers** in the oral cavity and esophagus. If these signs occur, therapy may be discontinued or lessened.

C. Innervation
  • **Peristalsis** depends on innervation to the smooth muscles of the digestive tract.
  1. Sympathetic postganglionic fibers from sympathetic chain pass through gut wall to glands and smooth muscle.
  2. Parasympathetic preganglionic fibers arrive on cell bodies of parasympathetic postganglionic neurons in ganglia in the gut wall; **postganglionic fibers** pass to glands and smooth muscle.
    a. Meissner's (submucosal) plexuses regulate local secretions, blood flow, and absorption.
    b. Auerbach's (myenteric) plexuses coordinate muscular activity of gut wall.

D. Gut-associated lymphoid tissue (GALT)
  • **Luminal surface** of lining epithelium is **coated with secretory IgA**, forming a first line of defense against antigens in the GI tract.
  1. Isolated lymph follicles (nodules)
    a. M cells, specialized squamous epithelial cells interspersed within the luminal epithelium, **take up dietary antigens** from the lumen and **transport them to lymph follicles** in the underlying lamina propria (Figure 14-2).
    b. Antigen-stimulated B cells within follicles differentiate into **IgA-secreting plasma cells,** which move through the adjacent lamina propria.

Secretory IgA, the intra-gut antibody, is produced by Peyer's patches and other GALT, then transported across the intestinal epithelium to protect against intraluminal antigens.

        2. Diffuse lymphatic tissue of the lamina propria (lymphocytes, macrophages, and IgA-secreting plasma cells)

        3. Aggregated lymph follicles

        a. Waldeyer's ring of tonsils of the oropharynx

        b. Peyer's patches in submucosa of ileum

II. Oral Cavity

- The histology of the oral cavity (lips → pharynx) is highly modified from the basic plan described above.

A. Lips

    1. Core of skeletal muscle, the **orbicularis oris**

    2. Anterior surface, covered by dermis and epidermis (e.g., hair follicles)

    3. Posterior surface, covered by **nonkeratinized stratified squamous epithelium**, or **oral epithelium**, and lamina propria (no muscularis mucosae)

B. Teeth

- From the inside to outside, a tooth contains the following structural components:

    1. Pulp: connective tissue containing blood vessels and nerves located within the pulp cavity

    - **Inflammation** of the pulp produces classic "**toothache.**"

    2. Dentin: mineralized layer around the pulp cavity that forms the bulk of the tooth; harder than bone but not as hard as enamel

    3. Enamel: relatively thin mineralized layer that forms **external surface of tooth crown;** hardest substance in the body, containing 98% **hydroxyapatite** by weight

    - Acid injury from self-induced vomiting wears away enamel layer.

    4. Cementum: mineralized layer that forms **external surface of root** of the tooth (part within bony socket) and is similar in composition to bone.

    - Like bone, cementum layer extends connective tissue fibers (**Sharpey's fibers**) into adjacent tissue.

C. Tongue

    1. Skeletal muscle core with fibers running in **three different geometric planes** is characteristic of the tongue.

    2. Mucosa of tongue lacks underlying submucosa on dorsal surface and muscularis mucosa throughout.

    a. Ventral (inferior) surface is covered by oral epithelium (nonkeratinized stratified squamous epithelium).

    b. Dorsal (superior) surface is covered by stratified squamous epithelium that contains some keratin (**parakeratinized**).

    3. Lingual papillae are variously shaped structures with a connective tissue core that **project from dorsal surface** of the anterior two thirds of the tongue.

    a. Taste buds are present in fungiform and circumvallate papillae but not in filiform papillae (see Chapter 19).

    b. Glands of von Ebner produce serous secretion that continuously rinses out the trenches surrounding circumvallate papillae, so that any change in ingested food can be detected quickly by cleansed taste buds.

D. Hard palate
- The mucosa of the hard palate is firmly attached to the palatine bone.
  1. **Superior/nasal mucosa** is lined by **respiratory epithelium** (pseudostratified ciliated columnar epithelium).
     - Contains considerable adipose tissue and **seromucous glands**
  2. **Lingual mucosa** is lined by parakeratinized stratified squamous epithelium.
     - Contains purely **mucous glands**

E. Soft palate
  1. **Contraction of skeletal muscle core** raises soft palate against wall of the pharynx, closing the choanae (posterior nares) and thereby **preventing food from entering nasal cavity** during swallowing.
  2. **Mucosa** is similar to that of lingual mucosa of the hard palate.
  3. **Uvula**, the posterior tip of the soft palate, is surfaced by oral epithelium.

F. Pharynx
- A common chamber for food and air, the pharynx is continuous with the nasal and oral cavities and with the lumen of the esophagus.
  1. **Pharyngeal mucosa**
     a. Respiratory epithelium where only air is present
     b. Oral epithelium where food may be present
  2. **Pharyngeal constrictor muscles** consist of skeletal muscle beneath mucosa.

G. Disorders of the oral cavity
  1. **Oral leukoplakia** is marked by **thickened, slightly raised white patches** in the mucous membrane of the lips, tongue, and lining of the cheeks.
     - Use of **smokeless tobacco** and **pipe smoking** are risk factors.
     - Patches should be biopsied to rule out squamous cell dysplasia or cancer.
  2. **Oral cancer**, most commonly **squamous cell carcinoma**, usually develops on the lips, tongue, and floor of the mouth and can spread to lymph nodes.
  3. **Herpetic stomatitis** is characterized by **fluid-filled, painful blisters (cold sores)** on the lips or near nostrils.
     - Outbreaks result from acute infection of oral mucosa by **herpes simplex virus type I (HSV1)**, which remains latent in trigeminal ganglion.
  4. **Aphthous stomatitis** is characterized by small, whitish ulcers with a red border (**canker sores**) in the mucosa of the lips, cheeks, and gums.

Squamous cell carcinoma: most common type of oral cancer; associated with smoking and excess alcohol intake.

Cold sores: fluid-filled blisters; usually on the lips or near nostrils; caused by HSV1.

Canker sores: whitish ulcers with red border; in mucosa of lips, cheeks, and gums; noninfectious etiology.

III. **Alimentary Canal**
  • The major regional specializations to the basic histologic plan of the alimentary canal are summarized in Table 14-1.
  A. **Esophagus**
    1. **Mucosa**
      • Is surfaced by **oral epithelium** (nonkeratinized stratified squamous epithelium) and has a **highly developed muscularis mucosae**
      • Exhibits **mucosal folds** when no food is passing through
    2. **Muscularis externa**
      a. **Upper third** of esophagus: **skeletal muscle only**
      b. **Middle third** of esophagus: mixture of **skeletal and smooth muscle**
      c. **Lower third** of esophagus: **smooth muscle only**
    3. **Mucous glands**
      a. **Esophageal glands proper** in submucosa
      b. **Esophageal cardiac glands** in lamina propria

TABLE 14-1 Selected Histologic Features of the Alimentary Canal

Region*	Surface Epithelial Cells	Glands	Regional Specializations
Esophagus	Stratified squamous nonkeratinized	Mucous glands in lamina propria and submucosa	• Skeletal and smooth muscle in muscularis externa
Stomach	Mucous columnar	Gastric glands in lamina propria open into gastric pits	• Rugae (mucosal folds) • Three smooth muscle layers in muscularis externa
Small intestine	Enterocytes (columnar with microvilli) and goblet cells	Brunner's submucosal mucous glands (only in duodenum); crypts of Lieberkühn in mucosa; mucus-secreting goblet cells	• Villi (mucosal folds) • Plicae circulares (large folds of mucosa and submucosa) • Peyer's patches in ileum
Large intestine: Cecum Colon Rectum	From cecum to rectum, number of enterocytes decreases and number of goblet cells increases	Mucus-secreting goblet cells	• Taeniae coli in muscularis externa of cecum and colon • Crypts with few secretory Paneth cells
Anal canal	Proximal: similar to rectum; distal: stratified squamous nonkeratinized; at anus: stratified squamous keratinized (skin)	Sebaceous glands; mucus-producing circumanal glands	• Anal columns of Morgagni (longitudinal mucosal folds) • Anal valves (transverse mucosal folds) • Anal sphincters

*All regions possess four basic tunics: mucosa, submucosa, muscularis externa, and serosa or adventitia.

4. Esophageal disorders
   a. Plummer-Vinson syndrome is marked by triad of **cervical esophageal webs, iron-deficiency anemia**, and **glossitis.**
      (1) Growth of webs, which makes swallowing solid foods difficult, is linked to **lack of iron**. Webs disappear when iron deficiency is corrected.
      (2) Carcinoma of the **oropharynx** and **upper esophagus** are possible complications.
   b. Esophageal varices occur in patients with **alcoholic cirrhosis**, which compromises venous return from liver to hepatic vein.
      (1) Blood uses alternate route, leading to distention of veins (varices) in submucosa of lower esophagus.
      (2) Vomiting may cause esophageal varices to rupture.
   c. GERD (gastroesophageal reflux disease) results from incompetent lower esophageal sphincter.
      (1) Heartburn is common early symptom of GERD; difficulty swallowing and bleeding occur in more advanced cases.
      (2) In chronic cases, back flow of acidic stomach contents may lead to metaplasia of normal esophageal squamous epithelium to gastric or intestinal type, producing **Barrett's esophagus.**
   d. Achalasia is the combined lack of peristalsis in the body of the esophagus and failure of lower esophageal sphincter to relax.
      • This condition results from degeneration of myenteric ganglion cells in the esophageal wall.
   e. Esophageal adenocarcinoma is the most common cancer of the esophagus. Barrett's esophagus is an important risk factor.
   f. Squamous cell carcinoma arises primarily in the **lower two thirds** of the organ and metastasizes to regional lymph nodes.
      • Risk factors include **cigarette smoking**, heavy **alcohol** use, achalasia, and esophageal webs.

B. Stomach
   • Bolus of **food** from esophagus **is acidified and broken down** in the stomach, forming **chyme**, a low pH viscous fluid that exits the pylorus into the duodenum.
   1. Gastric mucosa is surfaced by simple epithelium composed of **mucous columnar cells**.
      a. Insoluble mucus secreted from surface cells prevents damage to the lining from acidic luminal contents.
      b. Longitudinal mucosal folds (**rugae**) are most prominent in empty stomach.
      c. Gastric pits are epithelial recesses into which gastric glands open.
   2. Muscularis externa deviates from basic histologic plan by presence of **three** (not two) **layers** with addition of an inner **oblique** smooth muscle layer.

Chronic GERD may cause Barrett's esophagus, which predisposes to esophageal adeno-carcinoma of the distal esophagus.

3. **Gastric glands** are simple branched tubular glands.
   - These glands consist of an **isthmus**, which opens into the bottom of a gastric pit; a **neck;** and a **base (fundus)**, which traverses the lamina propria (Figure 14-3).
   a. **Mucous neck cells** secrete **soluble** mucus.
   b. **Stem cells** (in neck) proliferate and differentiate to replace all other cells of the gland, pit, and surface epithelium.
   c. **Chief (zymogenic) cells** (in base) are typical protein-secreting cells with basal rough endoplasmic reticulum (RER) and apical secretory granules.
      - Secrete **pepsinogen**, which is converted into the proteolytic enzyme **pepsin** on exposure to low pH of the stomach lumen
   d. **Parietal (oxyntic) cells** (in base) are large triangular cells with eosinophilic cytoplasm, extensive **intracellular canalicular system**, many microvilli at apical surface, and many mitochondria.
      (1) Secrete **intrinsic factor**, which is necessary for absorption of **vitamin B$_{12}$** by the terminal ileum

Parietal cells produce intrinsic factor and HCl; chief cells produce pepsinogen.

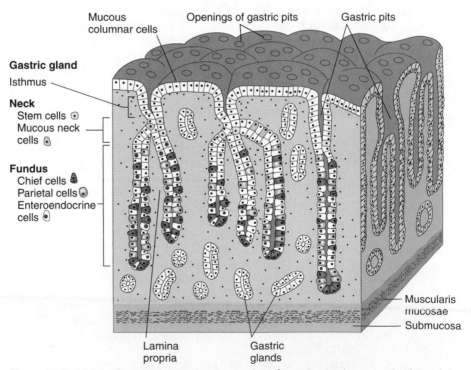

Figure 14-3 Lining of stomach showing the relation of gastric glands to gastric pits and the underlying muscularis mucosae. Glands are most developed in the fundic region where gastric pits form about a fifth of the mucosa and the glands themselves about four fifths. Fundic glands, shown here, possess all the different cell types found in gastric glands, whereas cardiac and pyloric glands contain only mucus-producing cells and stem cells.

(2) Manufacture **HCl** by transporting hydrogen and chloride ions across the canalicular membranes

(3) Located primarily in the **body** and **fundus** of the stomach

e. **Enteroendocrine cells** (in base) belong to the population of **diffuse neuroendocrine cells** found throughout the body.

(1) Also known as **APUD cells** (**a**mine **p**recursor **u**ptake and **d**ecarboxylation cells)

(2) Oriented with apex of cell directed toward the basal lamina and nucleus close to free (luminal) surface

(3) **Secrete hormones** toward capillaries in the lamina propria (Table 14-2)

C. **Small intestine** (Figure 14-4)

1. **Intestinal specializations that increase surface area for absorption**

a. **Microvilli:** projections from apical surface of columnar absorptive cells (**enterocytes**)

b. **Villi:** folds of the inner two mucosal layers (epithelium and lamina propria)

(1) Diffuse lymphatic tissue and **lacteals** (blind-ending lymphatic capillaries) are located within the lamina propria.

(2) **Absence of villi,** which greatly increase absorption area of the small bowel, leads to **malabsorption** of nutrients.

c. **Plicae circulares (valves of Kerkring):** large permanent folds of mucosa and submucosa

• Begin in lower duodenum with most found in jejunum; decrease in size and amount in ileum

TABLE 14-2 Some Hormones Secreted by Enteroendocrine Cells of the GI Tract

Hormone	Secretion Site	Function*
Cholecystokinin (CCK)	Small intestine	• Stimulates secretion of pancreatic enzymes and gallbladder contraction • Inhibits gastric emptying
Gastrin	Stomach and duodenum	• Stimulates secretion of HCl and pepsinogen
Motilin	Small intestine	• Increases gut motility
Secretin	Small intestine	• Stimulates bicarbonate secretion by pancreas
Serotonin	Stomach through colon	• Stimulates smooth muscle • Inhibits gastric secretion
Somatostatin	Stomach through colon	• Inhibits nearby neuro-endocrine cells
Vasoactive intestinal peptide (VIP)	Stomach through colon	• Increases gut motility and intestinal ion/water secretion

*Some of these substances have additional physiologic effects in other parts of the body.

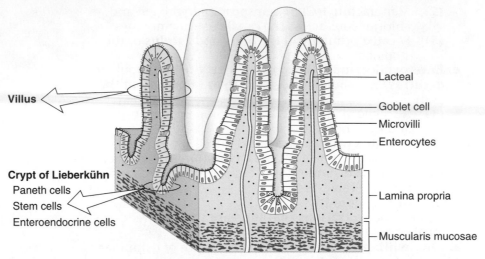

Figure 14-4 Lining of the small intestine. Intestinal villi are evaginations of the epithelium and lamina propria; each villus contains a single lacteal. Crypts of Lieberkühn are invaginations of the epithelium into the lamina propria.

2. **Glands whose secretions enter intestinal lumen**
   a. **Brunner's glands:** submucosal glands that secrete **alkaline mucus;** present only in the **duodenum**
   b. **Unicellular mucous glands** (goblet cells) within luminal epithelium
   c. **Crypts of Lieberkühn:** simple tubular glands within the intestinal mucosa that open between adjacent villi and extend to muscularis mucosae (see Figure 14-4)
   d. **Extramural glands:** pancreas, gallbladder, and liver
      • Empty their exocrine secretions into the duodenum
3. **Cells of the intestinal lining**
   a. **Enterocytes** are tall columnar, highly absorptive cells that constitute the primary cell type of surface epithelium
      (1) Covered with closely packed microvilli on apical surface facing intestinal lumen, forming the **brush border**, which contains disaccharidases (see Figure 4-4)
      (2) Possess **junctional complexes** that prevent paracellular movement of material across intestinal epithelium
   b. **Goblet cells**, which are interspersed among enterocytes, increase in number from duodenum to rectum.
      • Filled with **mucigen** granules in apical portion of cell
   c. **Enteroendocrine (APUD) cells** are hormone-producing cells similar to those in gastric lining (see Table 14-2).
   d. **Paneth cells**, at base of crypts of Lieberkühn, contain prominent **eosinophilic granules**.
      (1) Secrete **digestive enzymes** and **lysozyme**, an antibacterial enzyme
      (2) **Phagocytose** some microorganisms and help regulate intestinal flora

Enteroendocrine (APUD) cells located in the GI tract produce serotonin, gastrin, motilin, CCK, secretin, and VIP.

    e. Stem cells near base of crypts of Lieberkühn can replace all the other cells of the intestinal lining.
- Daughter cells migrate upward to tip of villus and then desquamate by the trillions.

4. Absorption of monosaccharides and amino acids

    a. Transport proteins in apical surface of enterocytes mediate uptake of monosaccharides and amino acids from intestinal lumen.

    b. Absorbed materials are actively transported across basal surface into lamina propria, where they enter the circulation.

5. Absorption of lipids

    a. Bile salts help organize lipid digestion products into **micelles,** which are endocytosed at apical surfaces of enterocytes.

    b. Within smooth endoplasmic reticulum (SER) of enterocytes, fatty acids and glycerol are resynthesized into triglycerides.

    c. Chylomicrons are formed in the Golgi and then released by exocytosis at the lateral cell membrane below the junctional complex.
- Contain diet-derived triglycerides, cholesterol, protein, and fat-soluble vitamins

    (1) Released chylomicrons pass between cells, cross the basal lamina, and enter lacteals in the lamina propria (see Figure 14-4).

    (2) Contents of lymphatic vessels eventually reach the thoracic duct, which joins the blood circulation.

6. Peptic ulcers: inflammatory lesions in the mucosal lining of the **stomach** or **duodenum** that penetrate the muscularis mucosae.

    a. *Helicobacter pylori,* the most common cause of peptic ulcers, produces **urease.**

    b. Ammonia, resulting from action of urease on urea, damages the mucous barrier, leading to acid injury of the mucosa, submucosa, and underlying muscle layer.

> Gastric and duodenal ulcers are most commonly caused by *Helicobacter pylori.*

D. Large intestine
- Primary functions are to absorb water and electrolytes and to lubricate feces with mucous.

1. Surface features

    a. From cecum to anal canal, **enterocytes decrease** and **goblet cells increase** in number.

    b. Crypts are present (few if any Paneth cells), but villi and plicae circulares are absent.

2. Muscularis externa in cecum and colon

    a. Outer longitudinal layer forms three strong, flat strips, the **taeniae coli.**

    b. Myenteric (Auerbach's) ganglia are located between taeniae coli and subjacent circular layer of smooth muscle.

3. **Hirschsprung's disease (congenital megacolon)** is caused by congenital absence of autonomic ganglia (**aganglionosis**).
- Paralysis in the aganglionic segment largely prevents passage of material through it, leading to distention of the bowel (**megacolon**) and possibly **perforation** if untreated.

E. Anal canal

1. **Upper portion** is continuous histologically and grossly with rectum.
  a. **Anal columns (of Morgagni):** longitudinal folds of anal mucosa
  b. **Anal valves:** small transverse folds connecting distal ends of anal columns; **pectinate line** of gross anatomy
  c. **Anal sinuses:** troughs between adjacent folds

2. **Lower portion** (distal to anal valves) is surfaced by nonkeratinized stratified squamous epithelium that is continuous with **skin** of anus.

3. **Anal sphincters**
  a. **Internal** sphincter = circular **smooth muscle** of muscularis externa
    - Is under **involuntary** feedback control
  b. **External** sphincter = **skeletal muscle**
    - Maintains continuous tonus, thus keeping orifice closed, but degree of tonus is under **voluntary** control

4. **Hemorrhoids:** varicosed veins either above or below the anorectal line.
  - External hemorrhoids thrombose; internal hemorrhoids bleed.

F. Ulcerative colitis and Crohn's disease are chronic inflammatory diseases that exhibit a familial tendency and affect various portions of the GI tract.
- They are of unknown etiology but may result from cytokines and inflammatory mediators released subsequent to inappropriate activation of the immune system.

IV. **Extramural Glands of the Digestive System**
- Exocrine secretions critical to the digestive process enter the oral cavity from the salivary glands and the small intestine from the liver, gallbladder, and pancreas.

A. Major salivary glands

1. **Components of saliva**
  a. **Water and glycoproteins** clean and lubricate oral cavity.
  b. **IgA, lysozyme, and lactoferrin** provide defense against pathogens.
  c. **Salivary amylase** begins digestion of carbohydrates.

2. **Neoplasms of the salivary glands**
  a. **Pleomorphic (mixed) adenoma:** most common salivary gland tumor, occurring much more frequently in women than men
    - Presents as smooth, painless, hard, slow-growing mass, most often in **parotid gland**

Congenital megacolon (Hirschsprung's disease) is due to absence of autonomic ganglia; proximal, distended section is innervated.

Salivary gland acini:
- Parotid glands: mostly serous
- Sublingual glands: mostly mucous
- Submandibular: both (mixed)

    b. Mucoepidermoid carcinoma: most common malignant tumor of salivary glands; may be indolent or aggressive

B. Liver

  1. Hepatic functions

    a. Synthesis and release of bile into canaliculi between individual hepatocytes (exocrine function)

    b. Synthesis and release directly into blood of several **plasma proteins** (e.g., albumin, prothrombin, fibrinogen, lipoproteins) and **glucose** (gluconeogenesis)

    c. Storage of metabolites, particularly **glycogen** (stored carbohydrate) and **triglycerides** (stored lipid)

    d. Biochemical degradation of toxic substances (e.g., alcohol) and certain endogenous metabolites (e.g., estrogen)

    e. Metabolic activation of certain substances that are inactive in the body until chemically transformed by liver enzymes

      • Examples include **cyclophosphamide,** a chemotherapeutic drug, and indirect-acting **carcinogens** (e.g., vinyl chloride, aflatoxin B_1, and benzpyrene).

  2. Histophysiologic organization of the liver (Figure 14-5)

    • The basic structural-functional unit of liver parenchyma has been described in three ways.

    a. Classical hepatic lobule emphasizes release of plasma proteins and glucose into the blood.

      (1) Shape: **hexagon**

      (2) At center: single **central vein**

      (3) At periphery: six **portal tracts** (triads or canals), each containing branches of the hepatic artery, portal vein, and bile duct

    b. Portal lobule emphasizes release of bile.

      (1) Shape: **triangle**

      (2) At center: a **portal tract**

      (3) At periphery: **three** "surrounding" **central veins** at points of the triangle

    c. Acinus emphasizes gradient of **metabolic activity** within liver.

      (1) Shape: **diamond**

      (2) At periphery: **two central veins** at ends of long axis and **two portal tracts** at ends of short axis

      (3) At center: **vascular backbone** with contributions from vessels in each of the two portal tracts

  3. Blood flow to and from the liver

    a. Portal vein from small intestine, spleen, and pancreas brings **nutrient-rich blood** to liver.

    b. Common hepatic artery brings **oxygen-rich blood** to liver.

    c. Arterial and venous blood mix in hepatic **sinusoids.**

    d. Hepatic vein, formed by coalescence of central veins, carries blood from liver to inferior vena cava to right heart.

  4. Bile flow

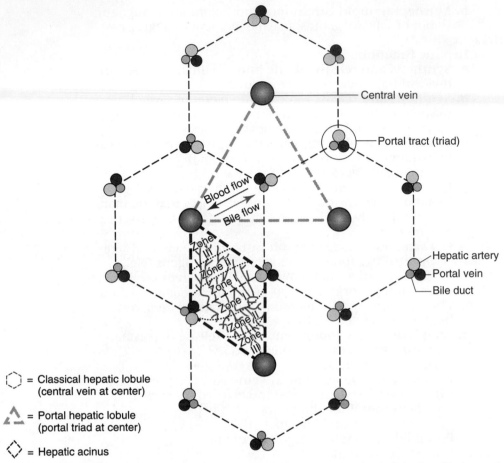

Central vein

Portal tract (triad)

Blood flow

Bile flow

Zone III
Zone II
Zone I
Zone I
Zone II
Zone III

Hepatic artery
Portal vein
Bile duct

= Classical hepatic lobule
(central vein at center)

= Portal hepatic lobule
(portal triad at center)

= Hepatic acinus

Figure 14-5 Schematic representation of the classic lobule, portal lobule, and acinus of the liver. Each portal tract, or triad, contains branches of the hepatic artery, portal vein, and bile duct. Note that blood flows from triads toward central veins, whereas bile drains in opposite directions toward triads.

    a. Direction of bile flow is toward periphery of classic hepatic lobule, **opposite to direction of blood flow** (see Figure 14-5).

    b. Bile flows through canaliculi between adjacent hepatocytes → ductules (**canals of Hering**) in portal canals → larger bile ducts.

5. Metabolic zones of hepatic acini

- Oxygen is lost from blood as it flows from branches of the hepatic artery through acinar sinusoids toward the two central veins associated with an acinus.

- Resulting **oxygen gradient divides each half of an acinus into three functional zones** (see Figure 14-5).

    a. Zone 1 (closest to arterial center): highest oxygen saturation, nutrient levels, and metabolic activity

- This zone is most resistant to insult and hepatocytes here are the first to begin regenerative process after partial hepatectomy.

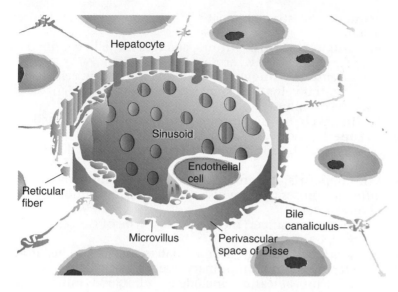

Figure 14-6 Three-dimensional depiction of liver ultrastructure showing the relation of hepatocytes to a blood sinusoid. Materials readily move from the sinusoidal lumen into the space of Disse because the endothelium contains paracellular gaps and is underlain by a discontinuous basement membrane (see Figure 11-3). Hepatocytes secrete bile into canaliculi, which drain toward triads at the periphery of a classic lobule.

    b. Zone 2: anatomically and physiologically intermediate between zones 1 and 3

    c. Zone 3 (closest to the central vein): lowest oxygen saturation, nutrient levels, and metabolic activity

  6. Hepatic ultrastructure (Figure 14-6)

    a. Hepatic sinusoids arise near periphery of classic lobule and course between cords of hepatocytes, draining toward the central vein.

      • Lined by **sinusoidal endothelial cells** and phagocytic **Kupffer cells**

    b. Space of Disse is perivascular space between sinusoid endothelium and adjacent hepatocytes.

      • Contains reticular fibers, lipocytes (Ito cells) that store vitamin A, and blood plasma minus formed elements

    c. Hepatocytes, the liver's parenchymal cells, **freely exchange material with contents of spaces of Disse.**

      (1) **Microvilli** are present on those surfaces facing spaces of Disse.

      (2) **Bile canaliculi** are delineated as tiny grooves between abutting surfaces of adjacent hepatocytes and are sealed laterally by zonulae occludens.

      (3) **Basophilic** cytoplasmic regions contain RER and free polysomes.

      (4) **Acidophilic** cytoplasmic regions contain mitochondria and **peroxisomes,** which break down hydrogen peroxide produced by normal metabolic activity.

      (5) Unstained cytoplasmic regions contain multiple Golgi bodies, glycogen inclusions (PAS positive), and lipid droplets.

  7. Cirrhosis of the liver: chronic disease marked by death of hepatocytes and their replacement by fibroblasts and collagen fibers, producing cirrhotic scarring and regenerative nodules, consisting of hepatocytes entrapped by the fibrous tissues

    a. Cardiac cirrhosis: cirrhotic changes initially confined to **zone 3** of acini (i.e., around central veins).

- Caused by **sluggish blood flow** in hepatic vein, central veins, and sinusoids resulting from right-sided heart failure

    b. Biliary cirrhosis: cirrhotic changes initially confined to **zone 1** of acini (i.e., in portal tract regions).

- Caused by autoimmune destruction of bile ducts in triads

8. Viral hepatitis: inflammation of the liver caused by several different viruses that are distinguished by immunologic tests

9. Liver cancers

    a. Metastatic cancer: most common type of cancer to involve the liver

    b. Hepatocellular carcinoma: malignancy of the hepatocyte; most common primary liver cancer

       (1) Clinical features include jaundice, abdominal distention, ascites, and increased α-fetoprotein.

       (2) Predisposing factors are cirrhosis associated with **chronic hepatitis B and C, hemochromatosis,** and cirrhosis associated with **alcoholism.**

C. Gallbladder

  1. Functions of the gallbladder

    a. Storage and concentration of **bile**

    b. Release of bile in response to presence of fat in the duodenum

- **Cholecystokinin** (CCK) secreted by enteroendocrine cells in the duodenum stimulates contraction of the gallbladder and release of its contents.

  2. Tunics of the gallbladder

- Muscularis mucosae and submucosa are absent.

    a. Mucosa

       (1) Simple columnar epithelium with microvilli and junctional complexes

       (2) Richly vascularized lamina propria

    b. Muscularis externa: thin with three indistinct layers

    c. Serosa on external surface facing peritoneal cavity; **fibrosa/adventitia** on external surface facing liver

  3. Gallstones (cholelithiasis): concretions, usually of **cholesterol,** that form in the gallbladder or bile duct

    a. Too much cholesterol in the bile and/or **too little bile salts** are primary causes.

    b. A common disorder, seen especially in women over age 40, gallstones generally are **asymptomatic.**

D. Exocrine pancreas

- The endocrine secretions of the pancreas, which have no role in digestion, are discussed in Chapter 18.

  1. Pancreatic acinar cells

- These **pyramidal serous cells** contain basally located nuclei and RER; prominent Golgi; and apical secretory granules.

2. **Duct system of the pancreas**
   a. **Centroacinar cells** located **within acini** form beginning of duct system.
   b. Main pancreatic duct converges with the common bile duct just before emptying into the duodenum.
3. **Pancreatic secretions**
   a. **Digestive enzymes** are synthesized and stored in **acinar cells.** Their release is stimulated by CCK.
   b. **Bicarbonate-rich, alkaline fluid** is released by **ductal epithelial cells** in response to **secretin.**
      - This fluid raises the pH of chyme to an optimal level for pancreatic enzyme function.
4. **Acute pancreatitis:** inflammation of pancreas most often occurring in middle-aged or older patients who abuse **alcohol** and have **biliary tract obstruction** (e.g., gallstones)
   a. Clinical features include **midepigastric pain radiating to the back** and elevated serum lipase and amylase.
   b. Histologic features include pancreatic edema and white areas containing saponified fatty acids released by action of excess lipase on adjacent adipose tissue (**enzymatic fat necrosis**).

Secretin stimulates release of sodium bicarbonate from pancreatic ductal epithelium, whereas CCK causes release of enzymes from serous acini.

Pancreatic enzymes delivered to the duodenum include lipase, amylase, trypsinogen, pepsinogen, DNAase, and RNAase.

15

Urinary System

Target Topics

▷ Gross structure of the kidney and relation to uriniferous tubules
▷ Histophysiology of different portions of the uriniferous tubule
▷ Components and selectivity of renal filtration barrier
▷ ADH and regulation of urine concentration
▷ Juxtaglomerular apparatus and renin-angiotensin-aldosterone system
▷ Diabetes insipidus, glomerulonephritis, polycystic kidney disease, nephrotic syndrome, bladder cancer

Uriniferous tubule (functional unit of the kidney) = nephron + collecting tubules.

I. **Introduction**
    • The **urinary system** comprises the paired **kidneys** and **ureters** and unpaired **bladder** and **urethra.**
    A. **Functions of the kidneys**
       1. **Production of urine**
       2. **Endocrine hormone synthesis**
          a. **Renin**, which participates in regulation of blood pressure
          b. **Erythropoietin**, which promotes erythrocyte production
          c. **Vitamin D**, which is involved in the mineralization of bone
             • Conversion of inactive 25-(OH) provitamin D to active 1,25-$(OH)_2$ vitamin D (**calcitriol**) in kidneys is **stimulated by parathyroid hormone**, which promotes synthesis of 1-α-hydroxylase in the proximal tubules.
       3. **Removal of metabolic waste products** (e.g., urea, NH_3, and creatinine)
       4. **Maintenance of volume and composition** (e.g., pH, electrolytes) **of blood and tissue fluid**

B. Uriniferous tubule: continuous tubular structure with regional specializations that constitutes the **functional unit** of the kidney

- Each uriniferous tubule consists of a nephron and the collecting tubules into which it drains.

1. **Nephron** includes a renal corpuscle, proximal convoluted tubule (PCT), loop of Henle, and distal convoluted tubule (DCT).

2. **Collecting tubules** extend from arched collecting tubules to the papillary duct.

Nephron components: renal (Malpighian) corpuscle → proximal convoluted tubule (PCT) → loop of Henle → distal convoluted tubule (DCT).

II. **Gross Anatomy of the Kidney** (Figure 15-1)

- The kidney is a bean-shaped organ that contains mostly parenchyma (little stroma) and is covered by a **fibrous capsule.**

A. Renal hilus: indentation on medial border of the kidney where the capsule is discontinuous

- Is site where blood vessels, nerves, and the ureter enter and leave
- Expands interiorly to form the **renal sinus**

B. Renal pelvis: expanded **upper end of ureter** located within the renal sinus

1. **Major calyces:** intercommunicating branches of the renal pelvis

2. **Minor calyces:** subdivisions of the major calyces

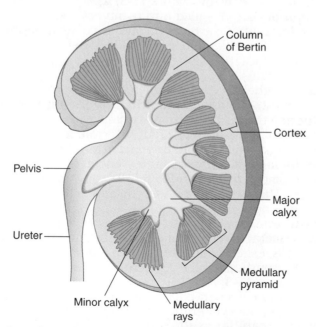

Figure 15-1 General organization of the kidney illustrating relation of ureter, pelvis, and calyces. Renal corpuscles, where filtrate is produced, are located in the outer cortical layer. Tubules in medullary rays carry the filtrate from the cortex into the medullary pyramids, which exit into minor calyces.

Renal corpuscles are located in the cortex. Tubules are located primarily in the medulla, which receives only 10% of the blood delivered to the kidneys.

C. **Renal cortex:** dark, highly vascular surface layer that contains **renal corpuscles** and has a granular appearance
D. **Renal medulla:** lighter interior layer that contains mostly **tubules,** giving it a striate appearance
   1. **Renal (medullary) pyramid:** pyramidal-shaped division of the medulla bordered by **renal columns of Bertin,** which are extensions of cortical tissue into the medulla
      • Each kidney has 10–18 renal pyramids.
      • Tips of two or three pyramids extend into a minor calyx as a **renal papilla.**
   2. **Medullary rays:** radial extensions of medullary tissue into the cortex
E. **Renal lobe:** a renal pyramid and its overlying cortex
F. **Renal lobule:** a central medullary ray and the surrounding nephrons that drain into it
   • Boundaries of lobules are imaginary lines located midway between adjacent medullary rays. Interlobular arteries and veins aid in defining boundaries of renal lobule.

III. **Uriniferous Tubules and Urine Production**
   • General structure of the uriniferous tubule and characteristics of the **simple epithelium** lining the wall are illustrated in Figure 15-2.
A. **Renal (Malpighian) corpuscle**

Juxtamedullary nephrons: long loop of Henle; renal corpuscle near medulla/cortex boundary; major role in establishing interstitial osmotic gradient.

   • Filtration of blood occurs in the renal corpuscle, which consists of a tuft of capillaries, the **glomerulus,** surrounded by **Bowman's capsule** (Figure 15-3, *A*).
   • Nephrons are classified into two types depending on the location of the renal corpuscle: **cortical nephrons** (≈85% of total) and **juxtamedullary nephrons** (≈15% of total).
   1. **Glomerulus**
      a. Endothelial cells of glomerular capillaries have **large fenestrae** but **lack the thin diaphragms** that typically span the openings in fenestrated capillaries.
      b. Blood flows from **afferent arteriole** through glomerular capillary network to **efferent arteriole.**

Cortical nephrons: relatively short loop of Henle; renal corpuscle in outer cortex; 85% of total nephrons.

      c. **Mesangial cells,** similar to pericytes, are located around glomerular capillaries.
         • These cells are phagocytic and help support capillary loops.
   2. **Bowman's capsule**
      a. **Visceral layer** is formed of highly modified epithelial cells, called **podocytes,** which are primarily responsible for synthesis of the glomerular basement membrane (Figure 15-3, *B*).
         (1) **Pedicels:** secondary (foot) processes extending from podocyte primary processes; **surround glomerular capillaries** and interdigitate with each other
         (2) **Filtration slits:** elongated spaces between adjacent pedicels; covered by a diaphragm (**slit membrane**)

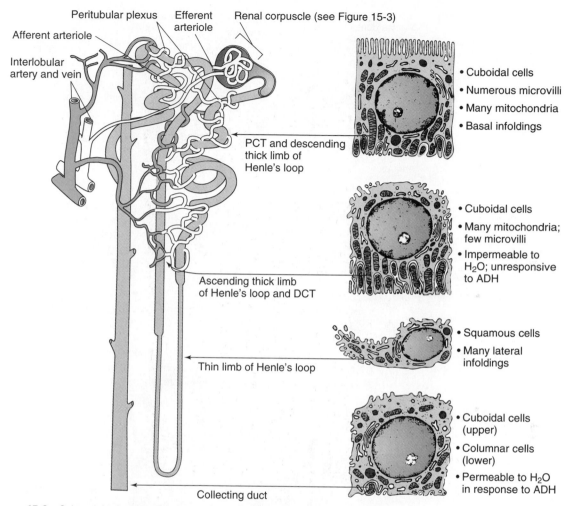

Figure 15-2 Schematic depiction of the uriniferous tubule and associated blood vessels. Microscopic appearance of the epithelial cells at various points reveals their characteristic ultrastructure. The long thin limb of Henle's loop in juxtamedullary nephrons is surrounded by small vessels (vasa recta), which are not shown.

(3) **Fused basal lamina of glomerular endothelium and podocytes:** the only continuous structure separating podocytes and endothelial cells

b. **Bowman's (urinary) space** is the narrow cavity between the visceral and parietal layers into which the glomerular filtrate drains.

•   This space is continuous with the proximal convoluted tubule at the **urinary pole.**

c. **Parietal layer** composed of simple squamous epithelium forms the outer wall of Bowman's capsule.

3. **Formation of glomerular filtrate**

•   Selective movement of substances from glomerular capillaries into Bowman's space forms the **glomerular filtrate.**

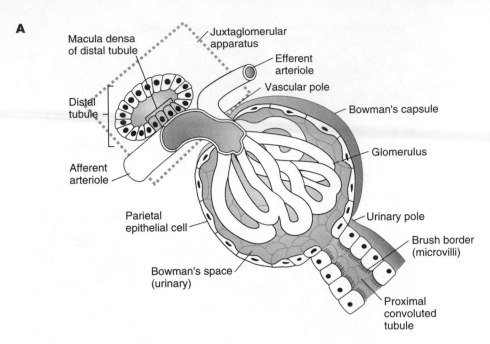

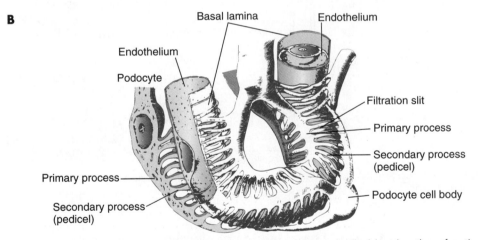

Figure 15-3 Renal (Malpighian) corpuscle. **A,** Schematic longitudinal hemisection of entire corpuscle illustrating its main structural features. Near the vascular pole, the distal convoluted tubule abuts the afferent arteriole in the juxtaglomerular apparatus. **B,** Three-dimensional reconstruction of the interface between the glomerular endothelium and podocytes in visceral layer of Bowman's capsule. This interface constitutes the urinary membrane (renal filtration barrier).

a. Components of renal filtration barrier (urinary membrane)

(1) Fenestrated endothelium

(2) Fused basal laminae of endothelial cells and podocytes

(3) Slit membrane

   b. Selectivity of renal filtration barrier
      (1) Water, ions, and most molecules with an MW <60–
         70 kDa pass into Bowman's space.
      (2) Molecules with an MW >60–70 kDa (e.g., albumin)
         are excluded and remain in the capillaries.
      (3) Molecules carrying a large negative charge (e.g.,
         albumin) also are excluded by **negatively charged
         heparan sulfate** in fused basal lamina.
   c. Factors promoting movement of fluid from glomerular
      capillaries into Bowman's space
      (1) Total cross-sectional area of efferent arteriole is less
         than that of afferent arteriole, leading to increased
         hydrostatic pressure in glomerulus.
      (2) Total hydrostatic pressure in capillary network is
         higher than that in Bowman's space.
   4. Rate of filtrate and urine production per day
      a. About **1700 liters of whole blood** pass through the
         kidneys per day.
      b. About **170 liters of glomerular filtrate** are formed daily.
      c. About **1.5 liters of urine** are produced daily from the fil-
         trate as it moves from Bowman's space through the re-
         mainder of the uriniferous tubules.
      • During production of urine, water and solutes move in
         and out of the tubules by diffusion or active transport.
         (1) **Reabsorption:** material in tubules (tubular fluid) →
            tissue fluid (interstitium) → blood in surrounding
            capillaries
         (2) **Secretion:** material in blood in capillaries → tissue
            fluid → lumen of tubules
B. Proximal convoluted tubule (PCT): ≈14 mm long
   • Distal portion, which is straight, also is called the **thick
      descending limb of Henle's loop.**
   1. Wall is composed of large **cuboidal epithelial cells** marked
      by the following structures (see Figure 15-2):
      a. Abundant **microvilli** (brush border), which contain **car-
         bonic anhydrase,** on apical surface facing the lumen
      b. Apical tubular invaginations (**canaculi**), **vesicles,** and
         granules, which function in transport of macromolecules
         into the cytoplasm
      c. Extensive **infoldings of basal plasmalemma,** which in-
         crease its surface area
      d. Numerous **mitochondria,** which are compartmentalized
         in basal portion of cells by basal infoldings and provide
         energy for active transport of Na^+ ions and other solutes
   2. Filtrate remains **isotonic** as it passes through the PCT and
      thick descending limb of Henle's loop, but is reduced to
      about one fourth of its initial volume.
      a. About two thirds of the water, Na^+, and Cl^- in the glo-
         merular filtrate is reabsorbed in the PCT (Figure 15-4).
      b. All of the glucose and amino acids in the filtrate nor-
         mally is reabsorbed with the aid of carrier proteins in the
         plasma membrane of tubular cells.

Filtrate remains iso-
tonic in proximal
convoluted tubule,
where much of
the H_2O, Na^+, K^+,
and Cl^- and all of
the glucose and
amino acids are
reabsorbed.

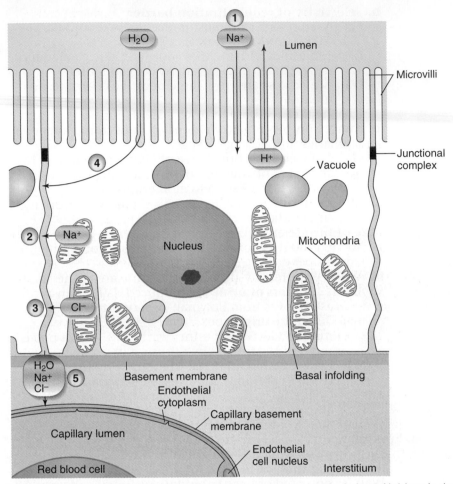

Figure 15-4 Reabsorption of salt and water in proximal convoluted tubule. *1,* Na$^+$ ions in the filtrate cross the apical surface of tubular cells in exchange for H$^+$ ions. *2,* Na$^+$/K$^+$ pumps in lateral membrane actively transport intracellular Na$^+$ ions into the spaces between adjacent tubule cells basal to junctional complexes; Cl$^-$ ions passively follow *(3).* Water reabsorption *(4)* is a consequence of osmotic draw caused by the active transport of Na$^+$ into the pericellular spaces. *5,* Water, salt, and other solutes that pass into the interstitium readily enter capillaries of the peritubular plexus, thus returning reabsorbed materials to the blood.

Filtrate becomes hypertonic in thin descending limb of Henle's loop.

    c. Larger metabolites (e.g., proteins, polysaccharides) in the filtrate are endocytosed at apical surface of tubular cells and released into the interstitium by exocytosis at basal surface.

C. Thin segment of Henle's loop: ≈2–10 mm in length

- Lengthy **thin segments in juxtamedullary nephrons** descend deeply into the medulla and are **critical in establishing a gradient of increasing tonicity** from the outer to inner medulla.

    1. Wall is composed of **squamous epithelial cells** (see Figure 15-2).

      a. **Many lateral interdigitations** between adjacent cells provide slits for passage of small molecules (especially H_2O) by diffusion.

      b. Apical surface possesses sparse microvilli.

    2. Filtrate becomes **hypertonic** as it passes through the thin **descending** limb of Henle's loop due to passive movement of H_2O into the interstitium.

D. **Thick ascending segment of Henle's loop:** ≈9 mm in length

    1. Wall is composed of **cuboidal epithelial cells** similar to those of the proximal convoluted tubule but with **few microvilli** (see Figure 15-2).

    2. Filtrate becomes **hypotonic** as it passes through the thick segment of Henle's loop.

      a. Cl^- is actively transported from lumen to interstitium and Na^+ and K^+ follow passively.

      b. Because the thick segment is **impermeable to H_2O**, reabsorption of Na^+, K^+, and Cl^- decreases the tonicity of the filtrate and increases the tonicity of the interstitium.

      c. Increased interstitial tonicity drives diffusion of H_2O out of the thin segment of Henle's loop.

E. **Distal convoluted tubule (DCT):** ≈5 mm in length

    1. Wall (simple cuboidal epithelium) is histologically similar to that of thick ascending segment of Henle's loop and also is **impermeable to H_2O.**

    2. Filtrate becomes increasingly **hypotonic** as it passes through the DCT.

      a. Na^+, Cl^-, Ca^{2+}, and PO_4^{3-} are **reabsorbed** from the DCT lumen.

      b. K^+, H^+, and NH_3 are **secreted** into the DCT lumen.

F. **Collecting tubules and ducts**

    1. **Arched collecting tubule:** short segment, lined by simple **cuboidal epithelium**, connecting distal convoluted tubule of a nephron and the collecting tubule into which it drains

    2. **Collecting duct:** straight tubule formed by convergence of arched tubules from multiple nephrons

      a. **Upper (cortical) portion** has **cuboidal epithelium** and lies within a medullary ray.

      b. **Lower (medullary) portion** has **columnar epithelium** and lies within a medullary pyramid.

    3. **Papillary ducts of Bellini:** large collecting tubules, with simple **columnar epithelium**, formed by convergence of smaller tubules within a pyramid.

      • Perforate surface of renal papilla at **area cribrosa**, emptying urine into a minor calyx

G. **Regulation of urine concentration in response to blood osmolarity** (Figure 15-5)

    • **Antidiuretic hormone (ADH)**, released from posterior pituitary gland, **increases the H_2O permeability** of the collecting tubules.

    • Because capillary networks surrounding tubules are freely permeable to H_2O and ions, changes in the tonicity of

ADH controls H_2O permeability of collecting tubules: ↑ blood tonicity causes ↑ ADH secretion, which leads to ↑ H_2O reabsorption, resulting in ↓ blood tonicity.

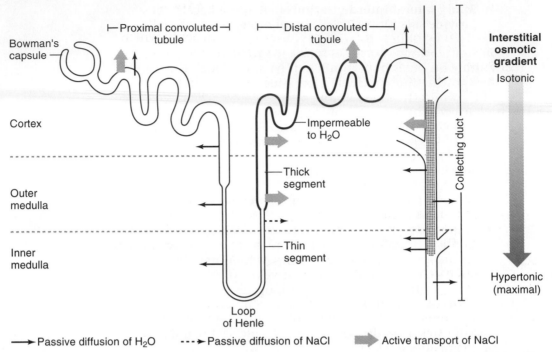

Figure 15-5 Overview of water and NaCl fluxes along uriniferous tubules. These fluxes largely determine the urine concentration. The interstitial osmotic gradient is established by differential permeability to H_2O and NaCl in the thin segment of Henle's loop and high permeability to urea in distal portion of collecting duct. The filtrate becomes hypotonic in the distal convoluted tubule due to active transport of NaCl out of the lumen and its impermeability to water. Antidiuretic hormone (ADH) controls the permeability of collecting tubules for H_2O (stippled area). In the presence of ADH, H_2O is drawn osmotically from fluid in the collecting tubules as it passes through the increasingly hypertonic medullary interstitium, thereby concentrating the urine.

tubular fluid leads to corresponding changes in blood tonicity.

1. **Increased tonicity of blood (hypertonic)** → increased ADH release → increased H_2O reabsorption from kidney tubules
   - Result: **more concentrated (hypertonic) urine** and decrease in tonicity of blood
2. **Decreased tonicity of blood (hypotonic)** → decreased ADH release → decreased H_2O reabsorption from kidney tubules
   - Result: **less concentrated (hypotonic) urine** and increase in tonicity of blood

H. **Diseases affecting kidney function**
   1. **Diabetes insipidus (DI): polyuria** leading to **dehydration** and **polydipsia**
      - **Decreased release of ADH (central** DI) or **decreased responsiveness** of renal tubules to ADH (**nephrogenic** DI) reduces water reabsorption by collecting tubules, resulting in large volume of dilute (low tonicity) urine.
   2. **Glomerulonephritis:** inflammation of the glomeruli, impairing their ability to filter plasma
      - Symptoms include **proteinuria, hematuria,** decreased urine production (**oliguria**), and **periorbital edema.**

Diabetes insipidus: decreased ADH release or decreased responsiveness of tubules to ADH; polyuria, dehydration, and polydipsia.

- Acute form may occur secondary to **group A strep-tococcal infection** (e.g., tonsillitis).
3. **Polycystic kidney disease:** an **inherited disorder** in which cystic dilation of the tubules develops throughout both kidneys.
    - Clinical manifestations include **hematuria, hypertension, bilaterally enlarged kidneys,** and pain in the lower back over the kidney area.
4. **Nephrotic syndrome:** any condition marked by massive **proteinuria** (>3.5 g in 24 hours), hypoalbuminemia, pitting edema, and hyperlipidemia resulting from damage to glomeruli
    - This condition occurs in several diseases including **minimal change disease** (lipoid nephrosis), a common childhood disorder in which the **negative charge on the urinary membrane is lost.**
5. **Alport's syndrome:** see Chapter 5, Section V

IV. **Juxtaglomerular Apparatus** (see Figure 15-3, *A*)
   - This structure, located near the vascular pole of the renal corpuscle, functions in **regulation of blood pressure.**
   A. Components of the juxtaglomerular apparatus
      1. **Macula densa:** specialized epithelial cells of the distal convoluted tubule where it contacts the afferent arteriole
      2. **Juxtaglomerular cells:** myoepithelial cells derived from smooth muscle in tunica media of afferent arteriole
   B. **Renin-angiotensin-aldosterone system** (Figure 15-6)
      1. **Renin,** an enzyme secreted by juxtaglomerular cells in response to a decrease in blood pressure, **converts angiotensinogen to angiotensin I** in the circulation.
      2. **ACE (angiotensin-converting enzyme),** located in endothelial cells of pulmonary capillaries, **hydrolyzes angiotensin I to angiotensin II.**
      3. **Angiotensin II** increases blood pressure directly by stimulating **vasoconstriction** and indirectly by stimulating **aldosterone secretion.**
         - In the kidneys, **aldosterone promotes Na^+ reabsorption,** increasing blood tonicity.

ACE inhibitors, which prevent formation of angiotensin II, reduce vasoconstriction and aldosterone secretion, thereby lowering blood pressure.

V. **Blood Supply of the Kidney**
   A. Arterial division
      - **Renal artery** → **interlobar arteries** (between pyramids) → **arcuate arteries** (between cortex and medulla) → **interlobular arteries** (between two medullary rays) → **afferent arterioles** → **glomerular capillaries** → **efferent arterioles** (see Figure 15-2)
   B. **Secondary capillary networks**
      1. **Peritubular plexuses,** which arise from efferent arterioles of cortical nephrons, **supply the cortical parenchyma** and then drain into interlobular veins.
      2. **Vasa recta,** which arise from efferent arterioles of juxtamedullary nephrons, **are important in reabsorption.**

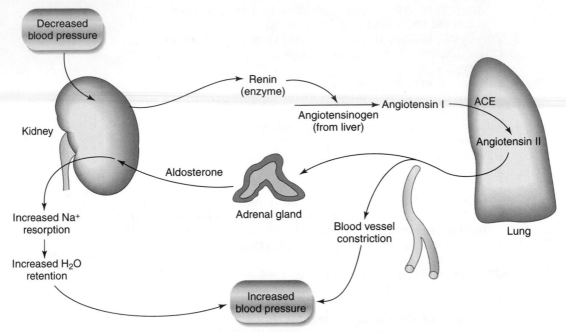

Figure 15-6 Renin-angiotensin-aldosterone system for regulating blood pressure. Secretion of the enzyme renin from the juxtaglomerular apparatus in response to a drop in renal blood flow leads to formation of angiotensin II in the lung. Angiotensin II is a vasoconstrictor and also promotes the synthesis and release of aldosterone, which increases Na$^+$ and H$_2$O reabsorption in the kidney. The angiotensin-converting enzyme *(ACE)*, which cleaves angiotensin I to angiotensin II, is found primarily in the lungs.

- **Arteriolae rectae** (descend into the medulla) → capillary network surrounding Henle's loop → **venulae rectae** (ascend toward arcuate veins at corticomedullary boundary)

C. Venous division
- **Stellate veins** (in outer cortex) → **interlobular veins** (midway between two medullary rays) → **arcuate veins** (between cortex and medulla) → **interlobar veins** (between pyramids) → **renal vein**

VI. Excretory Passages
- Distal to the renal papilla, a closed system of spaces and ducts collects, stores, and conveys urine to the body surface.
  A. Components
  1. **Inside kidneys:** minor calyx → major calyx → renal pelvis
  2. **Outside kidneys:** ureter → bladder → urethra
  B. Histology of urine-conducting system
  - With a few exceptions, the wall of the excretory passages is composed of the following layers:
  1. **Transitional epithelium** underlain by a **lamina propria**
     - From upper to lower portions of the urethra, epithelium changes from transitional to stratified squamous.

2. **Tunica muscularis** containing two or three smooth muscle layers
   - External sphincter of urethra is composed of striated muscle.
3. **Tunica adventitia** of fibroelastic tissue
   - This layer is absent in renal calyces and pelvis.

C. Bladder cancer
   - The most common cancer of the urinary tract, bladder cancer is a **transitional cell carcinoma** marked by **hematuria** and **multiple, recurring tumors.**
   - Risk factors include **cigarette smoking**, aniline dyes, cyclophosphamide, and infection with *Schistosoma haematobium,* which causes squamous cell carcinoma.

Bladder cancer: transitional cell carcinoma (most common urinary tract cancer); hematuria, multiple tumors that tend to recur.

16

Male Reproductive System

Target Topics

▷ Blood–testis barrier
▷ Stages in spermatogenesis
▷ Major changes during maturation of early spermatids into mature spermatozoa
▷ Sperm morphology
▷ Transport of sperm and formation of semen
▷ Effects of testosterone and other hormones on male reproductive system
▷ Cryptorchidism, testicular neoplasms, varicocele, hydrocele, benign prostatic hyperplasia, prostatic adenocarcinoma

I. **Introduction**
   A. **Testes** (paired gonads) elaborate male gametes (**spermatozoa**).
      1. **Tunica albuginea:** connective tissue capsule surrounding each testis
         • **Mediastinum testis** (thickened posterior region of the capsule) extends incomplete connective tissue septa that divide testis into numerous **lobules**, each containing two to four seminiferous tubules.
      2. **Seminiferous (germinal) tubules:** highly convoluted tubules (30–70 cm long)
         • **Seminiferous epithelium** lining the tubules is a specialized **glandlike** epithelium where **spermatogenesis** (formation of spermatozoa from spermatogonia) occurs.

    3. Intratesticular ducts that convey spermatozoa to surface of testis

      a. Tubuli recti: straight terminal portions of the seminiferous tubules lined by **simple columnar epithelium**

      b. Rete testis: anastomosing network of channels lined by **simple cuboidal epithelium** and located at the mediastinum

        • Tubuli recti drain into the rete testis.

B. Extratesticular ducts conduct spermatozoa outside the body.

C. Specialized glands release secretions that provide nutritive and lubricative elements to semen.

    1. Seminal vesicles

    2. Prostate gland

    3. Bulbourethral (Cowper's) glands

D. Glandular functions of the testes

    1. Exocrine function: production of holocrine cytogenic secretion containing spermatozoa occurs within the seminiferous epithelium.

    2. Endocrine function: synthesis and secretion of hormones is carried out by **Leydig cells** within the interstitium and by **Sertoli cells** within the seminiferous epithelium.

II. Spermatogenesis

A. Composition of the seminiferous epithelium (Figure 16-1)

    1. Spermatogenic cells

      a. Prior to puberty, the only spermatogenic cells present are undifferentiated, basally located **spermatogonia** that are **mitotically inactive.**

      b. Following puberty, when spermatogenesis begins, spermatogenic cells are present in a gradient from basal undifferentiated cells to differentiated spermatids ready for release as mature spermatozoa into the lumen.

    2. Sertoli cells are tall, columnar cells that extend from the basement membrane to the lumen.

      • **Support, protect, and nurture the germ cells** within the seminiferous epithelium; also **secrete inhibin** and **androgen-binding protein.**

      • Are **nondividing** cells that remain after degeneration of germ cells in senescent gonad

      a. Tight junctions (zonulae occludens) between adjacent Sertoli cells divide epithelium into a **basal compartment** containing spermatogonia and an **adluminal compartment** containing cells in later stages of spermatogenesis.

      b. Blood–testis barrier results from tight junctions between Sertoli cells.

        (1) Tissue fluid must pass through Sertoli cells to reach developing sperm in the adluminal compartment.

        (2) Proteins from developing sperm in adluminal compartment cannot reach bloodstream, thereby preventing possible immune response.

> Spermatogenesis = spermatocytogenesis + meiosis + spermiogenesis.

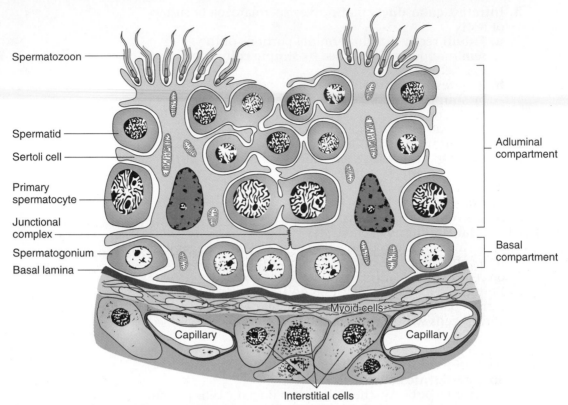

Spermatozoon

Spermatid

Sertoli cell

Primary
spermatocyte

Junctional
complex

Spermatogonium

Basal lamina

Adluminal
compartment

Basal
compartment

Myoid cells

Capillary

Capillary

Interstitial cells

Figure 16-1 Seminiferous epithelium and surrounding interstitial tissue. The spermatogenic cells are arranged in a basal → lumen gradient from the least differentiated (spermatogonia) to the most differentiated (spermatids). The epithelium is divided into two compartments by tight junctions between adjacent Sertoli cells, forming the blood–testis barrier. The basal compartment is occupied by spermatogonia and the adluminal compartment by developing spermatocytes, which are enveloped by Sertoli cells.

Before entering into cell division (mitosis or meiosis), spermatogonia or primary spermatocytes must replicate their DNA (S phase).

B. Stages in spermatogenesis (Figure 16-2)
- Formation of spermatozoa does **not** occur in synchrony in all tubules, but rather in wavelike **cycles of the seminiferous epithelium** involving the following stages:
  1. **Spermatocytogenesis:** spermatogonia → primary spermatocytes (mitotic divisions)
  2. **Meiosis:** primary spermatocytes → spermatids (meiotic divisions)
  3. **Spermiogenesis:** spermatids → mature spermatozoa (series of morphologic and physiologic changes)

C. Mitotic division of spermatogonia
  1. **Type A spermatogonia** (stem cells) occur in two forms.
     a. **Dark (Ad) cells** divide to replenish themselves or differentiate to form pale cells.
     b. **Pale (Ap) cells** undergo multiple mitotic divisions with **incomplete cytokinesis** and mature into type B spermatogonia (see Figure 16-2, *top*).

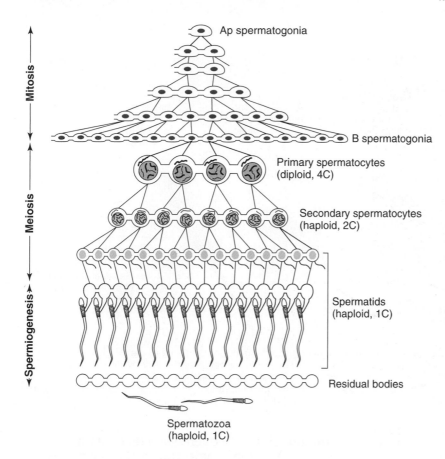

Ap spermatogonia

B spermatogonia

Primary spermatocytes
(diploid, 4C)

Secondary spermatocytes
(haploid, 2C)

Spermatids
(haploid, 1C)

Residual bodies

Spermatozoa
(haploid, 1C)

Mitosis

Meiosis

Spermiogenesis

Figure 16-2 Spermatogenesis. Mitotic division of the earliest spermatogonia committed to differentiation (Ap cells) yields daughter cells that are connected by intercellular bridges. These bridges, which persist through subsequent mitotic and meiotic divisions, are shed as part of residual bodies during the final phase of spermatid maturation to yield separate spermatozoa. Meiotic division of each primary spermatocyte, a diploid cell with 4C DNA, produces four haploid spermatids, each with 1C DNA.

   2. **Type B spermatogonia** undergo further mitotic divisions and then a cluster of linked cells, having replicated their DNA in the S phase, enter meiosis as primary spermatocytes.

D. Meiotic division of spermatocytes (see Figure 3-6, *B*)

- Each primary spermatocyte gives rise to four spermatids. **A group of primary spermatocytes** derived from a single type A spermatogonium and **linked by intercellular bridges undergo meiosis in synchrony** (see Figure 16-2, *middle*).

   1. **Primary spermatocytes:** these **diploid** cells with **4C DNA** content undergo **reductional division** to form secondary spermatocytes.
  - Crossing over and recombination of maternal and paternal chromatids can occur, producing new genetic combinations.

   2. **Secondary spermatocytes:** these **haploid** cells with **2C DNA** rapidly undergo **equational division** (without any intervening DNA synthesis) to form haploid **spermatids** with **1C DNA.**
  - Fusion of sperm and egg during fertilization restores the diploid chromosome number and 2C DNA in zygote.

B spermatogonia → spermatozoa takes about 64 days. Of total duration, about one fourth (16 days) is spent in spermiogenesis.

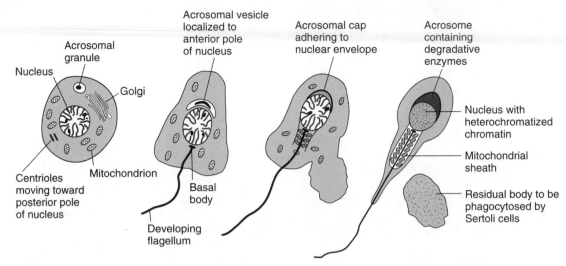

Figure 16-3 Principal changes that occur in a spermatid during spermiogenesis. Elements of the Golgi are incorporated into the acrosomal granule and the Golgi disappears. The centrioles initiate formation of the basal body and flagellum. The mitochondria gather as a sheath around upper portion of the flagellum. In the final stage, excess cytoplasm and intercellular bridges connecting spermatids are discarded, forming residual bodies that are phagocytosed. Finally, the morphologically mature but nonmotile spermatozoa are released tail first into lumen of the seminiferous tubule.

> - Each spermatid (and subsequent gamete) contains either an X or a Y chromosome; thus male gamete determines sex of zygote (see Figure 3-7).

E. Transformation of spermatids into mature spermatozoa
   - A group of spermatids linked by intercellular bridges and nestled within the apical cytoplasm of Sertoli cells undergo spermiogenesis in synchrony as depicted in Figure 16-3.

F. Characteristics of spermatozoa (Figure 16-4)
   1. Morphologically mature spermatozoa released into tubular lumen at the end of spermiogenesis are **immotile** and **incapable of fertilization**.
   2. Sperm motility is activated in the **epididymis**.
      - Males with **immotile cilia syndrome** or **Kartagener's syndrome** are infertile because their sperm are incapable of motility.
   3. Fertilization capability is acquired during **capacitation** of sperm within the uterine tube of the female.
   4. Enzymes within the acrosome that are released during fertilization facilitate entry of the sperm nucleus into the oocyte.

G. Temperature requirement for sperm production
   1. Temperature of 35° C, slightly below core body temperature, is necessary for spermatogenesis to occur. This is achieved by housing the testes within the scrotal chamber.

Before it is capable of fertilization, a spermatozoon must undergo capacitation and the acrosome reaction, which releases enzymes that assist entry into oocyte.

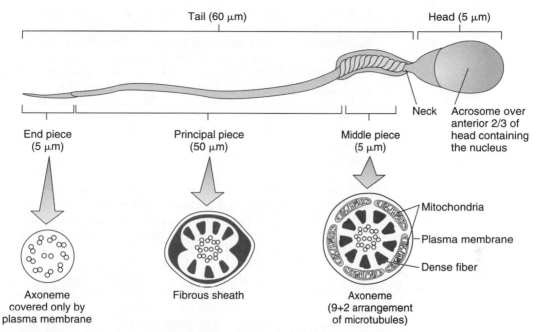

Figure 16-4 Morphology of a mammalian spermatozoon depicting features visible by light microscopy *(top)* and ultrastructure of the tail regions *(bottom)*. Note that the various regions are not to scale; the principal piece is much longer than other regions.

2. **Cryptorchidism**, failure of one or both the testes to descend, results in impaired spermatogenesis if the testis is not surgically moved into the scrotal sac before 2 years of age.

III. **Transport of Spermatozoa and Production of Semen**
   A. **Ducts through which sperm move from rete testis**
   • Ductuli efferentes → duct of epididymis → ductus (vas) deferens → ampulla of ductus deferens → ejaculatory duct → urethra
   B. **Mechanism of sperm movement**
   1. **Current** created by secretion of fluid by Sertoli cells into lumen of the seminiferous tubule and its reabsorption in ductuli efferentes **moves sperm** from rete testis **to ductus epididymis.**
   2. Ductus epididymis and ductus deferens are storage regions. Weak **peristaltic movements** in these ducts **move spermatozoa distally.**
   3. **Muscular contractions** of the ductus epididymis, ductus deferens, and urethra **force release of spermatozoa** during ejaculation.
   C. **Composition of semen**
   • **Semen = sperm + secretions** from the testis, ductal system, and accessory glands.

- Erotic stimulation promotes release of secretions from accessory glands.
1. **Seminal vesicles** secrete a viscous fluid rich in **fructose**, which provides energy for movement of sperm flagella.
   - Seminal fluid also contains factors that promote coagulation of semen and prevent agglutination of spermatozoa.
2. **Prostate gland** secretes a thin fluid rich in **acid phosphatase** and containing **prostaglandins**.
3. **Bulbourethral (Cowper's) glands** secrete a **mucuslike material** that lubricates the urethra, augmenting the mucous secretions of the **glands of Littre** within the penis.

D. **Penis**
- The male copulatory organ contains **three masses of erectile tissue** surrounded by **tunica albuginea**, a thick connective tissue sheath containing collagen and elastic fibers.
1. **Corpora cavernosae: paired dorsal** bodies containing **irregular vascular spaces**
   - Cavernous spaces are lined by **continuous endothelium** and separated by strands of **smooth muscle**.
   - **Engorgement** of spaces with blood during erection is under **parasympathetic control**.
2. **Corpus cavernosum urethrae (corpus spongiosum): single ventral** body surrounding the urethra and containing **regular vascular spaces**
   - Vascular spaces are lined by continuous endothelium and separated by septa that contain more elastic fibers and less smooth muscle than in corpora cavernosae
3. **Glans penis:** dilated distal end of corpus spongiosum lined by **stratified squamous epithelium**
   - Contains smooth muscle, sebaceous glands, and numerous sensory receptors

E. **Sequence of events at ejaculation**
- Secretion from Cowper's and Littre's glands → prostate secretion → release of spermatozoa from epididymis and vas deferens → secretion of seminal vesicles → release of semen.

IV. **Hormonal Control of Male Reproductive System** (Figure 16-5)
A. **Pituitary hormones** that promote testicular hormone production
- Release of these hormones is stimulated by **gonadotropin-releasing hormone (GnRH)** from the hypothalamus.
1. **Luteinizing hormone (LH)** stimulates **Leydig cells** to secrete **testosterone**.
   - Also known as **interstitial cell–stimulating hormone (ICSH)** in males.
2. **Follicle-stimulating hormone (FSH)** stimulates **Sertoli cells** to secrete **inhibin** and **androgen-binding protein**.

B. **Effects of testicular hormones**
1. **Testosterone**
   a. Promotes development of **secondary sex characteristics**
   b. Stimulates **spermatogenesis**
   c. Maintains **function** of **ducts** and **accessory glands**

Leydig cells in testicular interstitium secrete testosterone in response to stimulation by LH from the pituitary gland.

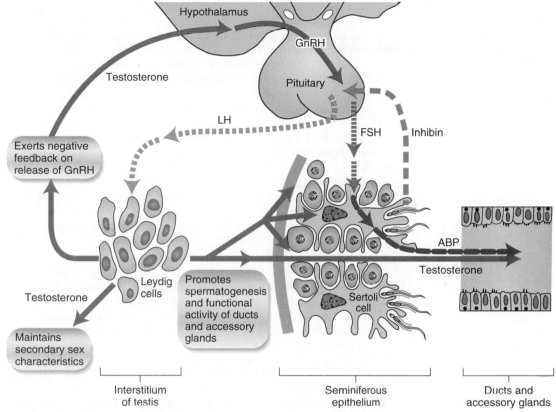

Figure 16-5 Regulation of testicular hormonal function. Gonadotropin-releasing hormone *(GnRH)* from the hypothalamus stimulates secretion of follicle-stimulating hormone *(FSH)* and luteinizing hormone *(LH)* from the anterior pituitary. FSH promotes secretion of androgen-binding protein *(ABP)* and inhibin by Sertoli cells. LH stimulates Leydig cells to secrete testosterone, which has several effects critical to male reproductive function and acts on the hypothalamus to inhibit GnRH secretion.

   d. Acts on hypothalamus to reduce release of GnRH, thereby exerting **negative feedback on LH and FSH secretion**
   2. Androgen-binding protein
      a. Binds testosterone and helps transport it across seminiferous epithelium to tubular lumen
      b. Helps maintain high local concentration of testosterone, which promotes spermatogenesis
   3. Inhibin
      • Acts on anterior pituitary to **decrease FSH secretion**

V. **Disorders of the Male Reproductive System**
    A. Testicular cancers
       1. Seminoma is one of several germ cell neoplasms, all of which are **malignant.**
          a. This neoplasm usually presents as **painless testicular enlargement;** may metastasize before original tumor can be felt.

Sertoli cells secrete androgen-binding protein and inhibin in response to FSH from the pituitary gland.

Most testicular cancers are malignant and derived from germ cells. These include seminoma, embryonal carcinoma, choriocarcinoma, yolk sac carcinoma, and teratoma.

Undescended testes (cryptorchidism) is the most common risk factor for a seminoma of the testis.

b. Highest incidence is between 35 and 40 years of age and in men with undescended (cryptorchid) testes.

c. Seminomas are **less aggressive** and **more sensitive to radiation** than other types of germ cell neoplasm.

2. **Leydig cell** and **Sertoli cell tumors** generally are **benign** but may cause endocrine abnormalities (e.g., gynecomastia, precocious puberty).

B. **Varicocele:** varicosity of the venous plexus of the spermatic cord (more common in left cord than in right cord)

- Marked by soft, elastic, often **painful swelling in the scrotum**
- Associated with reduced spermatogenesis due to increased temperature

C. **Hydrocele:** accumulation of fluid in scrotum or along spermatic cord

- May be caused by swelling of testis or obstruction in the cord
- Congenital form due to failure of the canal between the trunk cavity and scrotum to close completely before birth

D. **Benign prostatic hyperplasia:** usually hyperplasia of glandular cells and/or smooth muscle cells in **periurethral zone** of the prostrate gland

- Marked by **nocturia, difficulty initiating stream**, and **urinary frequency**
- Is **not** a precancerous disorder

E. **Prostatic adenocarcinoma:** origin usually in the **peripheral zone** of the prostrate; metastasis to bone common

- Marked clinically by an **enlarged, firm, nodular prostate** on digital rectal exam
- Often associated with elevated serum levels of **acid phosphatase** and **prostate-specific antigen (PSA)**

Benign prostatic hyperplasia is the most common cause of urinary tract obstruction in males.

Prostatic adenocarcinoma is the most common malignancy of men, with onset beginning after 50 years of age and reaching peak incidence about age 75 years. PSA (prostate-specific antigen) is a tumor marker.

17

Female Reproductive System

Target Topics

▸ Histology of maturing ovarian follicles
▸ Structure and function of corpus luteum
▸ Cyclical changes in endometrium during menstrual cycle
▸ Hormonal regulation of ovarian and endometrial cycles
▸ Fertilization and implantation of embryo
▸ Structure and function of the placenta
▸ Hormone-induced changes in mammary glands
▸ Ectopic pregnancy, endometriosis, uterine fibroid, endometrial carcinoma, Pap smear, cervical cancer, placental abnormalities, breast cancer

I. Introduction
   A. Organs of the female reproductive system
      1. Ovaries
         a. **Exocrine function:** maturation and release of developing ova
         b. **Endocrine function:** synthesis and secretion of several hormones (e.g., estrogen, progesterone)
      2. **Oviducts**
      3. **Uterus**
      4. **Vagina and external genitalia**
      5. **Breasts**
   B. **Menstrual cycle:** hormone-induced histophysiologic changes in the ovaries and uterus that accompany oocyte maturation
      1. **Menarche:** occurrence of the first menses
      2. **Menopause:** period during which cyclical changes become intermittent and eventually cease

- During postmenopausal period there is a slow, progressive involution of the female reproductive system.
  - **C. Pregnancy-induced changes**
    1. **Cessation of menstrual cycle**
    2. **Formation of the placenta,** a **temporary structure** that secretes hormones needed to maintain pregnancy and permits exchange of materials between maternal and fetal blood supply
    3. **Development of secretory cells in breasts** in preparation for postnatal lactation

II. **Ovaries**
  - **A. General histologic features of the ovary**
    1. **Simple squamous to cuboidal epithelium** (a continuation of the peritoneum) covers external surface.
       - **a.** This is sometimes incorrectly referred to as "germinal epithelium."
       - **b. Surface-derived tumors** of the ovary derive from this epithelium.
    2. **Tunica albuginea** of fibrous connective tissue lies under the surface epithelium.
    3. **Cortex** contains **ovarian follicles** in various stages of maturation.
    4. **Medulla,** a vascular, highly cellular connective tissue, is not well defined.
  - **B. Embryonic formation of primordial follicles**
    1. **Primordial germ cells (oogonia)** migrate from yolk-sac endoderm into the ovaries early in the embryonic period.
    2. **Oogonia** proliferate by mitosis until 20–28 weeks' gestation, resulting in 3 million oogonia per ovary.
       - **a.** After ceasing mitosis, oogonia enter and become arrested in **prophase I of meiosis;** called **primary oocytes,** these arrested cells are **diploid** ($2n$) and have **4C DNA** (46 chromosomes, 92 chromatids).
       - **b. No additional primary oocytes are formed later in life.**
    3. **Primordial follicles** consist of **one primary oocyte** surrounded by a single layer of **squamous epithelial (follicular) cells** and a **basal lamina.**
       - Apoptosis (programmed cell death) of primordial follicles reduces their number to ≈200,000 per ovary at menarche.
  - **C. Maturation of ovarian follicles** (Figure 17-1)
    - At menarche, groups of 10–15 primordial follicles begin to grow at the start of each menstrual cycle, although only **one of each cohort** develops into a mature (graafian) follicle and **ovulates.**
    - Follicle maturation is marked by progressive morphologic changes in the oocyte, surrounding follicular cells, and adjacent stroma.
    1. **Unilaminar primary follicle**
       - **a.** Simple squamous epithelium changes to **single layer of cuboidal follicular cells.**

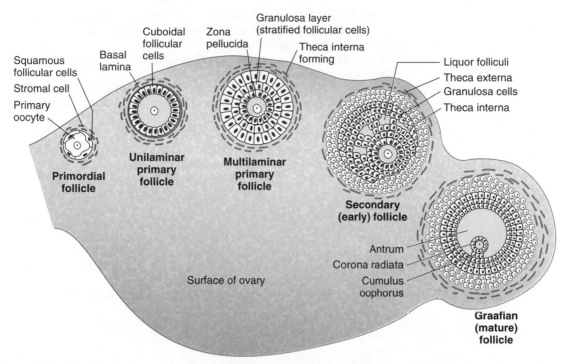

Figure 17-1 Maturation of ovarian follicles. Major features of developing follicle at different stages are depicted diagrammatically. The primary oocyte within a maturing follicle completes meiosis I and is arrested at metaphase II (haploid secondary oocyte) within a graafian follicle shortly before ovulation. Completion of the second meiotic division occurs during fertilization.

    b. Differentiation of primary oocyte begins, marked by increases in size and number of mitochondria, Golgi, rough endoplasmic reticulum (RER), and polysomes, which augment synthetic capacity of the oocyte.

    c. Zona pellucida, synthesized by both the oocyte and follicular cells, begins to form around the oocyte.

       • During fertilization, sperm bind to the zona pellucida.

2. Multilaminar primary follicle

    a. Stratification of cuboidal follicular cells occurs, forming **granulosa layer.**

    b. Stromal cells begin to form **thecal layer** around the follicle.

3. Secondary (antral) follicle

    a. Spaces filled with fluid (**liquor folliculi**) appear between granulosa cells and eventually coalesce into single large space, the **antrum.**

    b. Cumulus oophorus, a mound of granulosa cells extending into the antrum, attaches the oocyte to the follicular wall.

       • Granulosa cells adjacent to zona pellucida constitute the **corona radiata**, which accompanies the oocyte during ovulation.

    c. Theca interna, a secretory stromal layer adjacent to the granulosa cells, secretes **17-ketosteroids** (e.g., androstenedione).

        (1) Androstenedione is enzymatically converted to testosterone.

        (2) Follicle-stimulating hormone (FSH) stimulates enzymatic conversion of these androgens to **estrogen** in granulosa cells.

        (3) Subsequent rise in estrogen level induces expression of **receptors for luteinizing hormone (LH)** by granulosa cells.

    d. Theca externa, a fibrous, vascular stromal layer peripheral to theca interna, has no endocrine function.

4. Graafian follicle

- Mature ovarian follicle, which visibly bulges on ovarian surface, exists for 1–2 days before ovulation.

    a. Primary oocyte completes first meiotic division within mature follicle shortly before ovulation, forming a large secondary oocyte and small **polar body.**

    b. Secondary oocyte, a **haploid** cell (1*n*) with **2C DNA** (23 chromosomes, 46 chromatids), enters second meiotic division but is **arrested in metaphase II** at time of ovulation.

5. Atretic follicles

- Follicles in all stages are continually undergoing **atresia.**
- No scar is evident when atretic process is complete.

D. Ovulation and fate of secondary oocyte

- **Surge of LH,** induced by rising level of estrogen acting on the hypothalamo-hypophyseal system, triggers release of secondary oocyte surrounded by its corona radiata from graafian follicle (Figure 17-2).

1. Ovulated secondary oocyte is briefly contained in peritoneal cavity and normally is caught by **fimbria of oviduct.**

2. In the absence of fertilization, ovulated **oocyte dies** in about 24 hours.

3. During fertilization, the oocyte completes meiosis II.

E. Corpus luteum

- Collapsed remains of ovulated Graafian follicle (corpus hemorrhagicum) are transformed into the corpus luteum, a **temporary endocrine gland** whose cells become luteinized by exposure to **LH.**

1. Luteal cells

- Have abundant **smooth endoplasmic reticulum** and other cytoplasmic structures associated with **steroid secretion.**

    a. Granulosa lutein cells (derived from granulosa cells) produce most of the body's **progesterone.**

    b. Theca lutein cells (derived from theca interna cells) produce **estrogen** and some progesterone.

2. Fate of the corpus luteum in absence of fertilization

    a. Rising progesterone level progressively **inhibits LH production.**

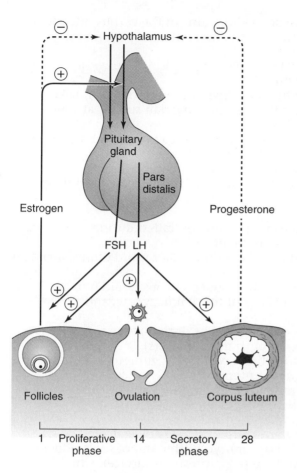

Figure 17-2 Hormonal control of ovarian function. Estrogen produced by developing follicle acts to inhibit follicle-stimulating hormone *(FSH)* and stimulate luteinizing hormone *(LH)* release, leading to surge of LH and proper FSH:LH ratio at mid-cycle that triggers ovulation. Progesterone produced by corpus luteum acts on the hypothalamus to decrease LH release. Scale at bottom refers to days in the menstrual cycle.

    b. Subsequent decrease in LH leads to **atrophy of the corpus luteum.**

    c. Resulting decrease in progesterone and estrogen sets the stage for **menstruation** and onset of another menstrual cycle.

  3. Fate of the corpus luteum in pregnancy

    a. Human chorionic gonadotropin (hCG), produced by syncytiotrophoblast cells of the implanting embryo, **maintains the corpus luteum** and its hormonal synthesis early in pregnancy.

      • Detection of hCG is basis of some pregnancy tests.

    b. Luteal-derived progesterone and estrogen sustain pregnancy for 2–3 months, after which the placenta becomes main source of these hormones.

      • Bilateral oophorectomy (ovariectomy) at this stage will not terminate a pregnancy.

    c. Relaxin, produced by the corpus luteum, relaxes uterine smooth muscle during pregnancy and facilitates parturition.

4. Corpus albicans: scarred remains of the corpus luteum after it degenerates following menstruation or pregnancy.

III. **Oviduct (Fallopian Tube)**
A. **Regions of the oviduct**
1. **Infundibulum:** funnel-shaped free end with fingerlike projections (**fimbria**) that "sweep" ovarian surface at time of ovulation
2. **Ampulla:** dilated region proximal to infundibulum where **fertilization** usually occurs
3. **Isthmus:** nondilated region proximal to ampulla
4. **Pars intramuralis:** part coursing through the uterine wall
B. **Oviduct wall**
1. **Mucosa**
a. **Simple columnar epithelium** (tallest during proliferative phase of menstrual cycle)
(1) **Ciliated cells** beat their cilia toward uterus, assisting in transport of zygote.
(2) **Secretory cells** produce viscous liquid film that supplies nourishment for ovum, zygote, and early embryo.
b. **Lamina propria:** edematous during premenstrual phase
2. **Muscularis** (two smooth muscle layers)
a. Contractions facilitate **contact of gametes** and **movement of zygote** to uterus.
b. **Estrogen stimulates** and **progesterone inhibits** contraction.
3. **Serosa**
C. **Ectopic pregnancy**
• Implantation of early embryo in the wall of the oviduct or other extrauterine site (e.g., intestinal surface), which cannot support fetal development
• Clinically marked by **amenorrhea**, pelvic pain and tenderness, tissue mass (usually in fallopian tube), **elevated hCG**, and hemorrhage into peritoneal cavity, if not surgically treated

IV. **Uterus**
A. **Uterine wall**
1. **Perimetrium:** external uterine covering that is serosa or adventitia depending on peritoneal reflections
2. **Myometrium:** vascularized smooth muscle tunic of uterus
a. **Thickness increases during pregnancy** due to estrogen-stimulated hypertrophy and hyperplasia of smooth muscle cells.
b. **Progesterone** and **relaxin depress** uterine contractions.
c. **Oxytocin** and **prostaglandin ($PGF_{2\alpha}$) stimulate** contractions, especially during parturition.
3. **Endometrium:** mucosal lining of the uterus composed of a **simple columnar epithelium**, highly vascular lamina propria, and **endometrial glands**

Layers of uterine wall:
• Perimetrium: external layer
• Myometrium: smooth muscle layer that thickens during pregnancy
• Endometrium: inner mucosal lining

    a. Functional layer (superficial 80%) undergoes hormone-induced changes during menstrual cycle and is **sloughed during menses.**
      • **Coiled (spiral) arteries** extend into this layer.
    b. Basal layer (deep 20%) is **never sloughed.**
      • Regeneration of functional layer occurs from intact bases of endometrial glands in the basal layer.
  B. Changes in endometrium during menstrual cycle
    (Figure 17-3, *left*)

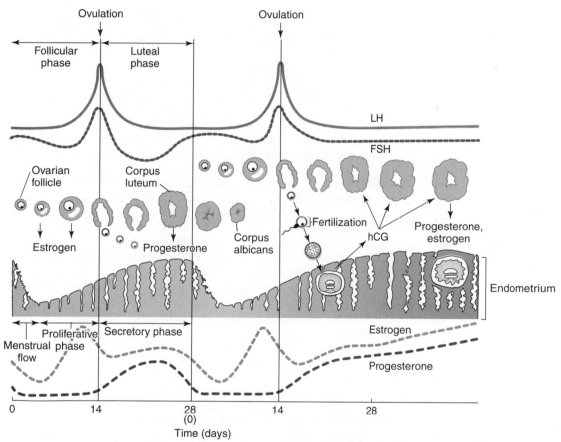

Figure 17-3 Correlation of ovarian and endometrial cycles regulated by changes in hormonal levels. Estrogen *(left)* secreted from developing ovarian follicles promotes rebuilding of functional layer of the endometrium (proliferative phase), which is sloughed during menstrual flow. High estrogen levels cause a surge of luteinizing hormone *(LH)*, triggering ovulation from one follicle. Rising level of progesterone secreted from corpus luteum mediates further changes in the endometrium (secretory phase). In the absence of fertilization and implantation *(left)*, the corpus luteum atrophies due to negative feedback by progesterone on LH release, causing a drop in progesterone and estrogen available to the endometrium. Degeneration of the functional layer occurs rapidly (ischemic phase), followed by menstruation. As progesterone and estrogen levels fall, pituitary secretion of follicle-stimulating hormone *(FSH)* and LH increases and the cycle begins again. If fertilization and implantation occur *(right)*, human chorionic gonadotropin *(hCG)* secreted by the implanted embryo "rescues" the corpus luteum. Continued secretion of progesterone and estrogen by the corpus luteum under stimulation of hCG maintains pregnancy for 2–3 months; placental estrogen and progesterone then take over.

1. **Menses:** days 1–4
   - Functional layer sloughs generating flow of **menstrual blood,** which **does not clot** due to fibrinolytic activity of **plasmin.**
2. **Proliferative phase:** days 5–14
   - This is the most variable phase of the cycle.
   a. **Estrogen** secreted from developing ovarian follicles **stimulates rebuilding of functional layer.**
   b. **Ovulation,** which **signals end** of this phase, is marked by a **rise in body temperature** (progesterone effect) and the presence of subnuclear vacuoles in the glandular cells.
3. **Secretory phase:** days 15–26
   - **Progesterone** secreted from corpus luteum **prepares** estrogen-primed **endometrium for implantation.**
   a. **Endometrial glands** become coiled, **secrete glycoprotein** material into lumen, and **accumulate glycogen** within their cells.
      - As secretory phase progresses, glycogen moves from base to apex of endometrial gland cells.
   b. **Spiral arteries** become more **highly coiled** and **elongate** to almost reach the endometrial surface.
   c. Endometrial **stroma** becomes **highly edematous** in late secretory phase in the absence of fertilization and implantation.
4. **Ischemic (premenstrual) phase:** days 27–28
   - Abrupt drop in estrogen and progesterone following atrophy of corpus luteum leads to progressive degeneration.
   a. Coiled arteries spasmodically contract.
   b. **Ischemia** is followed by necrosis of tissue distal to contracted segment.
   c. Hemorrhage of endometrial arteries marks beginning of menses.

C. **Cessation of menstrual cycle during pregnancy** (Figure 17-3, *right*)
   1. **Following fertilization and implantation** (usually on day 21), hCG maintains the corpus luteum.
      - Continued progesterone and estrogen secretion from the corpus luteum maintains the endometrium, which participates in formation of the placenta.
   2. **Feedback inhibition of FSH and LH release** from pituitary by progesterone and estrogen prevents development of ovarian follicles and ovulation during pregnancy.

D. **Uterine disorders**
   1. **Endometriosis:** ectopic presence of non-neoplastic endometrial tissue in extrauterine sites (commonly the ovaries or oviducts)
      a. Ectopic tissue undergoes hormone-induced changes during menstrual cycle.
      b. **Dysmenorrhea** (pain and excessive bleeding) occurs; **infertility** may result.

Endometrial phases: menses (days 1–4), proliferative (days 5–14), ending with ovulation, secretory (days 15–26), and premenstrual (days 27–28).

2. Uterine fibroid (leiomyoma): benign tumor of smooth muscle cells in uterine wall

   a. This is **most common tumor of women** with peak incidence at 35–45 years of age

   b. Clinical features, which are dependent on size, location, and number (multiple lesions are common), include abnormal uterine **bleeding,** pelvic discomfort, and infertility.

3. Endometrial carcinoma: most common malignancy of female genital tract with peak incidence in postmenopausal women (55–65 years)

   a. Usually causes irregular **vaginal bleeding**

   b. Associated with **hyperestrogenism** (nulliparity, early menarche), obesity, hypertension, and diabetes mellitus

Uterine leiomyoma (fibroid) is the most common benign tumor in women.

V. Uterine Cervix

- Lower cylindrical part of the uterus does **not** undergo extreme cyclical changes characteristic of the endometrium.

A. Endocervix (proximal end)

   1. Simple mucus-secreting columnar epithelium containing branched **cervical (mucous) glands**

   2. Variations in cervical mucus

   a. At mid-cycle, mucus is **watery and copious,** facilitating movement of sperm through the cervical os.

   b. **Postovulation and during pregnancy,** mucus is **viscous and less copious,** inhibiting entrance of sperm and microorganisms.

B. Portio vaginalis (distal end protruding into vagina)

   1. Stratified squamous parakeratinized epithelium contains five histologically distinct cell types.

   - Estrogen stimulates cytodifferentiation: basal cells → parabasal cells → intermediate cells → precornified cells → cornified cells (surface).

   2. Pap smear cytology of exfoliated cells reflects stage of menstrual cycle.

   a. During proliferative phase of cycle, more mature cells (**precornified** and **cornified**) predominate (estrogen effect).

   b. During secretory phase of cycle, **intermediate cells** predominate (progesterone effect).

C. Cervical cancer: invasive squamous cell carcinoma that evolves from **progression of cervical intraepithelial neoplasia** (CIN)

   - Preinvasive CIN changes can be detected on **Pap smear.**

   - **Risk factors** include infection with human papilloma virus (HPV16, HPV18), early age of first coitus, multiple high-risk sex partners, birth control pills, and cigarette smoking.

Pap smear of exfoliated cervical cells, which reflect stage of menstrual cycle, is useful in detecting cervical cancer but not very effective in detecting endometrial carcinoma.

Invasive cervical carcinoma is preceded by neoplastic changes (CIN) that can be detected in Pap smear. Infection with HPV (16, 18) is associated with CIN and invasive carcinoma in most cases.

VI. **Vagina**
   A. **Vaginal wall**
      1. **Mucosa**
         a. **Stratified squamous parakeratinized epithelium**
            (1) **Glycogen** accumulated by superficial cells is deposited in vaginal lumen as cells desquamate.
            (2) Epithelium is thickest during proliferative phase.
         b. **Lamina propria:** rich in elastic fibers; **no glands;** highly vascularized
      2. **Muscularis:** mostly longitudinal smooth muscle with some circular smooth muscle closest to lamina propria
      3. **Adventitia:** rich in elastic fibers
   B. **Vaginal lumen**
      1. **Lactobacilli** in normal bacterial flora **metabolize glycogen** from desquamated cells releasing lactic acid.
         • Resulting **low pH** of vaginal lumen **inhibits growth of pathogenic bacteria.**
      2. **Variations in glycogen content** during menstrual cycle cause changes in luminal pH.
         a. **Highest glycogen at mid-cycle** (lowest luminal pH; least susceptible to infection)
         b. **Lowest glycogen at late secretory phase** (highest luminal pH; most susceptible to infection)

VII. **External Genitalia**
   A. **Clitoris:** two bodies of **erectile tissue,** containing many sensory nerve endings and blood vessels, that terminate in rudimentary **glans clitoris**
      • Developmentally and structurally **homologous to penis**

Clitoromegaly is a sign of excess androgens in a woman.

   B. **Labia minora:** folds of skin with a core of dense irregular connective tissue
   C. **Labia majora:** longitudinal folds of skin containing considerable adipose tissue and a thin layer of smooth muscle
      • Developmentally **homologous to scrotum**
   D. **Vulvovaginal (Bartholin's) glands:** mucus-secreting glands that empty into each side of the vaginal vestibule
      • **Homologous to bulbourethral (Cowper's) glands** in male

VIII. **Fertilization**
   A. **Fusion of sperm and oocyte cytoplasm**
      1. Sperm penetrates **corona radiata** and binds to zona pellucida.
      2. Sperm plasma membrane fuses with acrosome membrane, forming channels through which acrosomal enzymes are released (**acrosomal reaction**).
      3. Released enzymes degrade acrosome, permitting the **acrosomal process,** an extension of the sperm head, to penetrate zona pellucida.
      4. Plasma membranes of oocyte and sperm head fuse and sperm nucleus enters the oocyte cytoplasm.

5. Oocyte exocytoses enzymes that reduce its sperm-binding capacity (**cortical reaction**), helping to prevent entry of multiple sperm.

B. Formation of zygote and initial cleavage

1. Following fertilization, **secondary oocyte completes meiosis II**, forming a second **polar body** and a large mature gamete, the **ovum**, containing female and male pronuclei.

    a. Female pronucleus: 1C DNA, haploid ($1n$), one sex chromosome (X)

    b. Male pronucleus: 1C DNA, haploid ($1n$), one sex chromosome (X or Y)

2. DNA replication occurs in each pronucleus, yielding a diploid **zygote** ($2n$, 4C DNA) with 46 chromosomes (92 chromatids) housed in the two pronuclei.

3. Membranes of the pronuclei break down and all the duplicated chromosomes align at the metaphase plate of the **first cleavage division.**

4. Completion of mitosis produces a **two-cell embryo** with 46 chromosomes in each cell ($2n$, 2C DNA).

    a. 22 autosomes from maternal parent

    b. 22 autosomes from paternal parent

    c. 1 sex chromosome from maternal parent (X)

    d. 1 sex chromosome from paternal parent (X *or* Y)

C. Errors of fertilization

1. Polyspermy results from entry of two sperm into oocyte

    a. Zygote has two male and one female pronuclei.

    b. Resulting **triploid embryo** is nonviable, and spontaneous abortion ensues.

2. Polygyny results from failure of a second polar body to form during meiotic division of secondary oocyte.

    a. Zygote has two female and one male pronuclei.

    b. Resulting **triploid embryo** is nonviable, and spontaneous abortion ensues.

> Two major errors of fertilization yield nonviable, triploid embryo:
> • Polyspermy = two sperm fertilize the egg (responsible for a partial mole)
> • Polygyny = failure of secondary oocyte to emit second polar body after fertilization

IX. Placenta

- A temporary organ consisting of **maternal and fetal components**, the placenta forms following successful implantation of the embryo into the uterine wall.
- **Maternal portion** synthesizes and secretes **estrogen** and **progesterone.**
- **Fetal portion** synthesizes and secretes hCG and **human placental lactogen (hPL).**

A. Implantation

1. Embryo travels through oviduct and reaches the uterus in about 3 days when it is at the **morula stage.**

2. Shedding of the zona pellucida at the **blastocyst stage** exposes **trophoblast cells**, which mediate penetration of the endometrium, usually at 7 days' postovulation (day 21 of menstrual cycle).

3. Trophoblast differentiates into two layers.

    a. Cytotrophoblast: inner **stem cell** layer

    b. Syncytiotrophoblast: outer layer, arising from cytotrophoblast; a true **syncytium** containing cell organelles for **hormone synthesis** (hCG and hPL)

  4. By **day 11** postovulation, the blastocyst is **deeply embedded** within the endometrium and the syncytiotrophoblast faces spaces (**lacunae**) filled with maternal blood.

B. Endometrium during pregnancy (Figure 17-4)

- In response to implantation, endometrial stromal cells enlarge and become filled with glycogen and lipid, forming **decidual cells.**

  1. Decidua basalis, which faces invading trophoblast in region of vascular apposition (**chorion frondosum**), constitutes the **maternal portion of the placenta.**

    - During 4th and 5th month, septa from decidua basalis grow into chorion frondosum, dividing placenta into 10–35 chambers (**cotyledons**).

  2. Decidua capsularis overlies embryo within uterine cavity.

  3. Decidua parietalis constitutes remainder of decidualized endometrium.

    - Fusion of decidua capsularis and decidua parietalis at mid-pregnancy obliterates the uterine cavity.

C. Fetal portion of the placenta (chorion frondosum)

- **Villi,** which develop as extensions from the chorionic plate, extend into the **intervillous space** (old lacunar spaces formed by syncytiotrophoblast at implantation).

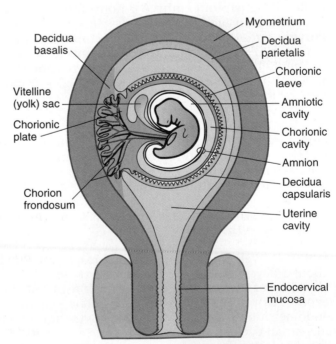

Figure 17-4 Overview of the pregnant uterus and the membranes and cavities associated with pregnancy. The portion of the chorion containing villi (chorion frondosum) and the decidua basalis of the endometrium form the placenta.

1. **Structure of mature (tertiary) villi**
   a. **Outer syncytiotrophoblast layer** has both **absorptive** and **secretory** functions.
      (1) Absorptive function indicated by numerous **pinocytic vessels** and **microvilli** on surface bathed in maternal blood.
      (2) Secretory function indicated by well-developed **endoplasmic reticulum** and **Golgi** complex and abundant **mitochondria**.
   b. **Inner cytotrophoblast layer** functions primarily to supply cells to syncytiotrophoblast.
      • This layer becomes discontinuous as pregnancy proceeds, allowing syncytiotrophoblast to sit on basement membrane.
   c. **Mesodermal connective tissue core** contains **fetal blood vessels** and macrophages (**Hofbauer cells**).
2. **Types and distribution of mature villi** (Figure 17-5)
   a. **Anchoring (stem) villi** are large villi attached to decidua basalis.
      • Cytotrophoblastic cells of anchoring villi form outer **cytotrophoblastic shell**, which is separated from maternal cells by a fibrinoid deposit.
   b. **Floating (free) villi** branch from anchoring villi and float in intervillous space, which is filled with maternal blood.
3. **Placental membrane**
   a. **Function**: a **sievelike barrier** through which substances can move **between maternal blood** in intervillous space **and fetal blood** within capillaries of villi.
   b. **Components in maternal to fetal direction:**
      • Syncytiotrophoblast → cytotrophoblast → basement membrane of trophoblast epithelium → basement membrane of fetal capillary → fetal capillary endothelium

D. **Metabolic exchange across placental membrane**
1. **Blood flow and gas exchange** (see Figure 17-5)
   a. Maternal arteries and veins open into intervillous space within each cotyledon.
   b. Highly oxygenated **maternal arterial blood** under high hydrostatic pressure spurts toward chorionic plate and **falls over villi.**
   c. **Fetal RBCs** in villi capillaries **take up oxygen** from maternal blood and **release carbon dioxide.**
      • High oxygen affinity of HbF facilitates gas exchange.
   d. Deoxygenated maternal blood enters veins and is returned to maternal lungs.
2. **Other substances transported**
   a. Nutrients, electrolytes, and hormones
   b. Metabolic waste products from fetus
   c. IgG maternal antibodies (**passive immunization of fetus**)
   d. Drugs and infectious agents
   e. Small amount of blood cells

Syncytiotrophoblast, the outer layer of the fetal portion of the placenta (chorion frondosum), produces hCG and hPL (human placental lactogen).

Fetal hemoglobin (HbF) has higher affinity for O_2 than adult hemoglobin, facilitating transfer of O_2 from maternal RBCs to fetal RBCs.

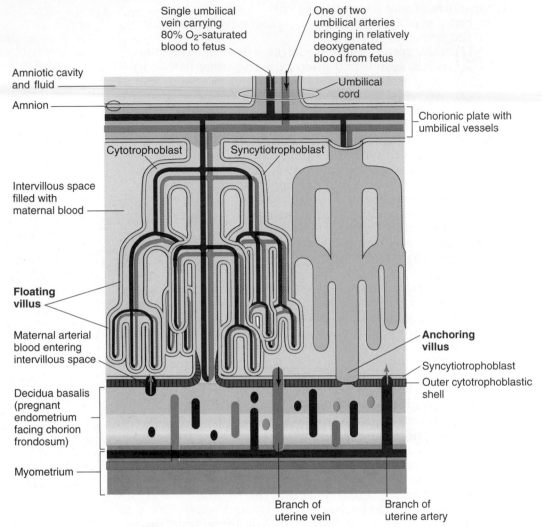

Figure 17-5 Schematic depiction of fetal blood vessels within chorionic villi and their relationships to maternal blood in the intervillous space and the decidua basalis of the endometrium. When an anchoring villus contacts the decidua basalis, the cytotrophoblast "breaks through" the syncytiotrophoblast to form the outer cytotrophoblastic shell. Note that branches of the two umbilical arteries carry deoxygenated blood into villi, whereas branches of the single umbilical vein carry oxygenated blood out of villi.

- Fetal blood cells can be separated from maternal blood and grown in vitro for **fetal karyotyping** as an alternative to amniocentesis or placental biopsy.
  3. **Mechanisms of transport across placental membrane**
     a. Simple and facilitated diffusion
     b. Active transport
     c. Pinocytosis
  E. **Placenta and fetal membranes in twins**
     1. **Fraternal (dizygotic) twins**
        - Two amnions, **two chorions**, two placentas (may be fused)

2. Identical (monozygotic) twins
  a. Division of embryonic disk or inner cell mass (96% of cases)
  • One or two amnions, **one chorion**, one placenta
  b. Earlier division of embryo at two-cell stage to morula (4% of cases)
  • Two amnions, two chorions, two placentas (same as for fraternal twins)
  c. Late but incomplete division of embryo (<0.2% of cases)
  • One amnion, one chorion, one placenta (**conjoined twins**)
F. Placental abnormalities
  1. Placenta accreta: trophoblastic invasion into uterine wall due to absence of a decidual layer.
  • Results in **massive hemorrhage** at parturition as result of improper separation
  2. Placenta previa: implantation in lower segment of uterus overlying the cervical os
  • Associated with **painless bleeding** during last trimester
  3. Abruptio placentae: premature detachment of the placenta with a retroplacental clot
  • Often causes shock, oliguria, and disseminated intravascular coagulation (**DIC**) in mother and may lead to **fetal death**
  4. Hydatidiform mole: abnormal enlargement of chorionic villi early in pregnancy resulting in mass of cysts resembling a **cluster of grapes**
  • Clinically manifests as marked **increase in hCG, vaginal bleeding, enlarged uterus, extreme nausea,** and **edema** during the first trimester
  • No embryo present in complete mole (46XX with both X chromosomes of paternal origin)
  • Triploid embryo present in partial mole (69XXY)
  5. Choriocarcinoma: malignancy arising from **trophoblast cells** of fetal membranes
  • May develop from complete hydatidiform mole or following a normal pregnancy or abortion

X. **Mammary Glands**
  A. Anatomy of mammary gland (Figure 17-6)
    1. Lobes
      a. Each gland consists of 15–25 **lobes**, separated by dense connective tissue septa.
      b. Each lobe houses **compound tubuloalveolar glands** draining into intralobular ducts → interlobular ducts → lactiferous sinus → lactiferous duct → nipple.
    2. Lactiferous sinuses and ducts
      a. Stratified cuboidal/columnar epithelium lines largest; simple cuboidal lines the smallest.
      b. Epithelium is surrounded by loose areolar connective tissue outside of which is dense irregular connective tissue with adipose cells.

Placenta accreta: connection between fetal placenta and uterine wall with partial or complete absence of decidua basalis. Hemorrhage on separation.

Placenta previa: attachment of placenta to lower uterus so it covers os. Painless bleeding.

Abruptio placentae: separation of placenta from uterine wall with retroplacental clot.

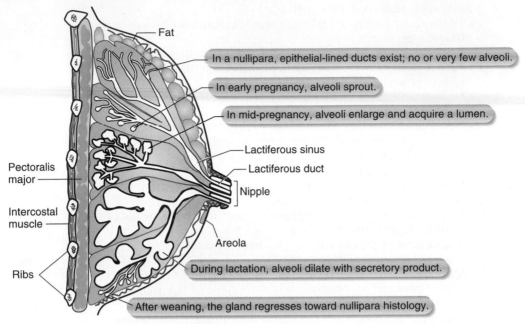

Fat

In a nullipara, epithelial-lined ducts exist; no or very few alveoli.

In early pregnancy, alveoli sprout.

In mid-pregnancy, alveoli enlarge and acquire a lumen.

Lactiferous sinus

Lactiferous duct

Nipple

Pectoralis major

Intercostal muscle

Ribs

Areola

During lactation, alveoli dilate with secretory product.

After weaning, the gland regresses toward nullipara histology.

Figure 17-6 Gross and microscopic anatomy of the breast illustrating hormone-induced changes in glandular morphology at different stages. Some sprouting of alveoli occurs during secretory phase of the menstrual cycle.

3. Alveoli
- Dilated ends of intralobular ducts are lined by **simple cuboidal epithelium** and surrounded by discontinuous layer of **stellate myoepithelial cells.**
  a. In nulliparous female
  - **Few,** if any, **alveoli** are present; some may develop and breast may enlarge during the secretory phase of menstrual cycle.
  b. During pregnancy
  - Alveoli undergo intense **growth and development** stimulated by **hormones** (estrogen, progesterone, and placental lactogen).
  c. During lactation
  - Alveolar epithelial cells contain **cytoplasmic fat droplets** and **secretory granules** filled with milk proteins. Lumens of alveoli are distended with secretion.
  d. During weaning
  - Alveoli revert to nulliparous state.
B. Production and secretion of milk
  1. Prolactin, secreted from anterior pituitary, stimulates **milk production.**
  - Breast feeding keeps prolactin levels high, thereby prolonging milk production in postpartum period.
  2. Oxytocin stimulates contraction of stellate myoepithelial cells, causing release of secretion into ducts.
  - Release of oxytocin from posterior pituitary is stimulated by **suckling.**

3. **Colostrum**, first secretion after birth, contains less fat and more protein (e.g., **antibodies**) than later milk.
4. **Milk secretion** occurs by two mechanisms.
   a. **Apocrine secretion:** lipid droplets
   b. **Merocrine secretion (exocytosis):** milk proteins, lactose, antibodies

C. **Breast cancer**
- 90% of cases arise in **ductal**, not glandular, epithelium.
- **Upper, outer quadrant** is most common location, since most breast tissue is located in that quadrant.

1. **Noninfiltrating intraductal carcinoma** is confined within basement membrane (carcinoma in situ).
2. **Infiltrating ductal carcinoma** involves penetration of basement membrane by malignant ductal epithelial cells.
   - Usually accompanied by reactive fibrosis (**scirrhous carcinoma**), even some calcification, giving mass a **stony, hard consistency**

Most breast cancers arise from ductal epithelium and are located in upper, outer quadrant.

18

Endocrine System

I. Introduction
   • **Endocrine signaling molecules** (hormones) **travel in the bloodstream** from their site of secretion to target cells.
   • **Binding of hormone molecules** to specific receptors expressed by target cells **elicits specific responses** within those cells.
   A. Components of the endocrine system
      1. **Several ductless glands** (e.g., thyroid, adrenal, pituitary)
      2. **Clusters of cells** within certain organs (e.g., pancreas, ovary, testis)
      3. **Scattered endocrine cells** within the digestive and respiratory systems (see Table 14-2)
   B. Major cytological specializations of endocrine cells
      1. **Polarity**
         • **Apex** of cell is oriented **toward** blood **vessel.**
      2. **Organelles**
         a. **Steroid hormone–producing cells:** prominence of **smooth** endoplasmic reticulum (SER)
         b. **Protein/polypeptide-producing cells:** prominence of **rough** endoplasmic reticulum (RER)
         c. **Glycoprotein-producing cells:** well-developed SER and RER
   C. **Hormone storage by endocrine cells**

1. **Little or no storage** (released immediately after synthesis): **steroid sex hormones** (e.g., estrogen, testosterone)
2. **Intracellular storage** (cytoplasmic granules): **protein and peptide hormones** (e.g., insulin, oxytocin, prolactin)
3. **Extracellular storage** (follicles): **thyroid hormones**

D. **Regulation of endocrine hormone secretion**
   1. **Neural control**
      - **Sensory input** to the brain triggers nerve impulse to endocrine cells and **stimulates secretion.**
      a. Infant **suckling** at nipple → **oxytocin** release
      b. Intense **emotions** (anger, fear) → **catecholamine** release
   2. **Direct feedback control** (nonneural)
      - Effect of hormone action regulates secretion by endocrine cells. Examples include:
      a. **Rise in blood glucose** → insulin secretion increases → blood sugar falls → insulin secretion decreases
      b. **Decline in blood glucose** → glucagon secretion increases → blood sugar rises → glucagon secretion decreases
      c. **Decline in blood Ca^{2+}** → parathyroid hormone secretion increases → blood Ca^{2+} rises → parathyroid hormone secretion decreases
   3. **Indirect feedback control** (nonneural)
      a. Effect of hormone action or hormone level controls release of **hypothalamic hormones**, which in turn regulate secretion by endocrine cells.
      b. **Hypothalamo-hypophyseal-ovary axis** is one example:
         - Estrogen level in blood falls → GnRH secretion from hypothalamus increases → LH secretion increases → estrogen secretion from ovaries increases → estrogen level in blood rises → GnRH secretion decreases (Box 18-1)

Mechanisms for controlling hormone secretion:
- Neural impulses to secreting cells (e.g., oxytocin, catecholamines)
- Direct feedback control on secreting cells (e.g., insulin, glucagon)
- Indirect feedback control via hypothalamus on secreting cells (e.g., estrogen, thyroid hormones)

BOX 18-1 Hormone Abbreviations

Hypothalamic Regulatory Hormones
CRH = corticotropin-releasing hormone
GnRH = gonadotropin-releasing hormone
PIF = prolactin-inhibiting factor (dopamine)
PSF = prolactin-stimulating factor
SRH = somatotropin-releasing hormone
TRH = thyrotropin-releasing hormone

Other Hormones
ACTH = adrenocorticotropic hormone
ADH = antidiuretic hormone (vasopressin)
FSH = follicle-stimulating hormone
GH = growth hormone
LH = luteinizing hormone
PTH = parathyroid hormone
T_3 = triiodothyronine
T_4 = thyroxine
TSH = thyroid-stimulating hormone

II. **Pituitary Gland (Hypophysis)**
    A. Structural/functional divisions of the hypophysis (Figure 18-1)
        1. **Adenohypophysis (anterior pituitary)** arises from **oral ectoderm** (Rathke's pouch) and is divided into three parts:
            a. **Pars distalis** contains several types of **endocrine cells.**
            b. **Pars tuberalis** surrounds infundibulum and carries **portal veins** of hypophyseal portal system.
            c. **Pars intermedia** is rudimentary in humans.
        2. **Neurohypophysis (posterior pituitary)** arises from **neural ectoderm** and is divided into two parts:
            a. **Pars nervosa** contains **axon terminals of neurosecretory cells** whose cell bodies lie in the hypothalamus.
            b. **Infundibulum** connects pars nervosa to the hypothalamus and carries **axons** of hypothalamic neurosecretory cells.
    B. Hypophyseal portal system
        1. **Components** (see Figure 18-1)
            a. **Primary capillary plexus** in **median eminence** arises from superior hypophyseal arteries.

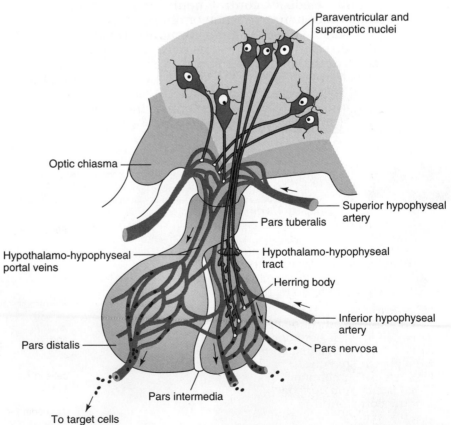

Figure 18-1 Drawing of the hypophysis showing its relation to the hypothalamus and vascularization.

b. Secondary capillary plexus surrounds endocrine cells of the **pars distalis.**

c. Portal veins (one to three) in **pars tuberalis** carry blood from primary to secondary plexus.

2. **Hypothalamic regulation of the anterior pituitary**
   - Finely tuned feedback regulatory systems, involving the hypophyseal portal system, control hormone secretion from the adenohypophysis.
   - **Hypothalamo-hypophyseal-thyroid axis** illustrated in Figure 18-2 is one example. Hypothalamo-hypophyseal-ovary axis is another example (see Figure 17-2).

   a. Releasing hormones, produced in cell bodies of hypothalamic neurosecretory cells, are released from axon terminals in the median eminence and enter the primary capillary plexus.

   b. After transport by portal veins to the secondary capillary plexus, **hormones** enter tissue fluid and act on **specific endocrine cells** in the anterior pituitary to control their secretion.

   c. Blood levels of hormones (or other physiologic factors) in turn control secretory activity of hypothalamic cells.

C. Secretory activity of the adenohypophysis
   - In humans, the **pars distalis** is the primary source of **anterior pituitary hormones,** although the pars tuberalis contains some endocrine cells.

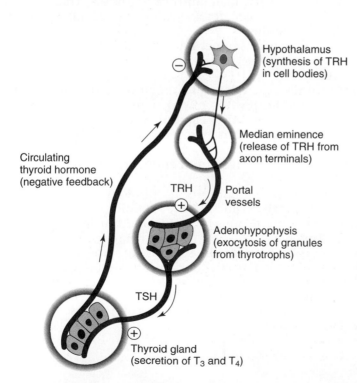

Hypothalamus
(synthesis of TRH
in cell bodies)

Median eminence
(release of TRH from
axon terminals)

Circulating
thyroid hormone
(negative feedback)

TRH

Portal
vessels

Adenohypophysis
(exocytosis of granules
from thyrotrophs)

TSH

Thyroid gland
(secretion of T_3 and T_4)

Figure 18-2 Hypothalamo-hypophyseal-thyroid axis, an example of indirect feedback control of hormone secretion from the adenohypophysis. Synthesis and secretion of thyrotropin-releasing hormone *(TRH)* is stimulated by low blood levels of thyroid hormones (T_3 and T_4). TRH promotes secretion (+) of thyroid-stimulating hormone *(TSH)* from endocrine cells in the adenohypophysis. TSH acts on the thyroid gland to stimulate secretion of T_3 and T_4, leading to a rise in the blood level of these hormones, which inhibits (−) TRH-producing hypothalamic cells.

- Secretory cells, classified as acidophils or basophils, are filled with hormone-containing **secretory granules** of varying size, abundance, and staining properties.
  1. **Acidophil secretions**
     a. **Mammotrophs** → prolactin
     b. **Somatotrophs** → GH (somatotropin)
  2. **Basophil secretions**
     a. **Corticotrophs** → ACTH
     b. **Gonadotrophs** → FSH and LH
     c. **Thyrotrophs** → TSH
  3. **Exocytosis** of secretory granules is stimulated or inhibited by **hypothalamic hormones** delivered by the hypophyseal portal system (see Box 18-1).
  4. **Actions of anterior pituitary hormones** (Table 18-1)
     - With the exception of prolactin and growth hormone, the anterior pituitary hormones directly or indirectly **promote the production of other hormones.**

D. **Secretory activity of the pars nervosa** (see Table 18-1)
  1. **Pituicytes** are stromal cells analogous to glial cells of the CNS.
  2. **Distal ends of hypothalamic neurosecretory cells** constitute parenchyma of pars distalis (see Figure 18-1).
     a. Cell bodies, located in the **paraventricular** and **supraoptic nuclei** of the hypothalamus, synthesize either **oxytocin** or **ADH** (vasopressin).
     b. Hormones are transported down long axons of these neurons, the **hypothalamo-hypophyseal tract**, to axon terminals where secretory granules accumulate, forming **Herring bodies.**
  3. **Hormone release** is under neural control.

III. **Thyroid Gland**
  A. **Thyroid follicles** are spherical structures lined by follicular epithelial cells and filled with **colloid**, a viscous gel composed primarily of **iodinated thyroglobulin.**
     - Colloid functions as an extracellular storage site for thyroid hormones.
  B. **Follicular cells** are derived from endoderm of the **thyroglossal duct.**
     1. **Low cuboidal to squamous** morphology when synthesizing and releasing thyroglobulin into colloid (Figure 18-3, *A*)
        a. **Iodide** from blood is imported and transported to follicular lumen.
        b. **Thyroid peroxidase** in apical membrane iodinates tyrosine residues of thyroglobulin extracellularly.
     2. **Tall columnar** morphology when liberating thyroid hormones from thyroglobulin (Figure 18-3, *B*)
        a. Under stimulus of TSH, colloid is endocytosed.
        b. Lysosomal enzymes degrade iodinated thyroglobulin, releasing primarily T_4, the prohormone form of the more biologically active T_3.

Anterior pituitary hormones and their target organs: ACTH (adrenal cortex); TSH (thyroid gland); FSH (ovary, testis); LH (ovary, testis); GH (all tissues); prolactin (breast).

Posterior pituitary hormones and their target organs: ADH (kidney, smooth muscle); oxytocin (breast, uterus).

TABLE 18-1   Major Hypophyseal Hormones in Humans

Hormone	Regulated by*	Target Organ/Tissue: Major Effects†
Anterior Pituitary (Pars Distalis)		
ACTH	↑ CRH ↓ Somatostatin	• Adrenal cortex: synthesis/secretion of glucocorticoids, androgens, estrogens
FSH	↑ GnRH ↓ Testosterone, estrogen, inhibin	• Ovary: maturation of follicle; synthesis of estrogen • Testis: secretion of androgen-binding protein and inhibin by Sertoli cells
LH	↑ LH, high estrogen ↓ Progesterone, testosterone	• Ovary: final maturation of follicles; ovulation; formation of corpus luteum • Testis: synthesis/secretion of testosterone by Leydig cells
TSH	↑ TRH ↓ Somatostatin	• Thyroid gland: synthesis/secretion of thyroid hormone (T_3, T_4)
GH (somatotropin)	↑ SRH, hypoglycemia, stress, exercise ↓ Somatostatin, hyperglycemia	• Liver: secretion of IGF-1, which stimulates growth (epiphyseal plates and soft tissue) • All tissues: RNA and protein synthesis, tissue growth, transport of glucose and amino acids into cells
Prolactin	↑ PSF ↓ PIF (dopamine)	• Mammary gland: production/secretion of milk; breast development
Posterior Pituitary (Pars Nervosa)		
ADH (vasopressin)	↑ High blood osmolarity ↓ Low blood osmolarity	• Kidney collecting ducts: water resorption • Vascular smooth muscle: contraction
Oxytocin	↑ Suckling, cervical dilation ↓ Progesterone, alcohol	• Mammary glands: milk ejection (milk letdown) • Uterine smooth muscle: contraction

ACTH, Adrenocorticotropic hormone; *CRH,* corticotropin-releasing hormone; *FSH,* follicle-stimulating hormone; *GH,* growth hormone; *LH,* luteinizing hormone; *PIF,* prolactin-inhibiting factor (dopamine); *PSF,* prolactin-stimulating factor; *TSH,* thyroid-stimulating hormone.
*↑, stimulation of hormone secretion; ↓, inhibition of secretion.
†In all cases, the indicated effect is stimulated by the corresponding hormone.

c. T_3 and T_4 (major fraction) are released from basal surface and enter capillaries.
   • T_4 is deiodinated in peripheral tissues (e.g., liver, kidney, heart) to T_3.
   • Major effect of thyroid hormones is to **accelerate basal metabolic rate (BMR)**, which leads to a rise in heat production.

TSH promotes production of thyroglobulin and release of T_3 and T_4.

A Synthetic/storage phase **B** Hormone-secreting phase

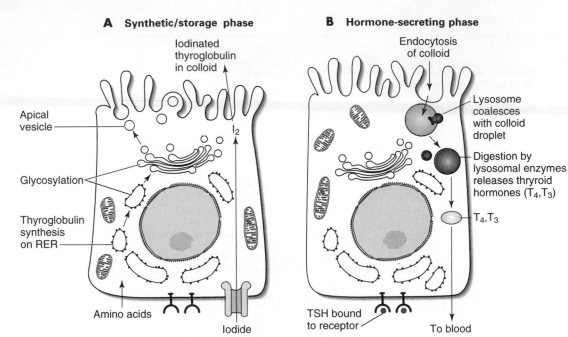

Figure 18-3 Synthesis, storage, and secretion of thyroid hormone by follicular cells. **A,** Follicular cells produce iodinated thyroglobulin, the major component of the viscous colloid that fills the lumen of thyroid follicles. Oxidation of iodide to iodine (I_2) and iodination of thyroglobulin are catalyzed by an enzyme localized near the apical membrane. **B,** In the presence of thyroid-stimulating hormone, follicular cells release thyroid hormones from thyroglobulin and secrete T_3 and T_4 (major fraction) from the basal surface into the blood. *RER,* Rough endoplasmic reticulum.

   C. Parafollicular cells, also known as **clear (C) cells**, are derived from endoderm of the **ultimobranchial body,** a diverticulum of the 5th pharyngeal pouch.
      1. Location: C cells are interspersed between follicular cells and the basal lamina at the periphery of follicles with their apex oriented away from the follicular lumen; they **never reach the lumen.**
      2. Secretion: in response to a **rise in blood Ca^{2+}** level, C cells secrete **calcitonin,** which suppresses bone reabsorption, leading to a **decrease in blood Ca^{2+}.**

 IV. Parathyroid Glands
   • Parenchyma of inferior and superior parathyroid glands is derived from endoderm of the **3rd and 4th pharyngeal pouches,** respectively.

PTH excess → hypercalcemia and hypophosphatemia

   A. Chief (principal) cells secrete PTH.
      1. Active cells have **dark cytoplasm** with numerous granules and well-developed Golgi and RER.
      2. Inactive cells have **light cytoplasm** with few granules and less prominent Golgi and RER.
        • Normal ratio of inactive to active cells is 3:1.
   B. PTH secretion is stimulated by a **decline in blood Ca^{2+}** level.
      • **PTH raises blood Ca^{2+} level** by promoting release of osteoclast-activating factor from osteoblasts, decreasing Ca^{2+}

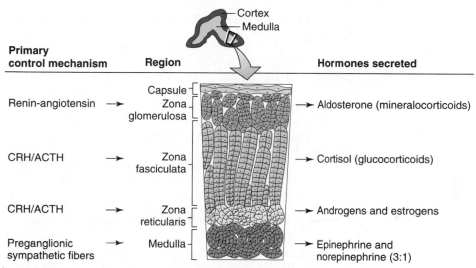

Figure 18-4 Schematic depiction of structural/functional divisions of the adrenal gland. Each of the three zones of the cortex secretes characteristic hormones, as does the medulla. CRH/ACTH refers to the hypothalamo-hypophyseal-adrenal axis involving corticotropin-releasing hormone *(CRH)* and adrenocorticotropic hormone *(ACTH)*. See Figure 15-6 for renin-angiotensin control of aldosterone secretion.

excretion by kidneys, and with vitamin D promoting intestinal absorption of Ca^{2+}.

PTH deficiency → hypocalcemia and hyperphosphatemia

V. Adrenal Glands

A. Structural/functional divisions of the adrenal glands

1. **Cortex** is derived from the **mesodermal** root of the dorsal mesentery.
   - Parenchyma is divided into three regions that synthesize and secrete different **steroid hormones.**
2. **Medulla** is derived from **neural crest cells.**
   - Parenchymal cells secrete **catecholamines** (epinephrine and norepinephrine).

B. Secretory activity of adrenal cortex (Figure 18-4)

1. **Zona glomerulosa:** superficial region constituting about 15% of cortical volume
   a. Parenchymal cells are arranged in **clumps/glomerular masses.**
   b. **Mineralocorticoids** secreted by these cells (e.g., **aldosterone**) **regulate electrolyte and water balance** via their action on renal tubules (see Figure 15-6).
      - **Atrial natriuretic peptide (ANP)** increases secretion of water and sodium in kidneys, antagonistic to the effect of aldosterone.
2. **Zona fasciculata:** middle region constituting about 78% of cortical volume

Regions of adrenal cortex from outside to inside:
- Zona glomerulosa → aldosterone (mineralocorticoids)
- Zona fasciculata → cortisol (glucocorticoids)
- Zona reticularis → androgens and estrogens

a. Parenchymal cells are arranged in **cords** that project radially inward from zona glomerulosa.

b. **Glucocorticoids** secreted by these cells (e.g., **cortisol**) primarily **regulate carbohydrate metabolism** but have numerous other effects.

3. **Zona reticularis:** deepest region constituting about 7% of cortical volume

a. Parenchymal cells are arranged in **anastomosing cords** between zona fasciculata and medulla.

b. **Androgens** and **estrogens** are produced in this zone in both sexes, supplementing those produced in the gonads.

C. **Secretory activity of adrenal medulla**

1. **Chromaffin cells** are **modified postganglionic sympathetic neurons** that synthesize, store, and secrete catecholamines.

a. **Norepinephrine-producing cells** (25% of total) contain heterogeneous granules with very electron-dense core surrounded by pale halo.

b. **Epinephrine-producing cells** (75% of total) contain small, homogeneous electron-dense granules.

2. **Catecholamine release** is triggered by stimulation from **preganglionic sympathetic axons** that synapse on chromaffin cells.

a. Neural stimulation, and hence secretion, increases in situations of **fear**, **anger**, and **stress**.

b. Subsequent **fight-or-flight response**, mediated by epinephrine and norepinephrine, is marked by **increased heart rate**, **blood pressure**, and **glycogenolysis**.

VI. **Pancreatic Islets of Langerhans**

• Pancreas contains clusters, or **islets**, of **endodermal-derived endocrine cells** scattered among its exocrine secretory acini (see Chapter 14).

• Islets are most numerous in the tail of the pancreas.

A. **Alpha (A, α) cells** secrete **glucagon**, which promotes breakdown of glycogen to glucose in the liver.

• Glucagon has **hyperglycemic effect** antagonistic to insulin.

B. **Beta (B, β) cells** secrete **insulin**, which acts on the plasma membrane of most cells to increase transport of glucose from the blood into cells.

• Insulin has **hypoglycemic effect** antagonistic to glucagon.

C. **Delta (D, δ) cells** secrete **somatostatin**, which acts in two ways.

1. **Paracrine effect:** inhibition of glucagon and insulin release from A and B cells of the pancreas.

2. **Endocrine effect:** inhibition of GH release from pars distalis.

VII. **Pineal Gland (Epiphysis Cerebri)**

A. **Pinealocytes** (parenchymal cells) are derived from **neural ectoderm.**

• Produce **melatonin** from serotonin

Adrenal medulla, derived from neural crest cells, produces epinephrine and norepinephrine in 3:1 ratio.

Flight-or-fight response mediated by epinephrine and norepinephrine: ↑ heart rate, ↑ blood pressure, ↑ glycogenolysis.

Secretions of pancreatic islet cells:
• α cells → glucagon
• β cells → insulin
• δ cells → somatostatin

- Possess long cellular processes that terminate in bulbous expansions near capillaries

B. Melatonin secretion is stimulated by neural impulses originating in areas of the central nervous system and reaching the pineal gland via postganglionic **sympathetic** fibers.

C. Circadian fluctuation in melatonin levels
- Under normal light/dark conditions, blood melatonin level is **threefold higher during the night** than during the day.

D. Antigonadotropic effect of melatonin
1. **Destruction of the pineal gland** during childhood causes **precocious sexual development.**
2. Administration of **melatonin** to a child **delays onset of puberty.**

VIII. **Summary of Major Nonpituitary Hormones (Table 18-2)**

Hypoglycemic effect of insulin is antagonistic to hyperglycemic effect of glucagon.

Melatonin level is highest during nocturnal phase; lowest, during diurnal phase.

TABLE 18-2   Major Nonpituitary Hormones

Origin/Hormone	Regulated by*	Target Organ/Tissue: Major Effects†
Thyroid Gland		
T_3, T_4	↑ TSH ↓ Somatostatin, high thyroid hormones (T_3, T_4)	• Most cells: ↑ basal metabolic rate, cardiac output, and nutrient utilization
Calcitonin	↑ High blood Ca^{2+} ↓ Low blood Ca^{2+}	• Bones: ↓ resorption
Parathyroid Glands		
PTH	↑ Low blood Ca^{2+} ↓ High blood Ca^{2+}, very low blood Mg^{2+}	• Bones: ↑ resorption • Kidneys: ↓ Ca^{2+} excretion • Intestine: ↑ Ca^2 absorption (with vitamin D)
Adrenal Glands		
Aldosterone (mineralocorticoids)	↑ Angiotensin II, low blood volume ↓ Fluid overload	• Distal kidney tubules: ↑ reabsorption of Na^+ (and thus of H_2O) and K^+ secretion
Cortisol (glucocorticoids)	↑ ACTH, stress ↓ High cortisol	• Liver: ↑ gluconeogenesis to raise blood sugar • Adipose tissue: ↑ breakdown of triglycerides • Various tissues: anti-inflammatory effects
Epinephrine and norepinephrine	↑ Sympathetic stimulation in response to fear, anger, stress	• Most tissues: ↑ cardiac output, vasoconstriction, glycogenolysis (hyperglycemic effect), and lipolysis

ACTH, Adrenocorticotropic hormone; *PTH,* parathyroid hormone; *TSH,* thyroid-stimulating hormone.
*↑, Stimulation of hormone secretion; ↓, inhibition of secretion.
†↑, Stimulation of indicated effect; ↓, inhibition of indicated effect.

Continued

TABLE 18-2 Major Nonpituitary Hormones—cont'd

Origin/Hormone	Regulated by*	Target Organ/Tissue: Major Effects†
Pancreatic Islets		
Glucagon (α cells)	↑ Low blood glucose ↓ High blood glucose, somatostatin	• Liver: ↑ glycogenolysis (hyperglycemic effect) and gluconeogenesis • Adipose tissue: ↑ lipolysis
Insulin (β cells)	↑ High blood glucose and amino acids ↓ Low blood glucose, somatostatin	• Muscle and adipose tissue: ↑ uptake of blood glucose (hypoglycemic effect) and amino acids into cells; ↑ protein synthesis • Adipose tissue: ↓ lipolysis; ↑ fat deposition
Somatostatin (δ cells)‡	↑ High hormone levels	• Pancreatic α and β cells: ↓ secretion of glucagon and insulin • Pars distalis: ↓ secretion of GH, TSH, and ACTH • GI tract: ↓ secretion of gastrin and secretin
Pineal Gland		
Melatonin	↑ Light exposure	• Gonads: ↓ development
Testis		
Testosterone (Leydig cells)	↑ LH ↓ High testosterone	• Seminiferous tubules: ↑ spermatogenesis • Other tissues: ↑ development and maintenance of male sex characteristics
Ovary		
Estrogen (follicles and corpus luteum)	↑ FSH ↓ High estrogen	• Uterus: ↑ rebuilding of endometrium following menses • Other tissues: ↑ development and maintenance of female sex characteristics
Progesterone (corpus luteum)	↑ LH ↓ High progesterone	• Uterus: ↑ secretory phase of menstrual cycle; ↓ uterine contractions • Breast: ↑ development of alveoli during pregnancy

GI Tract (see Chapter 14, Table 14-2)

FSH, Follicle-stimulating hormone; *GH,* growth hormone; *LH,* luteinizing hormone.
‡Also secreted by the hypothalamus.

Sense Organs

19

Target Topics

▸ Chambers and tunics of the eye

▸ Layers of the retina and their functions

▸ Accommodation for near and distant vision

▸ Structure and histophysiology of the vestibular organ

▸ Structure and histophysiology of the auditory organ

▸ Wilson's disease, glaucoma, lens defects, retinal disorders, Horner's syndrome, conjunctivitis, otitis media, hearing loss, Meniere's disease

I. **Eye**

   A. **Tunics of the eye** (Figure 19-1)

   1. **Retina** (innermost tunic)

      a. **Photosensitive region:** posterior to ora serrata

      (1) **Optic disc:** region on posterior aspect of eye where optic nerve exits

      • Possesses no photosensitive retina and constitutes the **blind spot**

      (2) **Fovea centralis:** located ≈2.5 mm lateral to optic disc in area of retina containing yellow pigment (**macula lutea**)

      • Contains **only cones** and exhibits **most acute vision**

      b. **Nonphotosensitive region:** anterior to ora serrata

      • Consists of two cell layers covering the iris, ciliary body, and ciliary processes

   2. **Uvea** (middle layer)

      a. **Choroid:** highly **vascular** connective tissue layer containing **melanocytes**

      (1) **Choriocapillaris,** the inner choroid zone, contains small blood vessels that supply the cells of the retina.

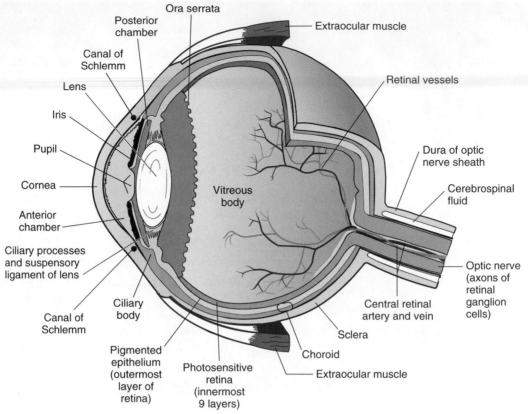

Figure 19-1 General anatomy of the eyeball including its tunics and chambers.

Sympathetic impulses → dilation of pupil. Parasympathetic impulses → constriction of pupil.

    (2) **Bruch's membrane**, composed of the **fused basal laminae** of the choriocapillaris and pigmented epithelium of the retina, constitutes the choroid's inner aspect.

  b. **Ciliary body:** wedge-shaped expansion of the choroid peripheral to the lens

    (1) **Ciliary processes** project toward the lens.

    (2) **Suspensory ligaments of Zinn** (zonula ciliaris) extend from ciliary processes to just behind equator of the lens, **anchoring the lens** in place.

    (3) **Ciliary muscle**, a circular mass of smooth muscle innervated by **parasympathetic** neurons, **changes shape of the lens** by relaxing and contracting.

  c. **Iris:** portion of uvea anterior to the lens that separates the anterior and posterior chambers and contains a central aperture, the **pupil**

    (1) Contraction of **dilator pupillae** muscle (**sympathetic** stimulation) **dilates** the pupil.

    (2) Contraction of **sphincter pupillae** muscle (**parasympathetic** stimulation) **constricts** the pupil.

3. **Fibrous tunic** (outer layer)
   a. **Sclera:** dense collagenous connective tissue that forms external layer of posterior five sixths of the eyeball and receives insertions of **extraocular muscles**
   b. **Cornea:** transparent **avascular** anterior portion of the fibrous tunic composed of the corneal epithelium, Bowman's (basement) membrane, substantia propria (fibroblasts and collagen fibers), Descemet's (basement) membrane, and corneal endothelium
   c. **Wilson's disease** (hepatolenticular degeneration): abnormality of copper processing that can lead to **Kayser-Fleischer ring** (brown or green **coloration of the cornea**), cirrhosis of the liver, and degeneration of neurons in the central nervous system

B. **Chambers of the eye**
   1. **Anterior chamber:** located posterior to cornea and anterior to iris
   2. **Posterior chamber:** located posterior to iris and anterior to lens
      a. Unpigmented epithelial cells of the ciliary retina secrete **aqueous humor,** a plasmalike fluid, into the posterior chamber.
      b. Aqueous humor flows through the pupil to the anterior chamber and then drains through a trabecular meshwork at the corneoscleral junction (**limbus**) into the **canal of Schlemm** and eventually into episcleral veins.
   3. **Vitreal cavity:** located posterior to lens and bordered by the retina
      • Contains the **vitreous body,** a structureless gelatinous mass that is 99% water
   4. **Glaucoma:** any condition characterized by **increased intraocular pressure**
      • **Compromised drainage of aqueous humor** from anterior chamber is associated with most types of glaucoma.

C. **Lens of the eye**
   • The lens, a **biconvex avascular** structure located behind the iris, receives nourishment from the aqueous humor and vitreous body.
   1. **Structural components**
      a. **Capsule,** the carbohydrate-rich external layer of the lens, contains **type IV collagen** and glycoproteins. It is underlain anteriorly by a simple cuboidal epithelium.
      b. **Lens fibers**—elongated, anucleated, six-sided cells (prisms)—fill the core of the lens.
      c. **Cataract,** an opacity of the lens or lens capsule that obstructs passage of light, results in impaired vision or blindness.
   2. **Accommodation of the lens**
      • Because of the natural elasticity of the lens, its shape can change to adjust to viewing objects at different distances.
      a. **Distant vision**

Congenital absence of the iris (aniridia) is commonly associated with Wilms' tumor, a rapidly developing carcinoma of the kidneys.

Kayser-Fleischer ring: golden brown or green discoloration at outer margin of the cornea seen in Wilson's disease.

Glaucoma is marked by increased intraocular pressure caused by excess aqueous humor.

Cataract: alteration in the lens core or capsule that interferes with light transmission. Most common type is associated with aging.

Near accommodation: ciliary and sphincter muscles contract, pupil smaller, lens thicker. Far accommodation: ciliary and sphincter muscles relax, pupil larger, lens thinner.

    (1) Thin, stretched lens can focus light rays from **distant objects** but not near objects.

    (2) When the ciliary muscle is **relaxed**, tension is placed on the suspensory ligament, causing the **lens to flatten** = accommodation for distant vision.

b. Near vision

    (1) Thick, unstretched lens can refract (bend) light rays enough to focus on **near objects.**

    (2) When the ciliary muscle is **contracted**, tension on the suspensory ligament is released and **lens becomes more spherical** = accommodation for near vision.

    (3) Reading for long periods requires **constant contraction** of ciliary muscle = **tired eyes.**

3. Lens defects affecting focusing of light

  a. Myopia (nearsightedness): inability to focus on distant objects.

    • Entering light rays are brought into **focus in front of the retina.** Corrected by concave lens.

  b. Hyperopia (farsightedness): inability to focus on near objects.

    • Entering light rays are brought into **focus behind the retina.** Corrected by convex lens.

  c. Presbyopia: inability to focus on near objects (hyperopia) due to **decreased elasticity** of the lens, which commonly occurs with **aging.** Corrected by convex lens.

D. Histology of the retina

1. Retinal layers

    • The **10 named layers** of the retina are depicted in Figure 19-2.

    • The **outer pigmented layer**, adjacent to the choroid, is derived from the **outer layer of the optic cup;** all the **other layers** are derived from the **inner layer of the optic cup.**

2. Photosensitive cells (first-order neurons)

    • **Cell bodies** of rods and cones are located in the **outer nuclear layer.**

    • Except in the region of the fovea centralis, **rods are much more numerous than cones.**

Rods for low-light, black-and-white vision; cones for high-light, acute vision and color perception.

  a. Rods are sensitive to **low-intensity light;** responsible for **black-and-white vision.**

    (1) Outer segment is filled with membranous **lamellae** that are **not continuous** with covering plasmalemma. Lamellae contain photosensitive **rhodopsin** (visual purple).

    (2) Inner segment, possessing numerous mitochondria, glycogen, rough endoplasmic reticulum, and Golgi, exhibits **metabolic activity** and **protein synthesis.**

    (3) Axons from as many as 100 rods **synapse** with a single bipolar cell in the **outer plexiform layer.**

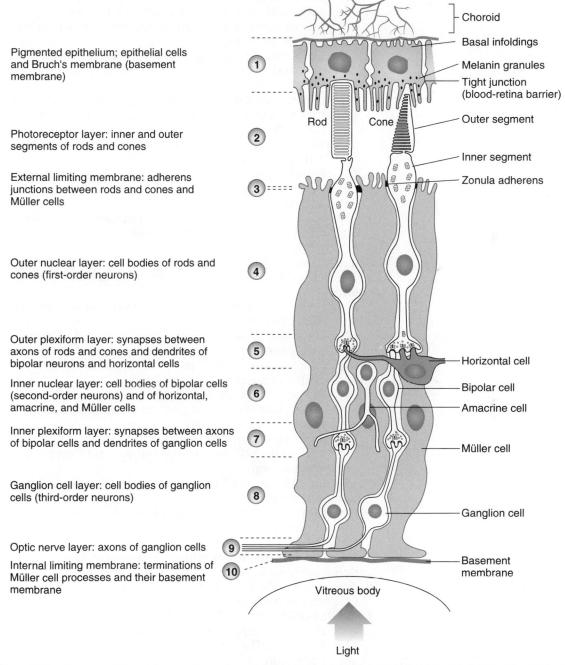

Choroid

Basal infoldings

Pigmented epithelium; epithelial cells
and Bruch's membrane (basement
membrane)

① Melanin granules

Tight junction
(blood-retina barrier)

Rod Cone

Outer segment

Photoreceptor layer: inner and outer
segments of rods and cones

② Inner segment

External limiting membrane: adherens
junctions between rods and cones and
Müller cells

③ Zonula adherens

Outer nuclear layer: cell bodies of rods and
cones (first-order neurons)

④

Outer plexiform layer: synapses between
axons of rods and cones and dendrites of
bipolar neurons and horizontal cells

⑤ Horizontal cell

Inner nuclear layer: cell bodies of bipolar cells
(second-order neurons) and of horizontal,
amacrine, and Müller cells

⑥ Bipolar cell

Amacrine cell

Inner plexiform layer: synapses between axons
of bipolar cells and dendrites of ganglion cells

⑦ Müller cell

Ganglion cell layer: cell bodies of ganglion
cells (third-order neurons)

⑧

Ganglion cell

Optic nerve layer: axons of ganglion cells

⑨

Internal limiting membrane: terminations of
Müller cell processes and their basement
membrane

⑩

Basement
membrane

Vitreous body

Light

Figure 19-2 Diagram of the 10 layers of the retina. Light enters through the internal limiting membrane, adjacent to the vitreous body, and passes through all the intervening layers to outer segments of rods and cones, which contain light-absorbing pigments. Absorption of light generates nerve impulses that are transmitted back through the layers via bipolar and ganglion cells, exiting the retina in axons of ganglion cells (layer 9).

        (4) **Dark adaptation** refers to the increase in photosensitivity of rhodopsin that occurs when an individual moves from bright light to dim light; this process takes some time.

    b. **Cones** are sensitive to **high-intensity light** and produce greater **visual acuity** than rods; responsible for **color vision.**

        (1) **Outer segment** is filled with membranous **lamellae** that are **continuous** with covering plasmalemma. Lamellae contain one of three different **iodopsins,** which **differ in their sensitivity to red, blue, and green light.**

        (2) **Inner segment,** as in rods, is **synthetic region** with many mitochondria and protein-synthesizing organelles.

        (3) Each cone synapses with a single bipolar cell (in contrast; each rod may synapse with several bipolar neurons).

  3. **Other retinal cells** (see Figure 19-2)

    a. **Pigmented epithelial cells:** outer layer adjacent to choroid

        (1) Synthesize **melanin,** which prevents reflection from uvea and sclera

        (2) Have apical processes that surround and **protect photosensitive outer segments** of rods and cones

        (3) **Phagocytose lamellae** shed from rods and cones and degrade them in lysosomes

        (4) Are connected by tight junctions, forming **blood–retina barrier,** which prevents blood from choroid reaching the retina

        (5) **Esterify vitamin A,** which is transported to rods and cones and used in the formation of photosensitive pigments

    b. **Bipolar cells: second-order neurons** with which rods and cones synapse

    c. **Ganglion cells:** multipolar **third-order neurons** whose long axons eventually are collected as the fibers of the **optic nerve**

    d. **Horizontal cells:** interneurons that connect rods and cones with each other and with bipolar neurons

    e. **Amacrine cells:** interneurons that connect ganglion cells and bipolar neurons

    f. **Müller cells:** irregularly branched, **neuroglial** cells that extend to most layers of retina

        (1) Zonulae adherens between Müller cells and rods/cones form **external limiting membrane.**

        (2) Innermost terminations of Müller cell processes and their basement membrane form **internal limiting membrane.**

  4. **Disorders of the retina**

    a. **Retinal detachment** can result from seepage of vitreous fluid or blood through the retina, leading to separation of the pigmented epithelial layer from all the sensory layers.

- Develops slowly, generally after age 40
- Often initially marked by appearance of numerous, **floating spots** in front of the affected eye, later progressing to a **shadow** that gradually comes over the eye

  b. Macular degeneration entails progressive breakdown of the macula lutea leading to gradual **loss of central vision** (fine detail) usually with preservation of peripheral vision.

- Initial symptoms include blurred vision, distortion of vertical straight lines, and worsening color vision.

  c. Retinoblastoma results from loss of function of the *RB* gene, a tumor-suppressor gene.

- Most cases occur in young children with initial symptoms including red, painful eye, **leukokoria** (cat's eye reflex), and squint.

E. Accessory structures of the eye

  1. Eyelid

    a. Anterior surface is covered with skin.

      (1) **Glands of Zeiss** are **sebaceous** glands associated with eyelashes.

      (2) **Glands of Moll** are **sweat** glands whose ducts open into eyelash follicles.

    b. Palpebral fascia constitutes fibrous core of eyelids.

      (1) **Sympathetic** stimulation causes **chronic contraction** of the superior tarsal muscle attached to fascia of the upper lid, causing **elevation of upper eyelid.**

      (2) **Meibomian glands** are **sebaceous** glands, not associated with hair follicles, that open in front of the free edge of the lid. Their secretion keeps **normal tear film** in the eye.

    c. Palpebral conjunctiva, a stratified columnar or squamous epithelium, containing many goblet cells, lines inner surface of eyelids.

      (1) **Bulbar conjunctiva**, covering the eyeball, is similar to and continuous with palpebral conjunctiva.

      (2) "Lost" contact lenses become lodged at junctions between two conjunctivae, the superior and inferior fornices.

    d. Horner's ptosis (drooping of upper lid) results from loss of sympathetic innervation to the superior tarsal muscle.

    e. Horner's syndrome includes **ptosis, miosis** (small pupil), and **anhydrosis** (loss of sweating) on affected side of the face.

- Both Horner's ptosis and syndrome may indicate invasion of lung carcinoma and destruction of cervical sympathetic chain on the ipsilateral side.

    f. Stye (hordeolum) is a localized inflammatory infection of one or more **sebaceous glands** (meibomian or zeisian) in the eyelid, commonly caused by **staphylococci.**

Margin notes:

Retinal detachment: separation of pigmented epithelium from remaining retinal layers. Patient senses floating spots and then gradually enlarging shadow over the eye.

Horner's syndrome: ptosis (droopy upper eyelid) + miosis (contracted pupil) + anhydrosis (lack of sweating); may be sign of metastatic lung carcinoma.

      g. Conjunctivitis, inflammation of palpebral and/or bulbar conjunctivae, is caused by infection or allergy.
- Common symptoms are **thick discharge**, sticky eyelids, and red eyes.

  2. Lacrimal apparatus
    a. Lacrimal gland is a tubuloalveolar exocrine gland.
- Serous acini produce tears, which contain **lysozyme** (a bactericidal substance).

    b. Ducts drain into fornices of superior conjunctival sac, so that tears wash anterior surface of eye, keeping the cornea and conjunctiva moist.

    c. Tears collected in lacrimal ducts → sac → naso-lacrimal duct.

II. **Ear**
  A. Outer Ear
    1. Auricle
- Core of elastic cartilage is covered by **thin skin** (keratinized stratified squamous epithelium).

    2. External auditory meatus/canal
      a. Wall is composed of **elastic cartilage** in its outer third and **bone** in its inner two thirds.
      b. Stratified squamous epithelium lining the canal contains **sebaceous glands** and modified sweat glands (**ceruminous glands**).
- Combined secretions form **ear wax**.

    3. Tympanic membrane (eardrum)
- The eardrum delimits the external auditory canal medially and separates it from the middle ear.

      a. Core is formed of connective tissue (from mesoderm) that is **vascularized** and **innervated**.
      b. External surface is covered by **thin skin** derived from ectoderm of **1st branchial groove**.
      c. Inner surface is covered by **simple cuboidal epithelium** derived from **1st pharyngeal pouch**.

  B. Middle ear (tympanic cavity)
    1. Auditory (eustachian) tube, derived from **1st pharyngeal pouch**, connects middle ear with the nasopharynx.
    2. Oval and **round windows** are membrane-covered regions in bony surface of the middle ear separating it from the inner ear.
    3. Auditory ossicles traverse tympanic cavity and transmit movements of tympanic membrane to the oval window. From lateral to medial:
      a. Malleus (attached to tympanic membrane)
      b. Incus
      c. Stapes (medial end inserted into oval window)
    4. Tensor tympani and **stapedius muscle** insert into the malleus and stapes, respectively.
- Reflex contraction of these muscles in response to loud sounds dampens vibrations of auditory ossicles.

  C. Inner ear

Surface layers of eardrum: external = thin skin derived from 1st branchial groove; internal = simple cuboidal epithelium derived from 1st pharyngeal pouch.

Ossicles from eardrum to oval window: malleus → incus → stapes. Fusion of the ossicles (otosclerosis) is one cause of conductive hearing loss.

1. **Bony labyrinth:** complicated system of canals and chambers in bone, including the **semicircular canals, cochlea, scala vestibuli,** and **scala tympani**
   • Is filled with **perilymph,** which is **high in sodium**
2. **Membranous labyrinth:** various membranous structures, suspended inside the bony labyrinth, that function as **auditory** or **vestibular** organs
   • Is filled with **endolymph,** which is **high in potassium**
3. **Vestibular organ:** patches of special **sensory epithelium** that **responds to changes in position** (Figure 19-3)
   a. Maculae of the saccule and utricle
      (1) Epithelium contains columnar supporting cells and vestibular **hair cells** with numerous **stereocilia** and a single **kinocilium** on their apical surface.
      (2) Afferent nerve endings contact hair cells.
      (3) **Otolithic membrane,** a gelatinous mass containing calcium carbonate crystals (**otoliths**), overlies the epithelium.
      (4) **Linear acceleration of the head** displaces the otolithic membrane causing bending of stereocilia, which triggers a sensory impulse.
   b. Cristae ampullares of semicircular ducts
      (1) Epithelium contains supporting cells, hair cells, and efferent nerve endings similar to those in maculae.
      (2) **Cupula,** a gelatinous layer lacking otoliths, overlies epithelium.
      (3) **Rotation of head** displaces cupula causing bending of stereocilia, which triggers a sensory impulse.
4. **Auditory organ**
   a. Cochlear duct (scala media) is an endolymph-filled triangular-shaped structure that divides the bony cochlea into two perilymph-filled spaces: **scala vestibuli** and **scala tympani** (Figure 19-4, *A*).
      (1) **Vestibular membrane** forms roof of the duct.
      (2) **Basilar membrane** forms floor of the duct.

Vestibular organ detects changes in position; comprises ampullae of semicircular canals and maculae of saccule and utricle.

Linear acceleration of the head causes movement of otolithic membrane in saccule and utricle → stimulation of sensory hair cells.

Rotation of the head causes movement of cupula in semicircular ducts → stimulation of sensory hair cells.

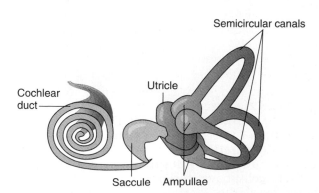

Figure 19-3 Components of the membranous labyrinth. Sensory receptors in the saccule, utricle, and cristae ampullares of the semicircular ducts form the vestibular organ. The organ of Corti within the cochlear duct is the auditory organ.

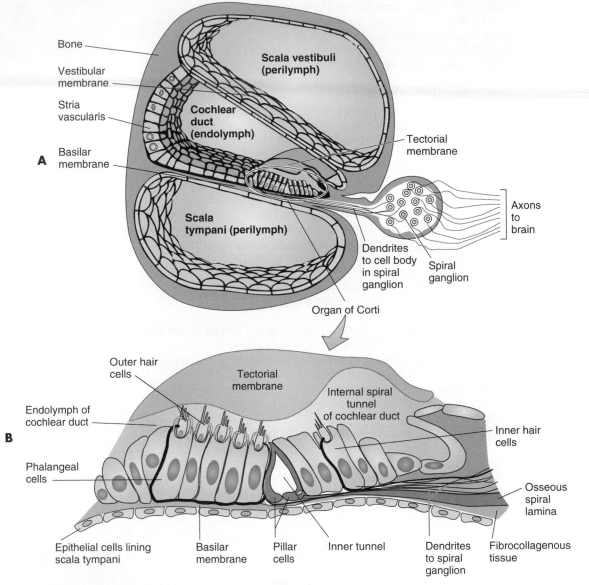

Figure 19-4 **A,** General structure of the inner ear showing location of the organ of Corti and its neural projection to the spiral ganglion and beyond. **B,** Detailed structure of the organ of Corti.

      (3) **Stria vascularis** forms lateral aspect and participates in formation of endolymph.

  b. Organ of Corti lies on basilar membrane of the cochlear duct (Figure 19-4, *B*).

      (1) **Inner** and **outer hair cells**, the auditory receptor cells, have **stereocilia** (but no kinocilium) on their apical border.

      (2) Supporting cells of several types are associated with hair cells.

(3) **Tectorial membrane**, a gelatinous mass, contacts stereocilia of the hair cells.

D. Histophysiology of hearing

1. **Sound transmission** from the environment to the organ of Corti occurs via the following pathway:
   - Air vibrations → external auditory canal → tympanic membrane → auditory ossicles → footplate of stapes in oval window → perilymph of scala vestibuli → vestibular membrane → endolymph of cochlear duct → basilar membrane/organ of Corti.

2. **Displacement of stereocilia** on hair cells of the organ of Corti, caused by deflection of the basilar membrane, is **converted into an electric impulse** (depolarization wave) that is conducted to cell bodies of neurons in spiral ganglion.

3. **High-frequency sounds** cause greatest deflection of the basilar membrane toward **base of the cochlea,** closer to oval window.

4. **Low-frequency sounds** cause greatest deflection of the basilar membrane toward **apex of cochlea** where scala vestibuli and scala tympani communicate via the **helicotrema.**
   - Thus, the lower the frequency of sound vibrations, the farther from the oval window is the deflection of the basilar membrane and stimulation of the organ of Corti.

E. Disorders of the ear

1. **Otitis media** (inflammation of the middle ear) commonly is caused by spread of bacterial pathogens (most commonly *Streptococcus pneumoniae*) from upper respiratory tract to the middle ear via the eustachian tube.
   - If the eustachian tube becomes blocked, **outward bulging or perforation of eardrum** may occur due to pressure buildup.

2. **Conductive hearing loss** is caused by a defect of the sound-conducting apparatus in the external auditory canal or middle ear.
   - **Otitis media** and **otosclerosis** (fusion of the ossicles) of the middle ear may cause this type of deafness.

3. **Neural deafness** results from a lesion in any of the neuronal segments carrying impulses from the organ of Corti to the brain.
   - **Disease, prolonged exposure to loud noises,** and exposure to certain **drugs** may cause nerve deafness.

4. **Meniere's disease,** a chronic disease of the inner ear, is caused by overproduction or decreased absorption of endolymph, leading to **distention of the membranous labyrinth.**
   - Hallmark symptoms are **tinnitus, recurrent vertigo, progressive hearing loss,** and feeling of fullness in the ear.

III. **Olfactory Mucosa**
   - The mucous membrane lining the roof of the nasal cavity consists of a **pseudostratified columnar epithelium** and an underlying lamina propria of loose areolar connective tissue.

Meniere's disease: tinnitus, recurrent vertigo, and progressive hearing loss due to excessive amounts of endolymph in membranous labyrinth.

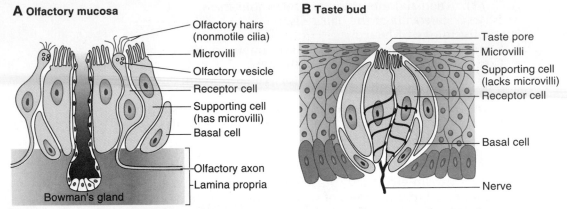

A Olfactory mucosa

- Olfactory hairs (nonmotile cilia)
- Microvilli
- Olfactory vesicle
- Receptor cell
- Supporting cell (has microvilli)
- Basal cell
- Olfactory axon
- Lamina propria

Bowman's gland

B Taste bud

- Taste pore
- Microvilli
- Supporting cell (lacks microvilli)
- Receptor cell
- Basal cell
- Nerve

Figure 19-5 **A,** Cellular components of the olfactory mucosa. Ducts from Bowman's glands in the lamina propria project between epithelial cells, delivering serous secretions to the surface. Olfactory hairs detect odoriferous substances dissolved in these secretions. **B,** Cellular components of taste buds. Microvilli on neuroepithelial receptor cells extend into the taste pore, which opens to the surface.

A. **Cells composing the olfactory epithelium** (Figure 19-5, *A*)
   1. **Olfactory receptor cells** are bipolar neurons.
      a. Single apical dendrite forms expanded knoblike **olfactory vesicle.**
      b. Several **modified cilia (olfactory hairs)** project from vesicle into layer of fluid covering the epithelium.
      c. Unmyelinated axon emerges from basal portion and enters the lamina propria. Bundles of axons join to form **olfactory nerve (CN I).**
   2. **Supporting (sustentacular) cells** have many apical **microvilli.**
   3. **Basal cells** are mitotically active, replacing themselves and other cells of the epithelium.
B. **Bowman's glands**
   - These branched tubuloalveolar glands release a **serous secretion** via narrow ducts to the surface.
   - Odoriferous substances dissolved in these secretions interact with receptors on olfactory hairs, generating an electric impulse.

IV. **Taste Buds**
   - Taste buds are oval structures that extend across the epithelium of **lingual papillae;** they are most numerous in fungiform and circumvallate papillae.
   A. **Cells composing taste buds** (Figure 19-5, *B*)
      1. **Neuroepithelial (receptor) cells** are elongated cells possessing numerous **microvilli,** which extend into the **taste pore,** a small opening to the surface.
         a. **Detect bitter, acid, sweet,** or **salt sensations** by direct contact of microvilli with dissolved substances
         b. Have **synaptic vesicles** near sites of apposition with nerve terminals

2. Supporting (sustentacular) cells lack microvilli.

3. Basal cells are mitotically active and replace all supporting and receptor cells, which are continually lost.

B. Nerve fibers

- Sensory nerve endings of **facial (CN VII), glossopharyngeal (CN IX),** or **vagus (CN X) nerves** enter base of taste bud and wind around receptor cells.

- Impulses from stimulated receptor cells are transmitted to nerve terminals across chemical synapses.

COMMON LABORATORY VALUES

Test	Conventional Units	SI Units
Blood, Plasma, Serum		
Alanine aminotransferase (ALT, GPT at 30° C)	8-20 U/L	8-20 U/L
Amylase, serum	25-125 U/L	25-125 U/L
Aspartate aminotransferase (AST, GOT at 30° C)	8-20 U/L	8-20 U/L
Bilirubin, serum (adult) Total // Direct	0.1-1.0 mg/dL // 0.0-0.3 mg/dL	2-17 µmol/L // 0-5 µmol/L
Calcium, serum (CA^{2+})	8.4-10.2 mg/dL	2.1-2.8 mmol/L
Cholesterol, serum	Rec: <200 mg/dL	<5.2 mmol/L
Cortisol, serum	8:00 AM: 6-23 µg/dL // 4:00 PM: 3-15 µg/dL	170-630 nmol/L // 80-410 nmol/L
	8:00 PM: ≤50% of 8:00 AM	Fraction of 8:00 AM: ≤0.50
Creatine kinase, serum	Male: 25-90 U/L	25-90 U/L
	Female: 10-70 U/L	10-70 U/L
Creatinine, serum	0.6-1.2 mg/dL	53-106 µmol/L
Electrolytes, serum		
Sodium (Na^+)	136-145 mEq/L	135-145 mmol/L
Chloride (Cl^-)	95-105 mEq/L	95-105 mmol/L
Potassium (K^+)	3.5-5.0 mEq/L	3.5-5.0 mmol/L
Bicarbonate (HCO_3^-)	22-28 mEq/L	22-28 mmol/L
Magnesium (Mg^{2+})	1.5-2.0 mEq/L	1.5-2.0 mmol/L
Estriol, total, serum (in pregnancy)		
24-28 wk // 32-36 wk	30-170 ng/mL // 60-280 ng/mL	104-590 // 208-970 nmol/L
28-32 wk // 36-40 wk	40-220 ng/mL // 80-350 ng/mL	140-760 // 280-1210 nmol/L
Ferritin, serum	Male: 15-200 ng/mL	15-200 µg/L
	Female: 12-150 ng/mL	12-150 µg/L
Follicle-stimulating hormone, serum/ plasma (FSH)	Male: 4-25 mIU/mL	4-25 U/L
	Female: premenopause 4-30 mIU/mL	4-30 U/L
	midcycle peak 10-90 mIU/mL	10-90 U/L
	postmenopause 40-250 mIU/mL	40-250 U/L
Gases, arterial blood (room air)		
pH	7.35-7.45	[H^+] 36-44 nmol/L
P_{CO_2}	33-45 mm Hg	4.4-5.9 kPa
P_{O_2}	75-105 mm Hg	10.0-14.0 kPa
Glucose, serum	Fasting: 70-110 mg/dL	3.8-6.1 mmol/L
	2 hr postprandial: <120 mg/dL	<6.6 mmol/L
Growth hormone–arginine stimulation	Fasting: <5 ng/mL provocative stimuli: >7 ng/mL	<5 µg/L >7 µg/L
Immunoglobulins, serum		
IgA	76-390 mg/dL	0.76-3.90 g/L
IgE	0-380 IU/mL	0-380 kIU/L
IgG	650-1500 mg/dL	6.5-15 g/L
IgM	40-345 mg/dL	0.4-3.45 g/L

COMMON LABORATORY VALUES—cont'd

Test	Conventional Units	SI Units
Blood, Plasma, Serum—cont'd		
Iron	50-170 µg/dL	9-30 µmol/L
Lactate dehydrogenase, serum (LDH)	45-90 U/L	45-90 U/L
Luteinizing hormone, serum/plasma (LH)	Male: 6-23 mIU/mL	6-23 U/L
	Female: follicular phase 5-30 mIU/mL	5-30 U/L
	midcycle 75-150 mIU/mL	75-150 U/L
	postmenopause 30-200 mIU/mL	30-200 U/L
Osmolality, serum	275-295 mOsm/kg	275-295 mOsm/kg
Parathyroid hormone, serum, N-terminal	230-630 pg/mL	230-630 ng/L
Phosphatase (alkaline), serum (p-NPP at 30° C)		
Phosphorus (inorganic), serum	3.0-4.5 mg/dL	1.0-1.5 mmol/L
Prolactin, serum (hPRL)	<20 ng/mL	<20 µg/L
Proteins, serum		
Total (recumbent)	6.0-8.0 g/dL	60-80 g/L
Albumin	3.5-5.5 g/dL	35-55 g/L
Globulin	2.3-3.5 g/dL	23-35 g/L
Thyroid-stimulating hormone, serum or plasma (TSH)	0.5-5.0 µU/mL	0.5-5.0 mU/L
Thyroidal iodine (^{123}I) uptake	8%-30% of administered dose/24 hr	0.08-0.30/24 hr
Thyroxine (T_4), serum	4.5-12 µg/dL	58-154 nmol/L
Triglycerides, serum	35-160 mg/dL	0.4-1.81 mmol/L
Triiodothyronine (T_3), serum (RIA)	115-190 ng/dL	1.8-2.9 nmol/L
Triiodothyronine (T_3) resin uptake	25%-38%	0.25-0.38
Urea nitrogen, serum (BUN)	7-18 mg/dL	1.2-3.0 mmol urea/L
Uric acid, serum	3.0-8.2 mg/dL	0.18-0.48 mmol/L
Cerebrospinal (CSF) Fluid		
Cell count	0-5 cells/mm³	$0-5 \times 10^6$/L
Chloride	118-132 mEq/L	118-132 mmol/L
Gamma globulin	3%-12% total proteins	0.03-0.12
Glucose	50-75 mg/dL	2.8-4.2 mmol/L
Pressure	70-180 mm H_2O	70-180 mm H_2O
Proteins, total	<40 mg/dL	<0.40 g/L
Hematology		
Bleeding time (template)	2-7 min	2-7 min
Erythrocyte count	Male: 4.3-5.9 million/mm³	$4.3-5.9 \times 10^{12}$/L
	Female: 3.5-5.5 million/mm³	$3.5-5.5 \times 10^{12}$/L
Erythrocyte sedimentation rate (Westergren)	Male: 0-15 mm/hr	0-15 mm/hr
	Female: 0-20 mm/hr	0-20 mm/hr

Continued

COMMON LABORATORY VALUES—cont'd

Test	Conventional Units	SI Units
Hematology—cont'd		
Hematocrit (Hct)	Male: 40%-54%	0.40-0.54
	Female: 37%-47%	0.37-0.47
Hemoglobin A$_{IC}$	≤6%	≤ 0.06%
Hemoglobin, blood (Hb)	Male: 13.5-17.5 g/dL	2.09-2.71 mmol/L
	Female: 12.0-16.0 g/dL	1.86-2.48 mmol/L
Hemoglobin, plasma	1-4 mg/dL	0.16-0.62 mmol/L
Leukocyte count and differential		
Leukocyte count	4500-11,000/mm^3	4.5-11.0 × 10^9/L
Segmented neutrophils	54%-62%	0.54-0.62
Bands	3%-5%	0.03-0.05
Eosinophils	1%-3%	0.01-0.03
Basophils	0%-0.75%	0-0.0075
Lymphocytes	25%-33%	0.25-0.33
Monocytes	3%-7%	0.03-0.07
Mean corpuscular hemoglobin (MCH)	25.4-34.6 pg/cell	0.39-0.54 fmol/cell
Mean corpuscular hemoglobin concentration (MCHC)	31%-37% Hb/cell	4.81-5.74 mmol Hb/L
Mean corpuscular volume (MCV)	80-100 μm^3	80-100 fl
Partial thromboplastin time (activated) (aPTT)	25-40 sec	25-40 sec
Platelet count	150,000-400,000/mm^3	150-400 × 10^9/L
Prothrombin time (PT)	12-14 sec	12-14 sec
Reticulocyte count	0.5%-1.5% of red cells	0.005-0.015
Thrombin time	<2 sec deviation from control	<2 sec deviation from control
Volume		
Plasma	Male: 25-43 mL/kg	0.025-0.043 L/kg
	Female: 28-45 mL/kg	0.028-0.045 L/kg
Red cell	Male: 20-36 mL/kg	0.020-0.036 L/kg
	Female: 19-31 mL/kg	0.019-0.031 L/kg
Sweat		
Chloride	0-35 mmol/L	0-35 mmol/L
Urine		
Calcium	100-300 mg/24 hr	2.5-7.5 mmol/24 hr
Creatinine clearance	Male: 97-137 mL/min	
	Female: 88-128 mL/min	
Estriol, total (in pregnancy)		
30 wk	6-18 mg/24 hr	21-62 μmol/24 hr
35 wk	9-28 mg/24 hr	31-97 μmol/24 hr
40 wk	13-42 mg/24 hr	45-146 μmol/24 hr
17-Hydroxycorticosteroids	Male: 3.0-9.0 mg/24 hr	8.2-25.0 μmol/24 hr
	Female: 2.0-8.0 mg/24 hr	5.5-22.0 μmol/24 hr
17-Ketosteroids, total	Male: 8-22 mg/24 hr	28-76 μmol/24 hr
	Female: 6-15 mg/24 hr	21-52 μmol/24 hr
Osmolality	50-1400 mOsm/kg	
Oxalate	8-40 μg/mL	90-445 μmol/L
Proteins, total	<150 mg/24 hr	<0.15 g/24 hr

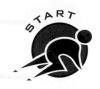

TEST 1

DIRECTIONS: Each numbered item or incomplete statement is followed by options arranged in alphabetical or logical order. Select the best answer to each question. Some options may be partially correct, but there is only **ONE BEST** answer.

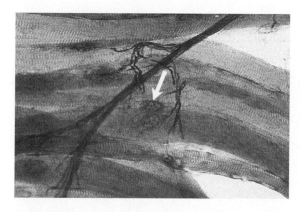

1. The arrow in this light micrograph is pointing to a structure that shows a defect that occurs in patients with myasthenia gravis. Which of the following correctly identifies this defect?

○ A. Decrease in acetylcholine (ACh) receptors
○ B. Increase in acetylcholinesterase
○ C. Number of synaptic vesicles
○ D. Reduction in junctional folds of sarcolemma
○ E. Schwann cell membrane

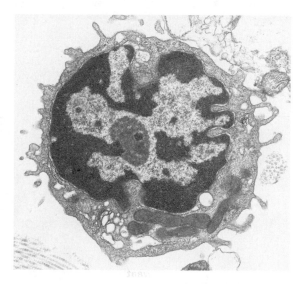

2. Which of the following is the main activity of the connective tissue cell shown in this transmission electron micrograph (TEM)?

○ A. Liberation of pharmacologically active substances
○ B. Phagocytosis of foreign substances
○ C. Production of fibers and ground substances
○ D. Production of immunocompetent cells
○ E. Release of major basic protein

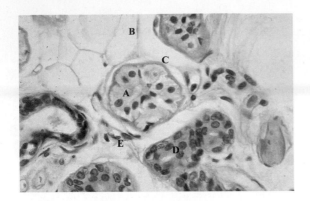

3. Which of the following cells of the dermis shown in this light micrograph fails to reabsorb chloride in patients with cystic fibrosis?

○ A. Cell at A
○ B. Cell at B
○ C. Cell at C
○ D. Cell at D
○ E. Cell at E

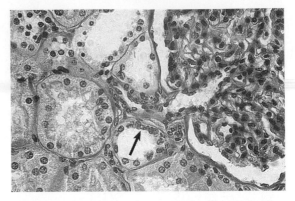

5. Which of the following functions is performed by the cells located at the tip of the arrow in this light micrograph (LM)?

○ A. Absorption of all glucose
○ B. Monitoring of chloride content
○ C. Production of angiotensin-converting enzyme
○ D. Secretion of erythropoietin
○ E. Secretion of renin

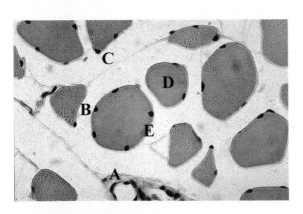

4. Duchenne muscular dystrophy (DMD) is expressed by the defect in which of the following locations shown in this light micrograph (LT)?

○ A. Site A
○ B. Site B (fiber numbers)
○ C. Site C (extracellular protein)
○ D. Site D
○ E. Site E

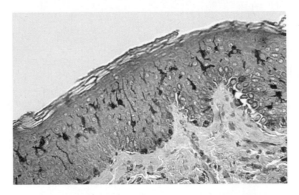

6. This section of skin has been stained immunohistochemically for S-100 protein, indicated by the dark brown cells showing the location of this cytoplasmic protein. Which of the following is the correct identification of these cells?

○ A. Keratinocytes and Langerhans' cells
○ B. Melanocytes and Langerhans' cells
○ C. Merkel cells

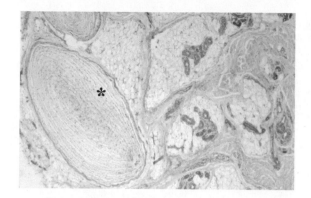

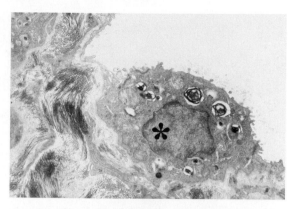

7. Which of the following receptors or nerve endings is indicated by the asterisk in this light micrograph (LM) of the dermis of the skin?

○ A. Krause end bulb
○ B. Meissner corpuscle
○ C. Merkel ending
○ D. Pacinian corpuscle
○ E. Ruffini corpuscle

9. The asterisk in this electron micrograph (EM) indicates an organelle of a cell located in the lung. Which of the following is the correct identity of the characteristic organelle of this cell?

○ A. Lamellar body
○ B. Mucous granule
○ C. Primary lysosome
○ D. Secondary lysosome

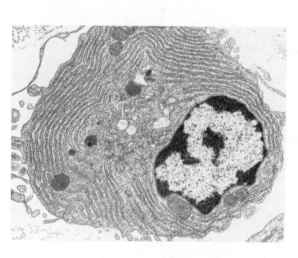

8. The cell shown in the accompanying electron micrograph (EM) is best recognized for production of which of the following substances?

○ A. Histamine
○ B. Hydrochloric acid
○ C. Immunoglobulins
○ D. Isoenzymes
○ E. Tropocollagen

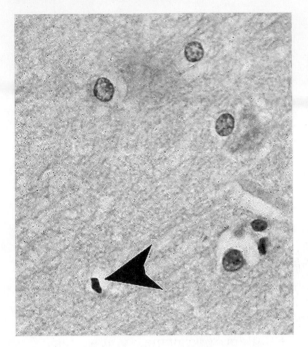

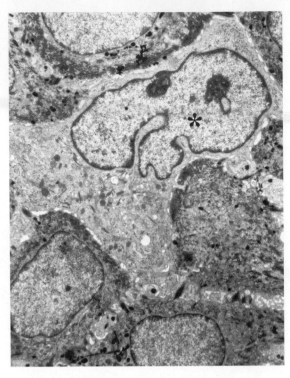

10. In the section of cerebrum shown in this light micrograph (LM), the cell at the tip of the arrow is responsible for which of the following actions?

○ A. Destruction of myelin in multiple sclerosis
○ B. Formation of gemistocytes
○ C. Formation of gliosis
○ D. HIV replication
○ E. Myelin synthesis

11. The cell located at the asterisk in this electron micrograph (EM) is positive for CD1 and is involved in the uptake and processing of antigens. Which of the following cells most accurately fits this description?

○ A. Helper T cell
○ B. Histiocyte
○ C. Kupffer's cell
○ D. Langerhans' cell
○ E. M cell

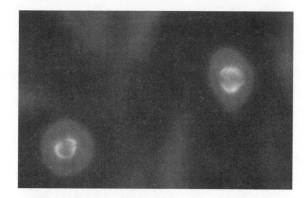

12. Which of the following drugs interacts with the fluorescent organelles shown in the accompanying light micrograph and causes a stabilization of microtubules?

○ A. Bleomycin
○ B. Cyclosporine
○ C. Methotrexate
○ D. Paclitaxel
○ E. Vinblastine

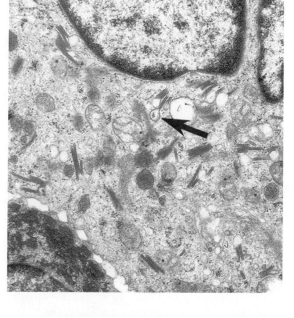

14. The accompanying electron micrograph (EM) shows cytoplasm of an epidermal cell. Which of the following is the correct identification of the characteristic, cell-specific organelle indicated by the arrow?

○ A. Beta granule
○ B. Birbeck granule
○ C. Melanosome
○ D. Weibel-Palade granule
○ E. Zebra body

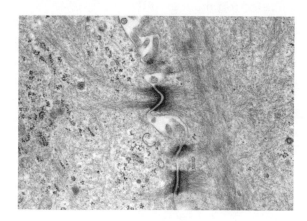

13. This electron micrograph (EM) shows several types of junctions and the filaments associated with them. Which of the following is the correct identification of this pair association?

○ A. Fascia adherens–actin
○ B. Macula densa–keratin
○ C. Macula densa–vimentin
○ D. Zonula adherens–actin
○ E. Zonula adherens–vimentin

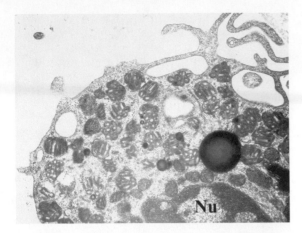

A. Alveolar macrophages
B. Neutrophils
C. Type I pneumocytes
D. Type II pneumocytes

15. Which of the following is the main activity of the connective tissue cell shown in this transmission electron micrograph (TEM)?

A. Liberation of pharmacologically active substances
B. Phagocytosis of foreign substances
C. Production of fibers and ground substances
D. Production of immunocompetent cells
E. Release of major basic protein

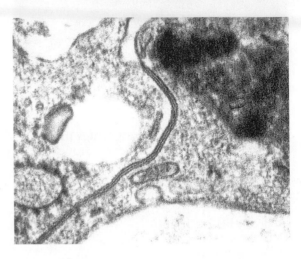

17. Which of the following is the means of communication between the cells seen in this electron micrograph?

A. Gap junction
B. Synapse
C. Zonula adherens
D. Zonula occludens

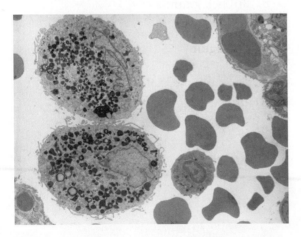

16. This electron micrograph (EM) shows a section of lung. Which of the following is the correct identification of the two large cells shown on the left-hand side of the EM?

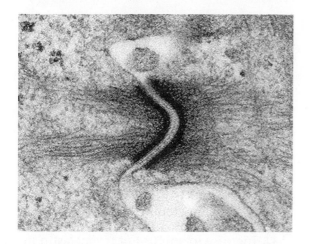

18. This electron micrograph (EM) shows a structure that contains a protein against which autoantibodies (IgG) are produced in patients with which of the following dermatologic diseases?

○ A. Bullous pemphigoid
○ B. Epidermolysis bullosa simplex
○ C. Ichthyosis
○ D. Pemphigus vulgaris
○ E. Vitiligo

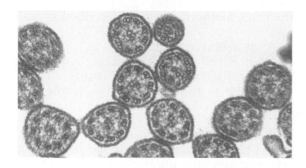

19. Which of the following is a molecular motor protein present in the structures shown in this electron micrograph (EM)?

○ A. Actinin
○ B. Clathrin
○ C. Dynein
○ D. Kinesin
○ E. Myosin

20. When stained immunohistochemically, a malignant fibrous histiocytoma of the connective tissue is found to be positive for keratin. Transmission electron microscopy (TEM) is ordered to confirm the presence of keratin in this tumor of mesodermal origin. Which of the following structures would be seen in or around these tumor cells?

○ A. Cells arranged like keratinocytes
○ B. Desmosomes
○ C. Granules filled with keratin
○ D. Intracytoplasmic inclusions filled with keratin
○ E. Tonofilaments

21. Which component of skeletal muscle is missing or abnormal in patients with Duchenne's muscular dystrophy?

○ A. Actin
○ B. Dystrophin
○ C. Myosin
○ D. Tropomyosin
○ E. Troponin

22. Which of the following hormones causes smooth muscle cells in the gallbladder to contract while concurrently causing the sphincter of Oddi to relax?

○ A. Cholecystokinin
○ B. Gastrin
○ C. Glucagon
○ D. Motilin
○ E. Secretin

23. In normal tissue, which of the following types of cellular specializations most effectively provides a permeability seal in the space between cells?

○ A. Macula adherens
○ B. Macula occludens
○ C. Nexus
○ D. Zonula adherens
○ E. Zonula occludens

24. At a site of inflammation, digestion of which of the following is considered an autophagic activity in the lysosome of parenchymal cells?

○ A. Bacteria
○ B. Centriole
○ C. Collagen fibers
○ D. Vesicular contents
○ E. Viral particle

25. A chromosomal analysis of various tissues taken from a woman shows XO, XX, and XXX. Cells from every tissue type contain 44 autosomes. It is assumed that a single abnormal division accounts for all of these aberrations. The division process that would account for these chromosome numbers is

○ A. meiotic anaphase lagging
○ B. meiotic nondisjunction
○ C. mitotic anaphase lagging
○ D. mitotic deletion
○ E. mitotic nondisjunction

26. Under normal conditions, a single secondary spermatocyte that has just completed meiosis I contains

○ A. either one X chromosome or one Y chromosome
○ B. either two X chromosomes or two Y chromosomes
○ C. one X chromosome and one Y chromosome
○ D. two X chromosomes and two Y chromosomes

27. Which cellular organelles are found in excessive amounts in tumor cells specialized to synthesize steroid hormones?

○ A. Golgi apparatus
○ B. Nucleus
○ C. Rough endoplasmic reticulum (RER)
○ D. Smooth endoplasmic reticulum (SER)

28. In normal stratified epithelia, most of the cells that replace surface cells that are lost through attrition or cell death originate in the

○ A. basal layer
○ B. intermediate layer
○ C. surface layer
○ D. underlying connective tissue

29. Drug X interferes with the cross-linking of tropoelastin but not with the synthesis of tropoelastin. After 2 months of treatment with drug X, which of the following changes is most likely to be seen?

○ A. Decrease in amount of tropoelastin in connective tissue
○ B. Increase in amount of elastin in connective tissue
○ C. Increase in amount of tropoelastin in connective tissue
○ D. Increase in elasticity of the tissue

30. A 32-year-old man is undergoing ionizing radiation treatment of a brain tumor. After 2 weeks of treatment, there will most likely be a decrease in the number of

○ A. astrocytes
○ B. microglia
○ C. neurons
○ D. oligodendrocytes

31. In a surgical biopsy of skeletal muscle, the thick filaments are best described as

○ A. attached to the Z line
○ B. localized in the A band
○ C. localized in the A and I bands
○ D. same as a single myosin molecule
○ E. shortened during muscle contraction

32. Chloramphenicol is an antibiotic that blocks mitochondrial protein synthesis. In a cell treated with chloramphenicol, synthesis of which of the following proteins will be diminished?

○ A. DNA polymerase
○ B. Electron transport system subunits
○ C. Enzymes of the tricarboxylic acid (TCA) cycle
○ D. Permeases of the inner mitochondrial membrane
○ E. Structural proteins of the outer mitochondrial membrane

33. Cells may be osmotically coupled when a change in the concentration of an ion in one cell causes a similar change in adjacent cells. Which type of cellular junction would facilitate this phenomenon?

- A. Macula adherens
- B. Macula occludens
- C. Nexus
- D. Zonula adherens
- E. Zonula occludens

34. Nondisjunction of all X chromosomes in a normal oocyte has occurred at the first and second meiotic division. During each division, the extra DNA passed to the cell that was to become the egg, which was fertilized by a normal Y-bearing sperm. The number of sex chromatin bodies that will be seen in interphase nuclei in the resulting fetus is

- A. 1
- B. 2
- C. 3
- D. 4
- E. 5

35. A patient with a rapidly growing tumor is treated with nitrogen mustard. Which type of cell will be most depleted 1 month after a week-long treatment with a sublethal dose of nitrogen mustard?

- A. Continuous replicators
- B. Nonreplicators with no stem cells
- C. Occasional replicators

36. An experimental antifertility drug enables meiotic cells to complete meiosis I but prevents them from entering meiosis II. After treatment with this drug, the blocked cells will contain the same amount of DNA as somatic cells in which stage of the cell cycle?

- A. G_1
- B. G_2
- C. Metaphase of mitosis
- D. Middle of the S phase
- E. Prophase of mitosis

37. Hurler syndrome is characterized by an accumulation of proteoglycans in connective tissue, macrophage lysosomes, and urine. Which of the following explains this condition?

- A. A proteoglycan-degrading hydrolase is missing
- B. The connective tissue lacks lysosomes
- C. The rate of proteoglycan degradation has increased
- D. The rate of proteoglycan synthesis has increased

38. In normal tissue, the zonula adherens functions to

- A. allow electronic coupling of adjacent cells
- B. encircle the cell completely
- C. fuse outer leaflets of the plasma membrane
- D. serve as a barrier to diffusion

39. Which of the following characteristics best describes thick filaments in skeletal muscle?

- A. They are found in the I band
- B. They contain actin
- C. They contain myosin
- D. They contain tropomyosin

40. A 32-year-old man is involved in an industrial accident and severs a peripheral nerve in his forearm. This injury may result in which of the following?

- A. Death of neurons in the dorsal horn of the spinal cord
- B. Degeneration of nerve processes proximal to the injury
- C. Proliferation of Schwann cells proximal to the injury
- D. Reactive changes in the lower thoracic dorsal root ganglia cells

41. Zellweger syndrome is characterized by craniofacial abnormalities, hypotonia, hepatomegaly, polycystic kidneys, jaundice, and death in early infancy. The liver, brain, and spleen of patients with this disorder do not produce adequate amounts of catalase and several oxidases. Which cellular organelle is responsible for this disorder?

○ A. Lysosome
○ B. Microtubule
○ C. Mitochondrion
○ D. Peroxisome

42. Which of the following structures is found on the E face of the plasma membrane?

○ A. Extrinsic membrane proteins
○ B. Glycocalyx
○ C. Nonpolar tails of phospholipids
○ D. Polar heads of phospholipids

43. The amount of rough endoplasmic reticulum (RER) exceeds the amount of smooth endoplasmic reticulum (SER) during which of the following cell functions?

○ A. Contraction of a skeletal muscle fiber
○ B. Fat absorption in a columnar epithelial cell
○ C. Peptide hormone production in a glandular cell
○ D. Steroid hormone production in a glandular cell

44. A characteristic that distinguishes white skeletal muscle fibers from red skeletal muscle fibers is that white fibers

○ A. are rich in myoglobin
○ B. have the greatest amount of glycogen per fiber
○ C. have the greatest number of mitochondria per fiber
○ D. have slow contractions and support continuous heavy work

45. Which of the following remains the same during muscle contraction or relaxation?

○ A. A band length during relaxation
○ B. H band length during contraction
○ C. I band length during contraction

46. A 7-year-old boy from a poor family has purpura and ecchymoses in the oral mucosa and skin, subperiosteal hematomas, and blood in several joints after minimal trauma. The child has a history of impaired wound healing. Which of the following should be considered when making a differential diagnosis?

○ A. Failure to maintain fully differentiated epithelia
○ B. Inadequate mineralization of cancellous bone
○ C. Increased intracellular levels of protein p53
○ D. Lack of prolyl and lysyl hydroxylase activity

47. Several Volkmann's canals appear in a bone section taken at the autopsy of a 92-year-old woman who died after a serious fall. These structures

○ A. are components of interstitial lamellae
○ B. contain the processes of osteocytes
○ C. interconnect haversian canals
○ D. interconnect lacunae

48. Hereditary spherocytosis involves a genetic defect that results in which of the following?

○ A. Change in the structure of spectrin
○ B. Decrease in the area of hyalomeres
○ C. Decrease in the diameter of the affected cell
○ D. Increase in intrinsic cell membrane proteins
○ E. Increase in the size of the granulomere region of a cell

49. An 8-year-old boy of African-American descent is diagnosed with homozygous sickle cell anemia. In which area of the body will the abnormal blood cells resulting from this condition be destroyed by erythrophagocytosis?

○ A. Cord of Billroth in the spleen
○ B. Hematopoietic cord in bone marrow
○ C. Marginal zone of the spleen
○ D. Medullary region of the thymus
○ E. Paratrabecular sinus in a lymph node

50. Many types of neoplasms, such as breast cancer, involve a defect in the ability of a cell to regulate its progression through the cell cycle. Which of the following defects is commonly seen in these types of neoplasms?

○ A. Lack of cyclin-dependent kinase (CDK) activity
○ B. Lack of retinoblastoma protein (pRB) phosphorylation
○ C. Overexpression of D cyclins
○ D. Underexpression of D cyclins
○ E. Up-regulation of p53

ANSWERS AND DISCUSSIONS

1. ***A*** (decrease in acetylcholine receptors) is correct. A reduction in the number of functionally active ACh receptors in the sarcolemma of the myoneural junction leads to myasthenia gravis, an autoimmune disorder characterized by progressive muscular weakness. Antibodies bind to the ACh receptors in the junctional folds and inhibit normal nerve-muscle communication. The cross-linking of the receptors by antibodies increases the rate of endocytosis of the receptors, and they cannot be replaced quickly enough by the muscle. The structure seen at the arrow tip is a motor end plate or myoneural junction. Branches are seen extending from the axon, and each terminates in a motor end plate on a muscle fiber.

B (increase in acetylcholinesterase) is incorrect. Acetylcholinesterase breaks down the neurotransmitter ACh, but this enzyme is not affected in myasthenia gravis.
C (number of synaptic vesicles) is incorrect. The number of synaptic vesicles in the terminal bouton of the motor end plate is not affected in myasthenia gravis.
D (reduction in junctional folds of sarcolemma) is incorrect. The junctional folds are the site of ACh binding and of internalization of the receptor-ACh complex, but reduction in the number of folds does not occur in myasthenia gravis.
E (Schwann cell membrane) is incorrect. The Schwann cell membrane wraps around the axon and extends to the muscle cell surface. It is not affected in myasthenia gravis.

2. ***D*** (production of immunocompetent cells) is correct. This TEM shows a lymphocyte, with its characteristic spherical shape, rim of ribosome-filled cytoplasm, spherical nucleus, and microvilli. Some undulation of the nucleus is apparent, and it is not unusual to see a deeply infolded nucleus. Lymphocytes usually contain a considerable amount of heterochromatin. Collagen fibers are visible around the cell, indicating its presence in connective tissue. Transmission electron microscopy cannot determine the type of lymphocyte from morphology; this cell could be a T, B, or null cell. B lymphocytes develop into immunocompetent plasma cells that produce immunoglobulins. T cells can be divided in groups, depending on the expression of receptors, and become immunologically activated as helper T cells, cytotoxic T cells, or T suppressor cells.

A (liberation of pharmacologically active substances) is incorrect. This connective tissue cell does not have organelles that contain pharmacologically active substances. An example of such a connective cell is the mast cell, which would be packed with granules.

B (phagocytosis of foreign substances) is incorrect. This connective tissue cell does not have the features of a macrophage, which phagocytizes foreign substances.

C (production of fibers and ground substances) is incorrect. This connective tissue cell does not produce connective fibers or ground substance components. The fibroblast performs that function, but it would have extensive rough endoplasmic reticulum and a different shape.

E (release of major basic protein) is incorrect. Major basic protein is produced by eosinophils. This connective tissue cell does not have a bilobed nucleus and granules, which are two visible characteristics of the eosinophil.

3. *D* (cell at D) is correct. In patients with cystic fibrosis, the sweat gland ducts fail to reabsorb chloride ions, leading to the accumulation of sodium chloride in sweat. This membrane transport failure is caused by a mutation in the cystic fibrosis transmembrane conductance regulator (CFTR). Sweat gland ducts are recognized by their darker-staining characteristics when compared with the secretory portions (cell at A) of the gland. Secretory cells and duct cells are located close to one another in this area of the dermis because the sweat gland is a simple coiled tubular gland. The coiled termination of the gland presents several profiles of the gland, which appear in cross section or longitudinal section in a circumscribed area.

A (cell at A) is incorrect. The cells at A are secretory cells of the sweat gland. The greatest volume of sweat is made by these cells and then modified by the duct cells.

B (cell at B) is incorrect. The cell at B is an adipocyte, which is not affected in cystic fibrosis.

C (cell at C) is incorrect. The cell at C is a myoepithelial cell, which has contractile properties and squeezes the secretory portion of the sweat gland. It is recognized by its position near the secretory cells and its eosinophilic or darker-staining properties, indicative of a cytoplasm filled with contractile microfilaments.

E (cell at E) is incorrect. The cell at E is an endothelial cell; it is not affected in cystic fibrosis.

4. *E* (site E) is correct. Site E identifies the cell membrane-lamina interactions. DMD is caused by a deficiency of dystrophin, an actin-associated protein. Dystrophin links the cytoplasmic actin filaments with laminin through a transmembrane dystrophin-associated glycoprotein complex. This network helps maintain the structural rigidity of the muscle fiber. It is also thought that the loss of dystrophin leads to sarcolemmal damage and then to necrosis of the muscle cell. Laminin completes the interaction with the extracellular matrix as it becomes associated with collagen in the endomysium. The DMD gene is located on the short arm of the X chromosome.

A   (site A) is incorrect. Vessels such as those seen at site A in the connective tissue perimysium are not affected in DMD. Endothelial cells are visible lining the vessel lumen.

B   (site B) is incorrect. Site B represents fibroblasts. Muscle fibers or cells are eventually lost in DMD, and this loss is accompanied by fibrosis and replacement with fat cells. The accumulation of fat cells accounts grossly for the pseudohypertrophy of muscles.

C   (site C) is incorrect. Site C indicates the extracellular protein. Extracellular proteins such as collagen and laminin, seen in this area of the endomysium, are not defective in DMD.

D   (site D) is incorrect. Site D indicates the myofibril filaments. The filaments of actin and myosin are not affected in DMD until the disease progresses and more myocyte necrosis occurs.

5. *B*   (monitoring of chloride content) is correct. The tip of the arrow points to the modified cells of the distal convoluted tubule, the macula densa. The section is readily identifiable as kidney because of the presence of the glomerulus at the upper right in the LM. The PAS stain accentuates the microvillous border of the proximal convoluted tubules and the basal laminae of tubules and glomerular epithelium. Macula densa cells are noted at the light microscope level by their close proximity, especially evident here by the compactness of the nuclei. These cells are able to detect decreases in the filtrate concentration of Na^+ and Cl^- and transfer this information to other cells of the juxtaglomerular apparatus, the renin-containing or juxtaglomerular (JG) cells. The cells nearest the afferent arteriole within the distal convoluted tubule wall make up the dense spot (macula densa). The JG cells, which are modified smooth muscle cells of the afferent arteriole, respond by secreting renin.

A   (absorption of all glucose) is incorrect. As discussed for Option B, absorption occurs along the distal convoluted tubule, and the cells located here perform an important function in cooperation with the JG cells and the extraglomerular mesangial cells. However, it is sodium that is absorbed along the distal convoluted tubule. Most glucose in absorbed in the proximal convoluted tubule.

C   (production of angiotensin-converting enzyme) is incorrect. Angiotensin-converting enzyme is primarily produced by endothelial cells of the lung. This enzyme works on the substrate (angiotensin II) produced from the reaction of renin (angiotensinogen) with angiotensin I.

D   (secretion of erythropoietin) is incorrect. Erythropoietin is produced by endothelial cells of the peritubular capillaries in the kidney cortex and perhaps by the extraglomerular mesangial cells.

E   (secretion of renin) is incorrect. The cells shown in the LM are located within the wall of the distal convoluted tubule. Renin-secreting cells would be located within the wall of the afferent arteriole.

6. **B** (melanocytes and Langerhans' cells) is correct. The darkly stained cells show the positive reaction for the S-100 protein. The Langerhans' cells make up about 4% of the epidermal cells and are the cells with long processes distributed through the stratum spinosum layer. The melanocytes are seen along the basal layer of the epidermis. Antibodies to S-100 are used to differentiate neural crest derivatives and their tumors, glial cell and ependymal cell tumors, and tumors of Schwann cells. The pattern of Langerhans' cells in the epidermis is especially noticeable in this section of human skin. The cells have long processes that extend through the epidermis and are useful in their function as antigen presenters.

A   (keratinocytes and Langerhans' cells) is incorrect. Most of the cells seen in the epidermis are keratinocytes, but they do not stain positively for S-100 (as indicated by a dark brown reaction). The nuclei of keratinocytes are visible throughout the stratum spinosum.
C   (Merkel cells) is incorrect. Merkel cells are found along the basal surface of the skin and may be modified keratinocytes, which contain neurosecretory granules and may function as mechanoreceptors. Such cells lack processes, unlike those seen in this section of skin.

7. **D**   (pacinian corpuscle) is correct. The pacinian corpuscle has the appearance of an onion in cross section, as seen here in the dermis of the skin. Sweat glands are present at the right of the LM, visible as tubular structures surrounded by adipose tissue. Pacinian corpuscles are also located in the periosteum and in connective tissue stroma of some organs and respond to touch and pressure. An axon is located in the center of the thin sheets of connective tissue lamellae.

A   (Krause end bulb) is incorrect. The asterisk indicates a pacinian corpuscle. Krause end bulbs are smaller than pacinian corpuscles, and the axon within has several branches. Like the pacinian corpuscle, the Krause end bulb is a type of mechanoreceptor.
B   (Meissner corpuscle) is incorrect. The asterisk indicates a pacinian corpuscle. Meissner corpuscles are pear-shaped or tornado-shaped structures located in the dermal papillae. A myelinated nerve fiber zigzags through the middle of this mechanoreceptor, which responds to slight deformation in the skin.
C   (Merkel ending) is incorrect. The asterisk indicates a pacinian corpuscle. Merkel endings are myelinated afferent fibers that terminate in contact with a Merkel cell near the stratum basale.
E   (Ruffini corpuscle) is incorrect. The asterisk indicates a pacinian corpuscle. Ruffini corpuscles are a different type of mechanoreceptor. They are usually oriented parallel to the skin, and bundles of collagen run through the core of the corpuscle.

8. *C* (immunoglobulins) is correct. The eccentric nucleus with marginal clumped chromatin, the abundance of rough endoplasmic reticulum (RER), and the paranuclear Golgi seen in this cell are characteristics of a plasma cell. Mitochondria are randomly distributed through the folds of RER, and lysosomes make up the organelles. Plasma cells manufacture the antibodies or immunoglobulins in the RER; the Golgi cross-links, attaches carbohydrate molecules, and packages the antibody. A directional signal is given to the small secretory vesicle as it travels through the Golgi, and it then moves to the cell membrane and is released by exocytosis. Some collagen fibrils are seen around the plasma cell.

A (histamine) is incorrect. Histamine is the main product of mast cells, which would not have as much RER as the plasma cell shown in the EM. Mast cells would also be packed with secretory granules.
B (hydrochloric acid) is incorrect. Hydrochloric acid is produced by parietal cells, which would not have as much RER as the plasma cell shown in the EM. Also, parietal cells would be packed with mitochondria.
D (isoenzymes) is incorrect. Although cells that secrete isoenzymes would contain the abundance of RER seen in the plasma cell in this EM, they would also contain large secretory granules.
E (tropocollagen) is incorrect. Tropocollagen is secreted by fibroblasts, which are elongated and have a different nuclear shape than the plasma cell seen in this EM. A fibroblast would also be surrounded by collagen, its secretory product.

9. *A* (lamellar body) is correct. The cell seen in this EM is a type II pneumocyte or great alveolar cell of the alveolar lining. The lamellar bodies are visible as dark, spherical granules with a concentric lamellar or myelin-figure appearance. The cell borders a lumen, which is the alveolar space, and rests on a basal lamina with collagen fibers in the interstitium. The cell is united to type I pneumocytes or squamous alveolar cells on either side by junctions. The lamellar bodies contain surfactant, which relieves surface tension as it spreads out over the surface of the type I cells and becomes a part of the blood–air barrier.

B (mucous granule) is incorrect. The asterisk indicates a lamellar body. Mucous granules would appear as clear or grayish structures on electron microscopy.
C (primary lysosome) is incorrect. The asterisk indicates a lamellar body. Primary lysosomes are homogeneous or contain a crystalline array of material.
D (secondary lysosomes) is incorrect. The asterisk indicates a lamellar body. Secondary lysosomes are heterogeneous. If this were a secondary lysosome, other types of secondary lysosomes would also be present. Although secondary lysosomes may appear as myelin figures and resemble lamellar bodies, the cell shown

here is a type II pneumocyte; thus the organelle is a lamellar body. Refer to the explanation for Option A.

10. *D* (HIV replication) is correct. The tip of the arrow points to the small, heterochromatic nucleus of a microglial cell. These cells can be recognized by their dense, irregularly shaped nuclei, when compared with the much larger, spherical, euchromatic nuclei of the astrocytes seen elsewhere in the LM. These cells are phagocytic and are derived from precursors in the bone marrow; thus they are considered the macrophage of the central nervous system. In patients infected with HIV-1, the microglia contain the virus and thus assist with its replication.

A (destruction of myelin in multiple sclerosis) is incorrect. The tip of the arrow points to a microglial cell. Destruction of myelin in patients with multiple sclerosis occurs as the result of an autoimmune process. The microglia then move into these areas and phagocytize the degraded myelin; however, they are not responsible for the initial destruction of myelin.
B (formation of gemistocytes) is incorrect. Gemistocytes are astrocytes with a prominent eosinophilic cytoplasm.
C (formation of gliosis) is incorrect. The multiplication of astrocytes around sites of tissue injury is referred to as gliosis. Astrocyte nuclei are spherical, euchromatic, and much larger than the nucleus seen at the tip of the arrow, which is a microglial cell.
E (myelin synthesis) is incorrect. Synthesis of myelin in the central nervous system is performed by oligodendrocytes. These cells have a spherical, heterochromatic nucleus that is smaller than the nucleus of astrocytes (seen elsewhere in the LM).

11. *D* (Langerhans' cell) is correct. Features of the Langerhans' cell include a convoluted nucleus with deep infoldings and a clear cytoplasm with scattered organelles. The Langerhans' cell is surrounded by keratinocytes with spherical nuclei that are much darker or electron dense. Most of this dense material consists of bundles of intermediate filaments or tonofibrils. Langerhans' cells do not form desmosomes with the keratinocytes but merely make contact with them along their periphery. Thus, no desmosomes would be seen between the Langerhans' cell and the keratinocytes. The pale cytoplasm indicates the absence of melanosomes. The Langerhans' cell plays a significant role in immunologic reactions; is capable of binding, processing, and presenting antigens; and is CD1 positive. None of the other cells listed in Options A, B, C, and E is CD1 positive. Langerhans' cells have dendritic processes, although these cannot be seen in this EM.

A (helper T cell) is incorrect. The cell shown is a Langerhans' cell. A helper T cell does not have a convoluted nucleus, and it is positive for CD3-5.

B (histiocyte) is incorrect. A histiocyte is the connective tissue macrophage and would have a more heterogeneous cytoplasm than is seen here. It would also be surrounded by collagen.

C (Kupffer's cell) is incorrect. A Kupffer's cell is the macrophage of the liver and lines a sinusoid. These features and the sinusoid lumen would be apparent in an EM.

E (M cell) is incorrect. An M cell is associated with lymphocytes in lymphoid aggregates called Peyer patches. M cells take up whole particles (bacteria, viruses) but transfer these foreign substances to neighboring lymphocytes. M cells have folds along the intestinal surface that distinguish them from the microvilli-covered enterocytes.

12. **D** (paclitaxel) is correct. The fluorescein-labeled organelles, which appear as bright structures in the cell center, are microtubules in the mitotic spindle of metaphase cells. The dark area in the center of the cells represents the chromosomes. Paclitaxel was originally isolated from the bark of the Pacific yew tree. Its mechanism was later found to be stabilization of microtubules, promoting the assembly of tubulin subunits and inhibiting depolymerization. This stabilization prevents chromosome movement and thus mitosis. It is known that microtubules are polar-oriented structures in the mitotic cell, adding tubulin subunits at one end and removing tubulin subunits at the other. Semisynthetic paclitaxel (Taxol) is more commonly used now as an anticancer agent.

A (bleomycin) is incorrect. Bleomycin is a cytostatic antibiotic that inserts into double-stranded DNA, leading to strand breakage.

B (cyclosporine) is incorrect. Cyclosporine inhibits the production of cytotoxic T lymphocytes by inhibiting transcription in precursors to these cells.

C (methotrexate) is incorrect. Methotrexate inhibits synthesis of DNA and RNA by inhibiting dihydrofolate reductase, an enzyme important in the synthesis of purines and thymidine.

E (vinblastine) is incorrect. Vinblastine, which is derived from the periwinkle plant, acts to prevent the polymerization of tubulin subunits into microtubules. The end result, however, is the same as occurs with paclitaxel—the prevention of mitosis.

13. **B** (macula densa–keratin) is correct. All of the junctions seen are macula densa junctions or desmosomes joining epithelial cells. They are recognized by a central linear density and distinct filaments that enter a darker region (intracellular plaque) from the cellular side. Keratin filaments of 10 nm or intermediate size are always associated with the macula densa junction. A bundle of microfilaments or actin filaments is also apparent in the EM, but these microfilaments run at a right angle to the intermediate filaments.

A   (fascia adherens–actin) is incorrect. The fascia adherens is a junction found in the transverse portion of the intercalated disk. It is anchored by actin filaments. No sarcomeres or myofibrils are visible in this EM.
C   (macula densa–vimentin) is incorrect. Vimentin filaments are characteristic of mesenchymal-derived cells and are not associated with the macula densa or desmosome. Keratin is the characteristic filament of epithelial-derived cells.
D   (zonula adherens–actin) and E (zonula adherens–vimentin) are incorrect. The zonula adherens does not have intercellular or transmembrane proteins in the junction. Actin filaments are associated with the zonula adherens, but the filaments seen in this EM are bigger than microfilaments. The filaments can be seen individually at this power; thus they are intermediate in type (keratin, vimentin, etc.). Vimentin filaments are not associated with any junctional type.

14. *B*   (Birbeck granule) is correct. Tennis racquet–shaped Birbeck granules are seen near both the nucleus and the cell membrane of this Langerhans' cell. The handle of the racquet has a linear density down the middle that is faintly visible in the EM. It is thought that these structures react with antigen being processed by the Langerhans' cell. Note the convoluted nucleus and otherwise lightly staining cytoplasm of this cell. The cell at the lower left is a keratinocyte, which contains darkly stained tonofilaments. The two cells are closely apposed but do not form desmosomes.

A   (beta granule) is incorrect. Beta granules of the pancreatic islet contain a characteristic small, round granule that has a crystal (or crystals) lying in flocculent matrix. They are sometimes called insulin granules.
C   (melanosome) is incorrect. Melanosomes are ellipsoid organelles that, in the later stages of development, become dense. In early stages they have a herringbone appearance. Melanosomes are the characteristic organelle of melanocytes and keratinocytes.
D   (Weibel-Palade granule) is incorrect. Weibel-Palade granules are cylindrical structures with tubular inclusions that are characteristic of endothelial cells.
E   (zebra body) is incorrect. Zebra bodies are lysosomes with accumulations of glycolipids that appear as stacks of osmiophilic material membranes and are characteristic of Fabry's disease.

15. *A*   (liberation of pharmacologically active substances) is correct. This TEM shows a mast cell. The whorled or scroll like arrangement of the granules and their dense numbers are the primary identification factors for this cell at the ultrastructural level. The nucleus is usually centrally located in such a cell but only a portion of the nucleus (Nu) is seen here. Mast cells quite often have elaborate cell borders with long microvilli for interaction with the environment. Histamine and other vasoactive mediators are contained in the granules.

B (phagocytosis of foreign substances) is incorrect. The connective tissue cell seen in this TEM does not have the features (secondary lysosomes, heterogeneous cytoplasm) of a macrophage that phagocytizes foreign substances.

C (production of fibers and ground substances) is incorrect. This connective tissue cell does not produce connective fibers or ground substance components. The fibroblast, which performs that function, would have extensive rough endoplasmic reticulum without the large number of granules seen in this TEM.

D (production of immunocompetent cells) is incorrect. This connective tissue cell contains granules, which indicates an end-stage differentiation or a cell other than those associated with the lymphoid cell line.

E (releasing of major basic protein) is incorrect. Major basic protein is produced by eosinophils. The connective tissue cell shown in this TEM does not have the characteristic crystal-containing granules of an eosinophil.

16. A (alveolar macrophages) is correct. These alveolar macrophages appear to be floating in the alveolar space but may be associated with the alveolar epithelium out of the plane. However, alveolar macrophages are free cells that migrate over the luminal surface. The thin alveolar epithelium can be seen at the top right and the bottom left of the EM. The ultrastructural features of alveolar macrophages as seen here include a large size (when compared with the red blood cells [RBCs] and neutrophil seen at the right of the center), irregular nuclei, many primary and secondary lysosomes, and a surface with prominent filopodia. Some congestion is present in this lung tissue, as indicated by the large number of RBCs in the alveolar space.

B (neutrophils) is incorrect. These cells are too large to be neutrophils. In addition, they have an irregular, convoluted nucleus instead of the lobed nucleus characteristic of neutrophils.

C (type I pneumocytes) is incorrect. Type I pneumocytes are flat cells, also called squamous alveolar cells, that are associated with the alveolar lining. They are seen lining the lumen at the top right in this EM.

D (type II pneumocytes) is incorrect. Type II pneumocytes are associated with the alveolar wall, forming junctions with type I pneumocytes. They contain lamellar bodies.

17. A (gap junction) is correct. The gap junction permits communication between these two cells by allowing passage of small molecules, thus permitting metabolic coupling. Gap junctions are longer than the other types of junctions, and the cell membranes are closely apposed with gaps along the membranes. The intercellular transmembrane channels or pores are made up of a protein called connexin. The dotlike connexin can be seen between the cell membranes.

B   (synapse) is incorrect. In a synapse, a number of vesicles are associated with one side of the two membranes. The cell membranes are not closely apposed, as seen here; instead, there is a space or cleft between the two membranes.
C   (zonula adherens) is incorrect. In a zonula adherens, the membranes are not connected with channels between cells.
D   (zonula occludens) is incorrect. In a zonula occludens, the membranes fuse; there is no communication between the cells.

18. *D*   (pemphigus vulgaris) is correct. In pemphigus vulgaris, the body produces IgG autoantibodies to the transmembrane adhesion protein of the desmosome, desmoglein. The intercellular plaque seen in the micrograph represents the desmoglein. Identification of this structure as a desmosome is confirmed by the presence of intermediate filaments entering into the cytoplasmic dense plaque on either side. The reaction of the antibody with the desmoglein results in dyshesion: The desmosome deteriorates, keratin filaments or tonofilaments are released and clump around the nucleus, and the cells separate. This process leads to intraepidermal vesicle formation, which can contain detached keratinocytes.

A   (bullous pemphigoid) is incorrect. Although bullous pemphigoid involves the production of IgG autoantibodies, these autoantibodies are made against a component of the basal lamina found just beneath the stratum basale.
B   (epidermolysis bullosa simplex) is incorrect. In epidermolysis bullosa simplex, a defect in keratin genes occurs. Production of intermediate filaments is responsible for changes in the epidermis.
C   (ichthyosis) is incorrect. Ichthyosis is characterized by a thickening of the stratum corneum (the external epidermal layer). It can have several causes, but none of them involves production of autoantibodies.
E   (vitiligo) is incorrect. In vitiligo, melanocytes are destroyed by what is thought to be an autoimmune mechanism. Melanocytes are not seen in this EM. Furthermore, melanocytes are not joined by desmosomes, nor are they joined to keratinocytes by desmosomes.

19. *C*   (dynein) is correct. These cross sections of cilia show the characteristic 9 + 2 arrangement of microtubules. Axonemal dynein is the molecular motor protein associated with cilia and flagella. (A flagellum will have the same 9 + 2 arrangement.) Motor proteins generate the sliding or moving forces in various cytoskeletal systems. An active ATPase is associated with these motor proteins. Axonemal dynein moves one microtubule across the surface of its neighboring microtubule, resulting in the bending of cilia or flagella.

A   (actinin) is incorrect. Actinin is not a molecular motor protein; it is an actin cross-linking protein found in filopodia, lamellipodia (ruffles), stress fibers, and adhesion plaques.

B (clathrin) is incorrect. Clathrin is a protein associated with coated vesicles. It forms a complex on the cytoplasmic side of endocytotic vesicles that lends stability to the vesicle.

D (kinesin) is incorrect. Kinesin is a molecular motor protein, but it is associated with cytoplasmic microtubules and not with axonemal microtubules. Vesicles move along microtubules with the aid of kinesin.

E (myosin) is incorrect. Myosin is a molecular motor protein, but it is not associated with cilia. It is associated with actin in both muscle and nonmuscle filamentous systems.

20. **E** (tonofilaments) is correct. Keratin is an intracellular protein arranged in a fibrillar or filamentous pattern. Keratin filaments are usually bundled into larger groups, which are then referred to as tonofilaments. These filaments may extend throughout the cell, giving structural support and mechanical stability to the cell. They may weave close to the nucleus, and they may end in junctions or desmosomes at the cell surface. Desmosomes may not be formed in some tissues, especially tumors.

A (cells arranged like keratinocytes) is incorrect. A cellular arrangement would not necessarily occur in a cell, and the arrangement of the cells does not guarantee the appearance of an intracellular protein.

B (desmosomes) is incorrect. As discussed for Option E, desmosomes may not be formed in some tissues, even though keratin filaments are present in the cell. Some tumor cells do not make contact and thus do not form desmosomes.

C (granules filled with keratin) and D (intracytoplasmic inclusions filled with keratin) are incorrect. Keratin is not packaged into granules but is arranged as a fibrillar protein in the form of intermediate filaments. If keratin filaments are disrupted, they usually coil throughout the cell in a random arrangement.

21. **B** (dystrophin) is correct. Dystrophin is a structural protein found in striated muscle and binds the cytoplasmic side of the sarcolemma to actin. Duchenne's muscular dystrophy (DMD) is characterized by a progressive degeneration of skeletal muscle fibers. The severity of the dystrophy depends upon the extent of damage to the gene that carries the code for dystrophin. In Duchenne type dystrophy, an X-linked gene results in the absence of dystrophin. In the Becker type of dystrophy, the same X-linked gene is not as severely damaged; as a result, dystrophin is produced by the cell, but it is abnormal. For this reason, the Becker type of dystrophy is not as severe as DMD.

A (actin) is incorrect. Actin is one of the main components of thin filaments in muscle fibers. In patients with DMD, dystrophin is absent. This defect contributes to the progressive degeneration of skeletal muscle fibers seen in individuals with this disorder.

C (myosin) is incorrect. Myosin is one of the main components of thick filaments; it is *not* missing in patients with DMD.

D (tropomyosin) is incorrect. Tropomyosin consists of pencil-shaped molecules that lie in shallow grooves on the surface of the actin filaments. It is not missing in patients with DMD.

E (troponin) is incorrect. A single troponin molecule is bound to tropomyosin by one of its subunits (TnT). TnC, one of the other subunits of troponin, has a great affinity for calcium. The third type of troponin subunit, TnI, binds to actin and prevents an interaction between actin and myosin. When calcium binds to TnC, this subunit undergoes a conformational change that causes tropomyosin to expose previously blocked active sites on actin filaments. This allows myosin heads to bind with actin and results in the thick and thin filaments sliding by each other, shortening the length of the sarcomeres and mediating muscle contraction. These factors are not altered in patients with DMD. Serum troponin levels are increased in patients with an acute myocardial infarction.

22. *A* (cholecystokinin) is correct. Cholecystokinin (CCK) is released by enteroendocrine cells in the small intestine in the presence of lipids. CCK causes smooth muscle in the gallbladder to contract to move bile into the common bile duct to reach the intestine. It has the opposite effect on smooth muscle in the sphincter of Oddi, causing it to relax and allow bile to flow into the duodenum.

B (gastrin) is incorrect. Gastrin is secreted by the enteroendocrine cells of both the stomach and the small intestine. One effect of gastrin is stimulation of the secretion of HCl from the parietal cells in the gastric glands.

C (glucagon) is incorrect. Glucagon is produced by enteroendocrine cells in the stomach and small intestine and alpha cells in the pancreas. It primarily stimulates gluconeogenesis in the hepatocytes.

D (motilin) is incorrect. Motilin is synthesized and released by enteroendocrine cells in the small intestine. It increases peristaltic activity of the intestine.

E (secretin) is incorrect. Secretin is produced by enteroendocrine cells in the small intestine to induce the ductal epithelium of the pancreas to release a bicarbonate-rich watery fluid.

23. *E* (zonula occludens) is correct. The zonula occludens is a belt-like membrane that completely surrounds the cell, forming a permeability seal.

A (macula adherens) is incorrect. A macula adherens joins two cells at a discrete spot on the cell surface. Material can pass between the cells in other areas. Therefore a macula adherens does not provide a permeability seal around the entire cell.

B (macula occludens) is incorrect. A macula occludens is a belt-like region that does not completely surround the cell. Material can pass between two cells by avoiding this region.

C (nexus) is incorrect. A nexus (gap junction) provides channels that allow ions to flow between adjacent cells. It does not prevent the flow of material between cells.

D (zonula adherens) is incorrect. A zonula adherens is a discrete region in which two cells are held together. Material can pass between the cells by flowing around this zone.

24. *B* (centriole) is correct. Autophagia is the digestion of intracellular constituents by the cell's own lysosomes. The only structure listed that is intrinsic to the cell is the centriole.

A (bacteria) and E (viral particle) are incorrect. Bacteria and viruses enter the cell by direct invasion or endocytosis. Since they are not normal components of the cell, their destruction is not considered autophagic activity.

C (collagen fibers) is incorrect. Collagen is found in supporting tissue and hyaline cartilage.

D (vesicular contents) is incorrect. Intracellular vesicles are formed around ingested material, which is not a normal component of the cell. Therefore, the destruction of vesicular contents is not considered autophagic activity.

25. *E* (mitotic nondisjunction) is correct. Changes in the chromosomal constitution of a cell indicate that a mitotic event has occurred. Mitotic nondisjunction is the failure of sister chromatids to separate during anaphase. This process is responsible for a cell containing an extra chromosome.

A (meiotic anaphase lagging) and C (mitotic anaphase lagging) are incorrect. Anaphase lagging is the failure of a chromatid to move as quickly as the other chromatids during anaphase. This results in that chromatid (chromosome) being excluded from a daughter cell and in a cell with fewer (not extra) chromosomes.

B (meiotic nondisjunction) is incorrect. Meiotic nondisjunction is the failure of chromatids to separate during meiosis. It results in all cells having the same chromosomal constitution.

D (mitotic deletion) is incorrect. Mitotic deletion is the loss of part of a chromosome during mitosis. It does not change the number of chromosomes in the cell.

26. *A* (either one chromosome or one Y chromosome) is correct. The normal male gamete (sperm) contains one sex chromosome—either one X or one Y chromosome. When the primary spermatocyte enters meiosis I, the X chromosome and the Y chromosome pair up. At the end of meiosis I, each primary spermatocyte divides, producing two daughter cells, called *secondary spermatocytes*. Each secondary spermatocyte acquires either an X chromosome or a Y chromosome from the primary spermatocyte.

B (either two X chromosomes or two Y chromosomes) is incorrect. When the primary spermatocyte goes through anaphase I, its hemologous chromosome pairs separate, so that one sex chromosome ends up at one pole in the cell and the other ends up at the opposite pole. Even if nondisjunction were to occur (i.e., the chromosome pairs failed to separate during anaphase I), neither daughter cell would acquire two of the same chromosomes.

C (one X chromosome and one Y chromosome) is incorrect. During anaphase I, the sex chromosome pair in the primary spermatocyte separates and each member of the pair travels to opposite ends of the cell. Following telekinesis, each secondary spermatocyte will contain the single sex chromosome. The only way a single secondary spermatocyte can acquire both chromosomes from a primary spermatocyte is through nondisjunction (failure of a chromosome pair to separate during anaphase I). This is an abnormal condition, however.

D (two X chromosomes and two Y chromosomes) is incorrect. A primary spermatocyte only inherits a single X chromosome and a single Y chromosome from the spermatogonium. Therefore a secondary spermatocyte cannot acquire four chromosomes from a primary spermatocyte, especially since the secondary spermatocyte is a product of reductional division of a primary spermatocyte.

27. **D** (smooth endoplasmic reticulum) is correct. SER is a cytoplasmic organelle that contains enzymes required for steroid biosynthesis.

A (Golgi apparatus) is incorrect. The Golgi apparatus is a cytoplasmic organelle in which protein processing takes place.

B (nucleus) is incorrect. The synthesis of steroids takes place in the cytoplasm of the cell.

C (rough endoplasmic reticulum) is incorrect. RER is a cytoplasmic organelle in which protein synthesis takes place.

28. **A** (basal layer) is correct. Cells on the surface of normal stratified epithelia are replaced by continuously replicating vegetative intermitotic cells from the stem cell population in the basal layer.

B (intermediate layer) is incorrect. The intermediate layer in normal stratified epithelia contains differentiating intermitotic cells but no stem cells.

C (surface layer) is incorrect. The surface of normal stratified epithelia contains nonreplicating fixed postmitotic cells.

D (underlying connective tissue) is incorrect. Connective tissue lies beneath epithelia and does not contribute to the epithelial cell population.

29. *C* (increase in amount of tropoelastin in connective tissue) is correct. The amount of tropoelastin will increase because the drug does not interfere with tropoelastin synthesis. The elasticity of the tissue may decrease, however, because drug X prevents the cross-linking of tropoelastin fibers, which is necessary for the formation of elastin.

A (decrease in amount of tropoelastin in connective tissue) is incorrect. Tropoelastin continues to be synthesized during treatment with drug X. Therefore the amount of tropoelastin in connective tissue should increase (not decrease).
B (increase in amount of elastin in connective tissue) is incorrect. Although tropoelastin continues to be synthesized, drug X prevents it from forming cross links, and thus prevents the formation of elastin.
D (increase in the elasticity of the tissue) is incorrect. Elasticity will decrease because of decreased cross-linking of tropoelastin fibers.

30. *C* (neurons) is correct. Ionizing radiation kills cells in every stage of the cell cycle (i.e., both replicating and nonreplicating cells). Since neurons are fixed postmitotic cells, they cannot be replaced if they are destroyed.

A (astrocytes), B (microglia), and D (oligodendrocytes) are incorrect. These central nervous system glial cells are all reverting postmitotic cells. Although they can be damaged by ionizing radiation, they can be replaced.

31. *B* (localized in the A band) is correct. Thick filaments are found only in the A band.

A (attached to the Z line) is incorrect. Thin filaments (rather than thick filaments) are attached to the Z line.
C (localized in the A and I bands) is incorrect. Thin filaments are localized in both the A and I bands.
D (same as a single myosin molecule) is incorrect. Thick filaments are composed of hundreds of myosin molecules.
E (shortened during muscle contraction) is incorrect. Thick filaments do not shorten. The length of the sarcomere and the width of the I band shorten.

32. *B* (electron transport system subunits) is correct. Some of the subunits of the electron transport system and certain subunits of adenosine triphosphate (ATP) synthase are transcribed from the mitochondrial genome and translated on mitochondrial ribosomes. The other proteins listed are encoded in nuclear DNA and translated on cytoplasmic ribosomes.

A (DNA polymerase) is incorrect. DNA polymerase catalyzes the polymerization of nucleotides. It is encoded by nuclear (not mitochondrial) DNA.
C (enzymes of the tricarboxylic acid cycle) is incorrect. The TCA cycle is a metabolic pathway that catalyzes the production of ATP. These enzymes in this pathway are encoded by nuclear (not mitochondrial) DNA.
D (permeases of the inner mitochondrial membrane) is incorrect. Permeases are enzymes that enable substances to pass through a cell membrane. These enzymes are encoded by nuclear (not mitochondrial) DNA.
E (structural proteins of the outer mitochondrial membrane) is incorrect. These proteins are encoded by nuclear (not mitochondrial) DNA.

33. *C* (nexus) is correct. A nexus (gap junction) is a bridge between the membranes of adjacent cells. Nexi enable small ions to pass from a cell to an adjacent cell without passing through the extracellular space.

A (macula adherens), B (macula occludens), and D (zonula adherens) are incorrect. These structures hold cells together mechanically. They do not provide a passageway for communication between adjacent cells.
E (zonula occludens) is incorrect. A zonula occludens creates a permeability seal, which prevents particles from passing between cells.

34. *C* (3) is correct. The number of sex chromatin bodies is equal to the number of X chromosomes minus one. This cell will receive all four X chromatids from the ovum and no X chromosomes from the sperm.

A (1) is incorrect. A single sex chromatin body would be seen during interphase when two X chromosomes are present.
B (2) is incorrect. Two sex chromatin bodies would be seen during interphase when three X chromosomes are present.
D (4) is incorrect. Four sex chromatin bodies would be seen during interphase when five X chromosomes are present.
E (5) is incorrect. Five sex chromatin bodies would be seen during interphase when six X chromosomes are present.

35. *B* (nonreplicators with no stem cells) is correct. Nitrogen mustard is an alkylating agent that kills cells in every stage of the cell cycle. Cells in normal tissues are also affected by this therapy. Nonreplicators with no stem cell compartment will be destroyed and will not be replaced.

A (continuous replicators) is incorrect. Continuous replicators include stem cells for bone marrow and intestinal epithelium. These cells arrive from a sequence of increasingly differentiated

cells. As such, there is a pool of stem cells that can differentiate and replace the continuous replicators when they die or are destroyed.
C   (occasional replicators) is incorrect. These cells will be destroyed and will be replaced.

36. *A*   (G_1) is correct. The meiotic cells are blocked after having distributed half of their DNA content to each of two daughter cells. The DNA was previously duplicated during the S phase of the cell cycle. Therefore the meiotic cells contain the same amount of DNA as a G_1 somatic cell (i.e., before DNA is duplicated).

B   (G_2), C (metaphase of mitosis), D (middle of the S phase), and E (prophase of mitosis) are incorrect. A cell that completes meiosis I produces two daughter cells, each of which contains half as much DNA as the parent cell. Thus, each daughter cell contains the same amount of DNA as a somatic cell before it reaches the S phase of the cell cycle. Therefore these blocked cells will contain less DNA than a somatic cell in the S phase of subsequent G_2 phase or mitosis.

37. *A*   (a proteoglycan-degrading hydrolase is missing) is correct. Patients with Hurler syndrome lack an enzyme that is necessary for the breakdown of proteoglycans. Proteoglycan synthesis continues, however, and proteoglycans accumulate in body tissues.

B   (the connective tissue lacks lysosomes) is incorrect. Lack of a lysosome-specific hydrolase usually means that the lysosomes are not producing the enzyme in adequate amounts. It does not necessarily mean that the lysosomes themselves are in short supply.
C   (the rate of proteoglycan degradation has increased) is incorrect. The rate at which proteoglycans break down in patients with Hurler syndrome is slower than in normal patients.
D   (the rate of proteoglycan synthesis has increased) is incorrect. The rate of proteoglycan synthesis in patients with Hurler syndrome is the same as that in patients who do not have the disease.

38. *B*   (encircles the cell completely) is correct. The membranes of adjacent cells bind together within the zonula adherens.

A   (allows electronic coupling of adjacent cells) is incorrect. The gap junction (nexus) serves as a means of direct communication between adjacent cells. This allows electrons to flow from cell to cell, resulting in electronic coupling of adjacent cells.
C   (fuses outer leaflets of plasma membrane) is incorrect. The outer leaflets of the plasma membrane fuse in an occludens junction, not the zonula adherens.
D   (serves as a barrier to diffusion) is incorrect. The zonula occludens provides a permeability seal.

39. *C* (they contain myosin) is correct. The thick filaments contain the contractile protein myosin.

A (they are found in the I band) is incorrect. The thick filaments are found only in the A band.
B (they contain actin) and C (they contain tropomyosin) are incorrect. Actin and tropomyosin are found in the thin (not thick) filaments.

40. *C* (proliferation of Schwann cells proximal to the injury) is correct. Injury to a peripheral nerve axon results in a proliferation of Schwann cells, which guide the regenerating axon to its intended target.

A (death of neurons in the dorsal horn of the spinal cord) is incorrect. Injury to a peripheral nerve axon can result in the death of neurons in the dorsal root ganglion of sensory nerve fibers. It does not affect the dorsal horn, which contains the cell bodies of second-order sensory neurons.
B (degeneration of nerve processes proximal to the injury) is incorrect. Injury to a peripheral nerve axon can result in degeneration of the axon distal to the injury. This suggests that proteins are still being produced in the cell body and are still transported to the proximal segment of the axon; however, because of the injury, they are not transported to the distal segment of the axon.
D (reactive changes in the lower thoracic dorsal root ganglia cells) is incorrect. Reactive changes associated with damage to a peripheral nerve in the forearm would occur in dorsal root ganglia located in the lower cervical and upper thoracic regions, not the lower thoracic region of the spinal cord.

41. *D* (peroxisome) is correct. Peroxisomes contain various oxidative enzymes and catalase. A lack of peroxisomes is responsible for Zellweger syndrome.

A (lysosome) is incorrect. Lysosomes contain hydrolytic (not oxidative) enzymes. When these hydrolytic enzymes are lacking, the affected individual may develop Tay-Sachs disease or Gaucher's disease. Lysosomes do not play a role in Zellweger syndrome.
B (microtubule) is incorrect. Microtubules are essential for cell movement and maintaining the cell shape.
C (mitochondrion) is incorrect. Oxidative phosphorylation occurs in the mitochondria. A defect in the enzymes responsible for oxidative phosphorylation can interfere with the production of adenosine triphosphate.

42. *C* (nonpolar tails of phospholipids) is correct. Nonpolar tails of phospholipids are found on the P face and E face of the plasma membrane.

A (extrinsic membrane proteins), B (glycocalyx), and D (polar heads of phospholipids) are incorrect. These molecules are found on the extracellular surface of the plasma membrane.

43. *C* (peptide hormone production in a glandular cell) is correct. Cells that are in the process of producing large amounts of protein to export have more RER than SER.

A (contraction of a skeletal muscle fiber) is incorrect. The endoplasmic reticulum is replaced by the sarcoplasmic reticulum (SR) in muscle fibers. Skeletal muscle contains a large amount of SR, which stores much of the calcium that is used during contraction. The amount of SR does not change during contraction.
B (fat absorption in a columnar epithelial cell) is incorrect. Simple columnar epithelia is found along highly absorptive surfaces, including that of the small intestine (where fat is absorbed). Fat is degraded to monoglycerides, cholesterol, and fatty acids, all of which are absorbed. Medium-sized fatty acids are re-esterified to form triglycerides in mucosal cells, which occurs in the SER. Therefore SER will exceed RER in epithelial cells.
D (steroid hormone production in a glandular cell) is incorrect. Steroid synthesis takes place in the SER. Therefore this compartment will exceed the RER concentration during this process.

44. *B* (have the greatest amount of glycogen per fiber) is correct. White fibers in skeletal muscle show the greatest amount of glycogen.

A (are rich in myoglobin) is incorrect. Myoglobin is an oxygen-binding molecule. Red muscle fiber is rich in myoglobin.
C (have the greatest number of mitochondria per fiber) is incorrect. The mitochondrion is the "power house" of the cell, generating adenosine triphosphate molecules, which are used for energy. Red skeletal muscle fibers usually contain more mitochondria per fiber than white skeletal muscle fibers.
D (have slow contractions and support continuous heavy work) is incorrect. Red muscle fibers demonstrate slow contractions and support continuous heavy work.

45. *A* (A band length during relaxation) is correct. The length of the A band does not change during relaxation.

B (H band length during contraction) and C (I band length during contraction) are incorrect. The length of the H band and the I band both decrease during contraction.

46. *D*   (lack of prolyl and lysyl hydroxylase activity) is correct. Ascorbic acid is a cofactor in the catalysis of procollagen hydroxylation. Inadequate hydroxylation of procollagen results in inadequate cross-linking of collagen fibers, and consequently in weak collagen fibers or an inadequate number of normal collagen fibers. This defect causes weakened capillary and venule walls, which results in leakage of blood and leads to purpura and ecchymosis. It also results in weakened mucosa, which allows oral ulcers to develop. Sharpey's fibers, which attach the periosteum to bone, will also weaken, resulting in subperiosteal hemorrhages.

A   (failure to maintain fully differentiated epithelia) is incorrect. Epithelial differentiation is an important function of vitamin A. A deficiency in this vitamin can be ruled out in this patient, because his symptoms are not consistent with this problem. Much of the damage observed in the patient (particularly the ecchymoses and purpura) indicates the presence of leaky small blood vessels and suggests that the entire depth of the blood vessel wall has been breached—the endothelium as well as connective tissue surrounding these vessels. Vitamin A deficiency would not be responsible for this type of damage.
B   (inadequate mineralization of cancellous bone) is incorrect. The absorption of calcium from the intestine and its uptake into bone is diminished in individuals with hypovitaminosis D. Inadequate mineralization of bone can result in rickets (distortion of muscle-associated bones) or osteomalacia (softening of bone). Neither of these conditions was reported for this patient.
C   (increased intracellular levels of protein p53) is incorrect. The intracellular protein p53 accumulates in the cell in response to DNA damage (e.g., as a result of exposure to mutagenic agents or ionizing radiation). This type of exposure was not reported for this patient. Protein p53 causes the cell to arrest in the G_1 phase of the cell cycle, which gives the cell time to attempt to repair the damage before entering the S phase (when DNA is synthesized).

47. *C*   (interconnect haversian canals) is correct. Volkmann's canals run at various angles to the haversian systems, which run parallel to the long axis of long bones. Thus they interconnect haversian systems.

A   (are components of interstitial lamellae) is incorrect. Interstitial lamellae are small chunks of old, remodeled haversian systems. Volkmann's canal are not involved in the remodeling process and are not components of the interstitial lamellae.
B   (contain the processes of osteocytes) is incorrect. Volkmann's canals, like haversian canals, contain blood and lymph vessels. They do not contain the processes of osteocytes.
D   (interconnect lacunae) is incorrect. Lacunae are interconnected by canaliculi, not Volkmann's canals.

48. *A* (change in the structure of spectrin) is correct. Spectrin is a large, long microfilament with actin-binding sites on each end. These sites allow spectrin molecules to form a dense cytoskeletal meshwork adjacent to the P surface of the red blood cell (RBC) plasmalemma. A defect in the genetic code for spectrin results in a change in spectrin structure, hence, a change in the cytoskeleton of the RBC. Specifically, it causes RBCs to lose their normal biconcavity and take on a spherical shape.

   B (decrease in the area of hyalomere) is incorrect. Spherocytosis affects RBCs. The hyalomere is the peripheral part of platelets (not RBCs).
   C (decrease in the diameter of the affected cell) is incorrect. Spherocytosis affects an intracellular structural protein in RBCs. Damage to this protein affects the unique shape of the cell, not the overall diameter of the cell.
   D (increase in intrinsic cell membrane proteins) is incorrect. Spherocytosis affects the structure of an intracellular protein. It does not affect intrinsic proteins of the plasmalemma.
   E (increase in the size of the granulomere region of a cell) is incorrect. Spherocytosis affects an intercellular protein in RBCs. The granulomere is the granular central region of thrombocytes.

49. *A* (cord of Billroth in the spleen) is correct. The cords of Billroth are oblong aggregations of lymphatic tissue that lie between venous sinusoids in the red pulp of the spleen. Blood entering the spleen from the circulatory system passes through the cords of Billroth, where the formed elements of blood encounter macrophages that reside in these cords. The macrophages destroy damaged erythrocytes, including the sickle-shaped cells in this patient. Because of this activity, splenomegaly is a common finding in African-American patients with sickle cell anemia.

   B (hematopoietic cord of bone marrow) is incorrect. The hematopoietic cords of the bone marrow are the areas in which erythrocytopoiesis occurs.
   C (marginal zone of the spleen) is incorrect. The marginal zone lies between the red pulp and the white pulp of the spleen. Although it contains macrophages, the primary activity in this region is the presentation of antigens to T cells and B cells by dendritic cells in an attempt to trigger an immune response.
   D (medullary region of the thymus) is incorrect. The primary function of the thymus is to produce immunocompetent T cells. The medulla of the thymus contains mature T cells, which leave the thymus via venules and efferent lymphatic vessels to populate other lymphoid organs (e.g., the lymph nodes and spleen). Phagocytosis is not carried out by red blood cells.
   E (paratrabecular sinus in a lymph node) is incorrect. The subcapsular, medullary, and paratrabecular sinuses of the lymph node are bridged by phagocytic cells. These sinuses contain lymph (not blood).

50. *C* (overexpression of D cyclins) is correct. D cyclins are overexpressed in many types of tumors. An abnormally high level of D cyclins allows the phosphorylation of CDKs, which triggers CDK activity. CDKs then phosphorylate pRBs. Unphosphorylated pRBs block the progression of normal cells from the G_1 phase of the cell cycle (when cell proteins are made) to the S phase (when DNA is duplicated). Phosphorylation of pRBs removes this blockade, allowing the cell to "run" its cell cycle.

A (lack of cyclin-dependent kinase activity) is incorrect. Nonphosphorylated CDKs are inactive.
B (lack of retinoblastoma protein phosphorylation) is incorrect. Nonphosphorylated pRBs prevent normal cells from progressing from the G_1 to the S phase of the cell cycle. They are part of the cell's intrinsic mechanism for controlling cell growth and preventing the formation of tumors.
D (underexpression of D cyclins) is incorrect. As long as D cyclin levels are not excessive, pRB proteins will not be phosphorylated. The lack of phosphorylated pRBs prevents normal cells from progressing from the G_1 phase of the cell cycle to the S phase. It is part of the cell's intrinsic mechanism for controlling cell growth.
E (up-regulation of p53) is incorrect. p53 causes the cell to arrest in the G_1 phase of the cell cycle. This prevents the cell from preparing for replication.

TEST 2

DIRECTIONS: Each numbered item or incomplete statement is followed by options arranged in alphabetical or logical order. Select the best answer to each question. Some options may be partially correct, but there is only **ONE BEST** answer.

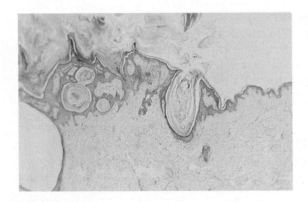

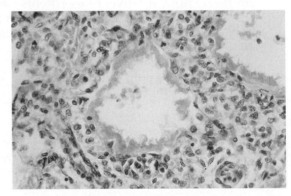

1. The photomicrograph shows tissue obtained by biopsy from a 32-year-old landscaper with a skin lesion in the axilla. Which of the following is the most likely diagnosis?

○ A. Basal cell carcinoma
○ B. Carcinoma of the sweat gland
○ C. Malignant melanoma
○ D. Seborrheic keratosis
○ E. Squamous cell carcinoma

2. The specimen in this photomicrograph was removed at autopsy from the lung of a neonate who was having difficulty breathing soon after birth. Which of the following is the most likely diagnosis?

○ A. Bronchopneumonia
○ B. Carcinoma of the lung
○ C. Hyaline membrane disease
○ D. Interstitial pulmonary fibrosis
○ E. Pulmonary edema

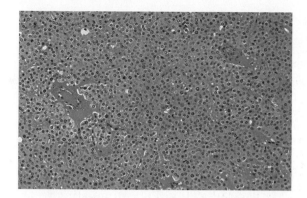

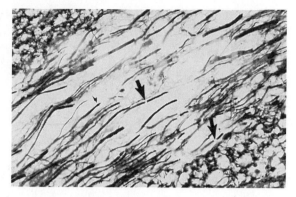

3. The benign tumor shown in the photomicrograph was removed from a 60-year-old woman with a renal calculus. Which of the following changes would you expect to find in results from this patient's laboratory studies?

○ A. Decrease in blood urea nitrogen (BUN)
○ B. Decrease in serum calcium levels
○ C. Decrease in triiodothyronine (T_3) and thyroxine (T_4) levels
○ D. Increase in serum calcium levels
○ E. Increase in T_3 and T_4 levels

5. The specimen in this photomicrograph was prepared with osmium stain. The arrows point to

○ A. adipose cells
○ B. H zone in skeletal muscle
○ C. I band in skeletal muscle
○ D. light collagen bands
○ E. nodes of Ranvier

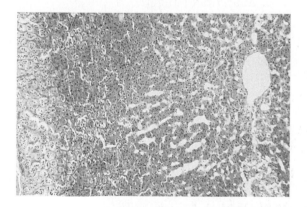

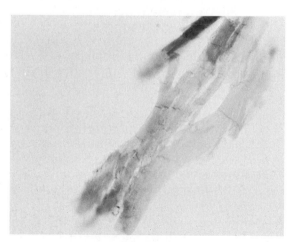

4. The surgical specimen shown above was removed from a young woman with severe cystic acne. Which of the following is the most likely diagnosis?

○ A. Adrenogenital syndrome
○ B. Alcoholic cirrhosis
○ C. Cholangiocarcinoma
○ D. Neoplasm of the Leydig cells
○ E. Right-sided cardiac failure

6. The black bands crossing at a right angle to the long axis of the fibers in this photomicrographs represent

○ A. A bands in skeletal muscle
○ B. crossbanding in collagen
○ C. I bands in skeletal muscle
○ D. intercalated disks in cardiac muscle
○ E. sarcomeres in cardiac muscle

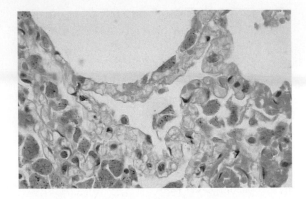

7. This photomicrograph shows a specimen taken from the lung of a 69-year-old man with a lengthy history of ischemic heart disease. The large cells with brown pigment are best classified as

○ A. alveolar macrophages with anthracotic pigment
○ B. eosinophils
○ C. hemosiderinophages
○ D. malignant melanoma cells
○ E. type II pneumocytes

8. A 92-year-old woman complains of hearing loss. Which of the following structures in the organ of Corti would be reduced in size in this patient?

○ A. Diameter of the inner ear tunnel
○ B. Hairs on the surface of inner hair cells
○ C. Thickness of the basilar membrane
○ D. Thickness of the tectorial membrane
○ E. Thickness of the vestibular membrane

9. Which of the following would correctly describe any B lymphocyte seen in a peripheral blood smear from a 33-year old man?

○ A. Actively producing humoral antibody
○ B. Differentiated in red bone marrow
○ C. Differentiated in the thymus
○ D. Well-developed Golgi apparatus
○ E. Well-developed rough endoplasmic reticulum (RER)

10. An 18-year-old woman undergoing chemotherapy for metastatic melanoma develops severe neutropenia. Which of the following agents would most likely be administered to treat this side effect of chemotherapy?

○ A. Colony-forming unit-erythrocyte (CFU-E)
○ B. Colony-forming unit-granulocyte macrophage (CFU-GM)
○ C. Erythropoietin (EPO)
○ D. Granulocyte colony-stimulating factor (G-CSF)
○ E. Monocyte colony-stimulating factor (M-CSF)

11. A 12-year-old Boy Scout developed a painful rash on his lower legs after walking through a patch of poison ivy during a camping trip. Which of the following cells would process and present the antigen introduced by the plant to initiate an immune response in the skin?

○ A. CD4 cell
○ B. Dendritic reticular cell
○ C. Epidermal Langerhans' cell
○ D. Histiocyte in a cord of Billroth
○ E. Kupffer cell

12. A 6-year-old boy who was being treated for otitis media in the pediatric section of a children's hospital acquired a staphylococcal infection. Some staphylococci are phagocytosed by neutrophils (PMNs). About 13 hours later when the PMNs are no longer viable, viable staphylococci are liberated from these cells. Which disease state is suggested by these findings?

○ A. Chédiak-Higashi disease
○ B. Chronic granulomatous disease of childhood
○ C. Chronic inflammation
○ D. Chronic myelogenous leukemia (CML)

13. A 31-year-old man complains of left unilateral ptosis and pupillary constriction in the left eye. Which of the following should be considered when developing a differential diagnosis?

○ A. Destruction of celiac ganglion
○ B. Destruction of postganglionic neurons in the ciliary ganglion
○ C. Loss of innervation of the superior tarsal muscle (Müller's muscle)
○ D. Mesothelioma of the diaphragmatic surface of the left lung
○ E. Papilledema of the left optic disk

14. Electron microscopy of a cell in the bone marrow shows a cell with many channels of smooth endoplasmic reticulum (SER) in the cytoplasm, many electron-dense cytoplasmic granules of uniform size, and a multilobulated nucleus. Which type of cell is being examined?

○ A. Basophilic erythroblast
○ B. Developing B lymphocyte
○ C. Megakaryocyte
○ D. Neutrophil (PMN)
○ E. Reticulocyte

15. As a man is walking past a construction site, he is startled by the sudden and repetitive loud noise of a jackhammer nearby. Which structure in the ear protects the inner ear from damage due to exposure to this type of noise?

○ A. Oval window
○ B. Round window
○ C. Stapedius muscle
○ D. Tectorial membrane
○ E. Vestibular membrane

16. In a patient with vitamin D deficiency, osteoblasts in the endosteal membrane line which component of a mature spicule of cancellous bone?

○ A. Calcified cartilage
○ B. Mineralized osteoid
○ C. Nonmineralized osteoid
○ D. Zone of hypertrophied chondrocytes

17. A biopsy of a section of the alveolar septa of the lung of a long-term smoker shows cells containing inhaled tar (carbon) particles. Which of the following cell types is most likely to contain such particles?

○ A. Ciliated cuboidal cells
○ B. Endothelial cells
○ C. Macrophages
○ D. Type I pneumocytes
○ E. Type II pneumocytes

18. A 28-year-old technician discovers that the drinking water in his laboratory has been contaminated with tritiated thymidine for the 2 months he worked around the clock in the laboratory. Almost all of the water he drank was from the laboratory. He is concerned about the effect this exposure may have on his ability to have children. The most advanced stage of spermatogenesis in which tritiated thymidine would be incorporated into DNA in this person would be

○ A. early spermatid
○ B. fully developed spermatozoa
○ C. primary spermatocyte
○ D. secondary spermatocyte
○ E. spermatogonia

19. A margin of normal tissue and a large, high-grade leiomyosarcoma are removed from the gastrointestinal (GI) tract of a 42-year-old man. The marginal tissue shows an abrupt transition between stratified squamous nonkeratinized or parakeratinized epithelium and simple columnar epithelium. This specimen was obtained from which segment of the GI tract?

○ A. Gastroduodenal junction
○ B. Gastroesophageal junction
○ C. Lip
○ D. Lower anal canal and skin
○ E. Oropharynx and esophagus

20. Which of the following cytokines activates macrophages so they can attack and destroy neoplastic cells?

○ A. Erythropoietin (EPO)
○ B. Granulocyte-colony stimulating factor (G-CSF)
○ C. Granulocyte-macrophage colony stimulating factor (GM-CSF)
○ D. Thrombopoietin

21. An 81-year-old man complains of difficulty breathing and undergoes a diagnostic bronchopulmonary lavage. Which of the following is removed in large numbers during the lavage of a bronchopulmonary segment?

○ A. Alveolar macrophage
○ B. Endothelial cell
○ C. Goblet cell
○ D. Type I pneumocyte
○ E. Type II pneumocyte

22. A B-cell lymphoma normally begins in which of the following sites where B cells are normally found?

○ A. Deep cortex of lymph node
○ B. Germinal centers of lymph nodes
○ C. Internodular connective tissue in the gastrointestinal (GI) tract
○ D. Parenchymal elements of the thymus
○ E. White pulp surrounding a splenic artery

23. During a routine examination, a 43-year-old man is found to have hypermobility of the joints and hyperelasticity of the skin. The patient's medical history includes a corneal rupture. Recent laboratory studies show that the patient has a deficiency of lysyl hydroxylase. Which of the following is the most likely diagnosis?

○ A. Cystic fibrosis
○ B. Ehlers-Danlos syndrome
○ C. Familial hypercholesterolemia
○ D. Fragile X syndrome
○ E. Marfan syndrome

24. Which of the following is a physiologic feature of every endocrine gland?

○ A. Dependence on autonomic innervation
○ B. Dependence on pituitary stimulation
○ C. Extensive local blood supply
○ D. Extensive smooth endoplasmic reticulum (SER)
○ E. Intracellular storage of large amounts of hormone

25. A 29-year-old woman bruises easily and has slight mucosal bleeding. The results of laboratory studies are as follows:

Complete blood count (CBC)
White blood cells (WBCs)	6300
Red blood cells (RBCs)	4.8 million/mm^3
Platelet count	92,000/mm^3

Differential count
Lymphocytes	23%
Neutrophils	67%
Basophils	0.5%
Monocytes	8%
Eosinophils	1.5%

Which of the following is the most likely diagnosis?

○ A. Leukocytosis
○ B. Neutropenia
○ C. Poikilocytosis
○ D. Polycythemia
○ E. Thrombocytopenia

26. Which of the following is responsible for maintaining the normal discoid shape of thrombocytes?

○ A. Fibrinogen
○ B. Glycogen
○ C. Hyalomere microfilaments
○ D. Open canalicular system
○ E. Serotonin in the granulomere

27. An analysis of the karyotype of a pediatric patient shows two cell populations, both of which are aneuploid. One has 2n + 1 chromosomes; the other has 2n − 1. Which single event is responsible for both types of aneuploidy seen in this patient?

○ A. Nondisjunction of a homologous pair of chromosomes (total of 4 chromatids) during anaphase I of meiosis
○ B. Nondisjunction of a sister pair of chromatids at anaphase II of meiosis
○ C. Nondisjunction of a sister pair of chromatids during mitotic anaphase of embryogenesis
○ D. Polygyny
○ E. Polyspermy

28. Microscopic examination of a surgical specimen taken from a small bowel resection shows varying degrees of pyknosis, karyorrhexis, and karyolysis in enterocytes located on the tips of the intestinal villi. Which of the following conditions is suggested by these findings?

○ A. Anaplasia
○ B. Apoptosis
○ C. Dysplasia
○ D. Inflammation

29. A 43-year-old man is diagnosed with poikilocytosis. Which of the following is an example of a poikilocyte?

○ A. Erythrocyte <6 m in diameter
○ B. Erythrocyte >9 m in diameter
○ C. Erythrocyte in a rouleaux formation
○ D. Spherocyte
○ E. Stab (band) eosinophil

30. A bronchopulmonary lavage produces a normal amount of surfactant. Which type of cell in the lung is the primary source of surfactant?

○ A. Bronchiolar gland cell
○ B. Dust cell
○ C. Goblet cell
○ D. Type I pneumocyte
○ E. Type II pneumocyte

31. Approximately 3 minutes after blood is drawn from a patient during a routine physical examination, it is placed in a 0.9% NaCl solution. Which of the following changes may take place?

○ A. Crenation
○ B. Hemolysis
○ C. Rise in oxyhemoglobin content
○ D. Spherocytosis
○ E. No change

32. Which of the following cell types is an important direct target for HIV?

○ A. CD4 T cell
○ B. CD8 T cell
○ C. CD20 B cell
○ D. Natural killer (NK) cell
○ E. Plasma cell

33. Renal allograft recipients who use immunosuppressive therapy are 25 times more likely to develop cancer than healthy people because of suppression of

○ A. basophils
○ B. dendritic reticular cells
○ C. natural killer (NK) cells
○ D. plasma cells
○ E. T suppressor cells

34. If the life span of osteoclasts remains constant with aging but the life span of osteoblasts is progressively shortened, which disease process is most likely to develop?

○ A. Osteoclastoma
○ B. Osteomalacia
○ C. Osteopetrosis
○ D. Osteoporosis
○ E. Scurvy

35. Two weeks after being tackled during football practice, a 20-year-old college student complains of frequent, severe headaches. A neuroradiologic examination shows several small radiopaque specks near the center of the brain suggesting calcification. Which of the following is most likely responsible for this finding?

○ A. Corpora amylacea in the pineal gland
○ B. Corpora arenacea in the pineal gland
○ C. Cupula of the crista ampullaris
○ D. Otoliths in the macula of the saccule
○ E. Otoliths in the macula of the utricle

36. A 29-year-old woman has been exposed to a large number of endotoxin-producing gram-negative bacteria, resulting in a large concentration of bacterial lipopolysaccharides in her blood. Which type of cell will respond to these changes by producing tumor necrosis factor (TNF)?

○ A. Basophil
○ B. Endothelial
○ C. Eosinophil
○ D. Monocyte
○ E. Platelet

37. A blood smear is prepared using a sample taken from a 12-year-old girl with chronic myelogenous leukemia (CML). Which of the following cell types will show the most prominent or largest nucleoli?

○ A. Basophilic myelocyte
○ B. Mature neutrophil (PMN)
○ C. Myeloblast
○ D. Neutrophilic metamyelocyte
○ E. Polychromatophilic normoblast

38. Assuming that a normal gamete contains 100 copies of ribosomal genes, how many copies of these genes are in a diploid cell during the G_2 phase of the intermitotic cell cycle?

○ A. 100
○ B. 200
○ C. 300
○ D. 400

39. Lipid-soluble high–molecular-weight alcohols readily enter the cell without using an energy-dependent process. When the alcohol concentration outside the cell increases, the rate at which it enters the cell increases; however, the concentration of alcohol inside the cell never exceeds the concentration of alcohol outside the cell. This indicates that these alcohols are transported across the cell membrane by

○ A. active transport
○ B. carrier-facilitated diffusion
○ B. exocytosis
○ D. non–carrier-mediated transport

40. Which of the following best describes a cardiac muscle fiber?

○ A. A nexus is found in the intercalated disk
○ B. Each fiber is innervated by an individual nerve ending
○ C. It lacks myofibrils
○ D. T tubules are found at the A-I intercept

41. Which of the following best describes the development of skeletal muscle?

○ A. A multinucleated cell is formed by repeated nuclear divisions in the absence of cytoplasmic division
○ B. A multinucleated cell results from the fusion of many single cells
○ C. After puberty, muscle mass grows by an increase in cell number
○ D. Skeletal muscle is derived from epithelial ectodermal and endodermal layers

42. A high–molecular-weight protein (500 amino acids) enters the cell without first being degraded by which mechanism?

○ A. Active transport
○ B. Carrier-facilitated diffusion
○ C. Endocytosis
○ D. Exocytosis
○ E. Non–carrier-mediated transport

43. In a particular organism, the nucleolar organizer is located on the short arm of a single chromosome pair. Deletion of both members of the chromosome pair would result in which of the following effects?

○ A. Increased hybridization of DNA with 18S and 28S rRNA
○ B. Increased number of nucleoli
○ C. Increased synthesis of 45S RNA
○ D. Loss of secondary constrictions

44. Which of the following is a distinguishing characteristic of synapses?

○ A. A myelin sheath must be present if synaptic transmission is to occur
○ B. Mitochondria and vesicles containing neurotransmitters accumulate in the presynaptic area
○ C. Most synapses exist between two dendritic processes
○ D. Occluding junctions hold the two neuronal processes together
○ E. Satellite cells intervene between the neuronal processes

45. The blood-brain barrier prevents certain substances from passing from the blood into the central nervous system. This function is primarily the responsibility of which of the following?

○ A. Accumulation of reactive astrocytes at the site of injury
○ B. Association of the choroid plexus with pia mater cells
○ C. Maintenance of the resting membrane potential
○ D. Presence of occluding junctions between capillary endothelial cells

46. The hypertonic quality of the interstitium of the renal medulla affects which of the following?

○ A. Resorption of water from the proximal convoluted tubule
○ B. Resorption of water from the straight collecting tubules
○ C. Resorption of water from the thick ascending portion of Henle's loop

47. A microscopic evaluation of a biopsy taken from the femur of a 3-year-old girl shows interstitial lamellae that appear on the most radiolucent areas of a photomicrograph. Interstitial lamellae are a consequence of which of the following events?

○ A. Failure of haversian systems to form correctly
○ B. Inadequate intake of vitamin C
○ C. Partial resorption of haversian systems by osteoclasts
○ D. Pulling apart of haversian systems by Sharpey's fibers
○ E. Stimulation of periosteum by parathyroid hormone (PTH)

48. Removal of the anterior lobe of the pituitary gland would have which of the following effects on the male reproductive system?

○ A. Decreased synthesis of androgen-binding protein
○ B. Increased production of testosterone
○ C. Increased spermatogenesis

49. Specimens taken from several parts of the gastrointestinal (GI) tract of a patient with cystic fibrosis are being prepared for microscopic study. In which structure will an epithelium be seen in which every surface cell is capable of secreting mucus?

○ A. Duodenum
○ B. Esophagus
○ C. Lower anal canal
○ D. Stomach
○ E. Transverse colon

50. A blood smear prepared from a sample obtained from a patient with leukemia contains many large cells. Each of the cells has a round nucleus containing several prominent nucleoli and a cytoplasm filled with small azurophilic granules. Using the description of the cells, which of the following is the most likely diagnosis?

○ A. Acute lymphoblastic leukemia (ALL)
○ B. Basophilic leukemia
○ C. Monoblastic leukemia
○ D. Promyelocytic leukemia
○ E. Stem cell leukemia

1. **D** (seborrheic keratosis) is correct. Normal epidermis can be seen to the right and hyperkeratosis to the left in the photomicrograph. Excessive keratin formation (entrapped in the epidermis) can also be seen. Seborrheic keratoses are benign lesions; however, when they suddenly increase in number, the patient may have an underlying stomach cancer (Leser-Trélat sign).

   A (basal cell carcinoma) is incorrect. Basal cell carcinoma normally arises from cells in the stratum basale layer of the epidermis. It invades the dermis, but usually does not affect the superficial layers of the epidermis.
   B (carcinoma of the sweat gland) is incorrect. Carcinoma of the sweat gland is a rare adenocarcinoma. It has a glandular appearance, not the sheetlike appearance of the tissue seen in this photomicrograph.
   C (malignant melanoma) is incorrect. Malignant melanoma arises from melanocytes, which usually are most easily seen near the border between the epidermis and dermis. It is not characterized by excessive keratin production (as shown), which normally occurs on the epidermal surface.
   E (squamous cell carcinoma) is incorrect. Squamous cell carcinoma is characterized by nests of squamous cells similar to those found in the stratum spinosum of the epidermis. Squamous pearls consisting of keratin may appear in the center of these nests. However, the excessive amounts of keratin on the epidermal surface that appear on the photomicrograph are not associated with this type of cancer.

2. **C** (hyaline membrane disease) is correct. An amorphous eosinophilic hyaline material lines the alveoli and bronchioles in the photomicrograph and forms a barrier between blood and air (diffusion defect). Hyaline membrane disease is due to a lack of surfactant, which leads to collapse of the alveoli and massive intrapulmonary shunting of blood.

   A (bronchopneumonia) is incorrect. Bronchopneumonia involves a suppurative inflammation that can fill the alveoli, bronchioles, and bronchi. Note that most of the nuclei in the photomicrograph are round-to-ovoid shaped, rather than multilobulated like neutrophils. Due to a lack of surfactant, the alveoli are collapsed; hence the nuclei are primarily those of type I pneumocytes.
   B (carcinoma of the lung) is incorrect. Several types of carcinomas arise in the lung, including squamous cell carcinoma, adenocarcinoma, small cell carcinoma, and mesothelioma. These tumors contain pleomorphic cells. Thus, if a carcinoma were

shown in the photomicrograph, discrete areas of the specimen would contain cells of the same type, but with variations in their appearance.

D (interstitial pulmonary fibrosis) is incorrect. Interstitial pulmonary fibrosis results in widespread fibrosis but with few inflammatory cells. It can be ruled out in this case because of the extensive number of inflammatory cells. There are no areas of fibrosis.

E (pulmonary edema) is incorrect. Pulmonary edema results in the alveoli being filled with fluid, which is usually a transudate (has a low protein and cell content). Pulmonary edema can be ruled out in this case because the alveoli are collapsed and do not contain fluid.

3. *D* (increase in serum calcium levels) is correct. The field of view in this photomicrograph is dominated by well-differentiated cells containing a prominent nucleus and a limited cytoplasm. These are characteristics of the chief cell, which is the dominant cell type in parathyroid tissue. The excessive number of chief cells without intervening adipose cells suggests an adenoma, a benign neoplasm. Chief cells produce parathyroid hormone, which raises calcium levels in the blood. Increased calcium in the urine predisposes an individual to calculus formation.

A (decrease in blood urea nitrogen) is incorrect. The BUN is an indication of the rate at which amino acids are metabolized in the liver. A decrease in BUN levels may indicate reduced activity of the liver enzymes in the urea cycle that convert toxic ammonia (a byproduct of deamination) into urea. This occurs in cirrhosis of the liver. The photomicrograph shows parathyroid tissue, which is not associated with urea metabolism.

B (decrease in serum calcium levels) is incorrect. The photomicrograph shows an overgrowth of chief cells, which indicates a parathyroid tumor. Chief cells secrete parathyroid hormone, which promotes the absorption of calcium from the kidneys and resorption of bone from increased osteoclastic activity. When the tumor is removed, the calcium levels will fall into the normal range.

C (decrease in triiodothyronine and thyroxine levels) and E (increase in T_3 and T_4 levels) are incorrect. The dominant cell in the photomicrograph is the chief cell of the parathyroid gland, which is identified by its prominent nucleus and limited cytoplasm. The overgrowth of these cells suggests a parathyroid adenoma. T_3 and T_4 are produced by the thyroid gland, not the parathyroid gland. Removal of the parathyroid tumor will not affect the production of thyroid hormones.

4. *A* (adrenogenital syndrome) is correct. The photomicrograph shows the three layers of the adrenal cortex; the vein to the right is in the adrenal medulla. The zona glomerulosa is the most lightly stained region (far left). This zone primarily synthesizes mineralocorticoids. Deep to the zona glomerulosa is the zona

fasciculata. This zone primarily synthe-sizes cortisol. Deep to the zona fasciculata is an area of hyperplasia in the zona reticularis. In females, the overproduction of androgens by the zona re-ticularis may result in a virilism syndrome (female pseudoher-maphroditism) if the patient has classic 21- or 11-hydroxylase enzyme deficiency. This patient most likely has the nonclassic type of 21-hydroxylase deficiency, in which the patient most often presents with severe acne.

B   (alcoholic cirrhosis) is incorrect. The left half of the photomi-crograph clearly shows three layers of tissue. In cirrhosis of the liver, sheets of hepatocytes are surrounded by bands of fibrous tissue, which are not evident in the photomicrograph.
C   (cholangiocarcinoma) is incorrect. Cholangiocarcinomas arise from the epithelial lining of the bile ducts. The structure of the epithelium lining the lumen of structures in the biliary tree ranges from a layer of hepatocyte plasma membranes lining bile cana-liculi to the highly twisted mucosa lining the cystic duct. None of the characteristic biliary lumina appear in the photomicrograph. The majority of cases of cholangiocarcinoma in the United States arise from primary sclerosing cholangitis associated with ul-cerative colitis.
D   (neoplasm of the Leydig cells) is incorrect. The Leydig cell has a large nucleus and is found alone or with a few other Leydig cells within the supporting tissue of the seminiferous tubules (i.e., along the periphery of the tubules) in the testis. Neither tubular cells nor tissue with a histology resembling that of Leydig cells appears in the photomicrograph. Also, the patient was female.
E   (right-sided cardiac failure) is incorrect. Right-sided cardiac failure produces an increase in venous hydrostatic pressure. In-creased pressure in the vena cava is transmitted back into the hepatic vein and eventually into the central vein of the liver. Congestion of blood in this vein causes a "nutmeg" gross appear-ance of the liver surface. Note that the vein in this photomicro-graph is not congested.

5. *E*   (nodes of Ranvier) is correct. The photomicrograph shows a segment of peripheral nerve stained with osmium, which stains myelin black. The nodes of Ranvier are discrete regions along the axon that are not covered by myelin. These unmyelinated regions serve as the anatomic basis for saltatory conduction.

A   (adipose cells) is incorrect. The adipose cell is round and filled with a lipid droplet that often presses the nucleus against the periphery of the cell. Adipose cells also react to the special stain (osmium) that was used to prepare the specimen in the photomi-crograph; their characteristic appearance is not seen here.
B   (H zone in skeletal muscle) is incorrect. The H zone is the region within the sarcomere of skeletal muscle fibers where the thick and thin myofilaments overlap. It can be viewed under a rel-atively high magnification (1000×). It would not be seen under the low-power magnification used in the photomicrograph.

C   (I band in skeletal tissue) is incorrect. The I band is the light area or isotropic band in the sarcomere of skeletal muscle. The Z line inserts in it. A much greater resolution is needed to see the I band than was used in the photomicrograph.

D   (light collagen bands) is incorrect. The light bands in collagen fibers alternate with dark bands. However, they can only be seen with the high resolution of an electron microscope.

6. ***D***   (intercalated disks in cardiac muscle) is correct. The photomicrograph shows cardiac muscle that has been teased to demonstrate how the cardiac muscle cells anastomose and branch with one another. The dark bands are intercalated disks. Adjacent cardiac muscle cells are held together in this region by various types of cell-to-cell junctions. Gap junctions allow intercellular ionic (electrical) communication.

A   (A bands in skeletal muscle) is incorrect. The A (anisotropic) band consists of the thick, myosin-rich myofilaments of the sarcomere. Although A bands cross the muscle fiber in skeletal and cardiac tissue, they are much thinner than intercalated disks. Also, thousands of A bands would be seen, instead of the dozen or so intercalated disks shown in this preparation.

B   (crossbanding in collagen) is incorrect. The alternating light-dark band pattern in collagen is an ultrastructural feature. It cannot be seen using light microscopy.

C   (I bands in skeletal muscle) is incorrect. The I bands of skeletal muscle are so called because they are isotropic (i.e., they allow light to pass through). Since they cannot appear as dark bands, they are ruled out in this preparation. As with A bands, I bands are much smaller than the intercalated disks seen here.

E   (sarcomeres in cardiac muscle) is incorrect. A sarcomere extends from one Z line to the next in both cardiac and skeletal muscle. Furthermore, it is much smaller than the intercalated disks shown in this preparation.

7. ***C***   (hemosiderinophages) is correct. Under certain circumstances, such as intra-alveolar hemorrhage in chronic heart failure, alveolar macrophages will phagocytose red blood cells (RBCs). One of the products of hemoglobin catabolism is hemosiderin, a substance that is stored within the macrophage where it appears as brown pigment. This most often occurs in patients with chronic passive congestion of the lung due to a heart problem, as seen in this patient. Because these macrophages store hemosiderin, they are often referred to as hemosiderinophages, or "heart failure cells."

A   (alveolar macrophages with anthracotic pigment) is incorrect. Anthracosis is a form of pneumoconiosis that is induced by coal dust deposits in the lungs. It can result in anthracotic pigment filling the alveoli and alveolar macrophages (black lung disease).

B   (eosinophils) is incorrect. Eosinophils contain granules that stain pink.

D   (malignant melanoma cells) is incorrect. Malignant melanoma arises from melanocytes. Melanin granules are black.

E   (type II pneumonocytes) is incorrect. Type II pneumonocytes (also known as greater alveolar cells) are found in the alveolar epithelium and secrete surfactant. These cells have large, round nuclei and a vacuolated cytoplasm that does not contain granules. Electron microscopy may show structures (lamellar bodies) indicating intracellular storage surfactant. Such cells do not appear in the photomicrograph.

8. *B*   (hairs on the surface of inner hair cells) is correct. The term "hairs" refers to stereocilia, which are microvilli, not cilia. The core of the stereocilium contains actin filaments cross-linked with fimbrin near the apical plasmalemma of the hair cell; this arrangement is responsible for its rigidity. When sound waves move the basilar membrane in the cochlea, the stereocilia are bent, causing the release of the content of the stereocilia into synaptic-like structures. This release excites the afferent nerve fibers that are closely associated with each hair cell. The hairs (stereocilia) on the surface of inner and outer hair cells decrease in number and size during the aging process, thereby reducing the ability to hear.

A   (diameter of the inner ear tunnel) is incorrect. The inner ear tunnel is filled with endolymph. The diameter of this tunnel has nothing to do with the process of hearing.

C   (thickness of the basilar membrane) is incorrect. The basilar membrane supports the organ of Corti in the inner ear. Vibrations in the basilar membrane cause the organ of Corti to move in relation to the overlying tectorial membrane. Hair cells (stereocilia) in the organ of Corti project into the tectorial membrane. The first step in the neurophysiology of hearing is movement of the basilar membrane, which causes the stereocilia to bend. The thickness of the basilar membrane is not as important in the hearing process as a decrease in the number of hairs on hair cells.

D   (thickness of the tectorial membrane) is incorrect. The tectorial membrane overlies the organ of Corti in the inner ear. Hair cells (stereocilia) in the organ of Corti project into the tectorial membrane. The first step in the neurophysiology of hearing occurs when the organ of Corti moves (as occurs when the underlying basilar membrane "vibrates"), causing these cells to bend. The thickness of the tectorial membrane is not as important in the hearing process as a decrease in the number of hairs on hair cells.

E   (thickness of the vestibular membrane) is incorrect. The vestibular membrane is the part of the cochlear duct that faces the scala vestibuli. It does not play a role in the process of hearing. Furthermore, this membrane is two cells thick throughout life.

9. **B** (differentiated in red bone marrow) is correct. B lymphocytes undergo differentiation from precursor cells in red bone marrow.

A (actively producing humoral antibody) is incorrect. Active production of humoral antibody is a function of plasma cells, which are terminally differentiated B cells.
C (differentiated in the thymus) is incorrect. T cells (not B cells) differentiate in the thymus gland.
D (well-developed Golgi apparatus) is incorrect. A well-developed Golgi apparatus would be found in the terminally differentiated descendant of a B lymphocyte (the plasma cell), but not in the B cell itself.
E (well-developed rough endoplasmic reticulum) is incorrect. A well-developed RER would be found in terminally differentiated descendants of B lymphocytes (plasma cells), but not in the B cell itself.

10. **D** (granulocyte colony-stimulating factor) is correct. G-CSF stimulates granulocytopoiesis (production of granulocytes), especially the production of neutrophils (PMNs). Thus it can cause the number of PMNs in the blood to rise from neutropenic to normal levels.

A (colony-forming unit-erythrocyte) is incorrect. Neutropenia is an abnormally low number of neutrophils in the blood. Patients with neutropenia require a factor that stimulates the production of neutrophils. CFU-E is a cell, not a growth factor.
B (colony-forming unit-granulocyte macrophage) is incorrect. Neutropenia is an abnormally low number of neutrophils in the blood. Patients with neutropenia require a factor that stimulates the production of neutrophils. CFU-GM is a cell, not a growth factor.
C (erythropoietin) is incorrect. Neutropenia is an abnormally low number of neutrophils in the blood. EPO stimulates erythrocytopoiesis, not granulocytopoiesis.
E (monocyte colony-stimulating factor) is incorrect. Neutropenia is an abnormally low number of neutrophils in the blood. M-CSF stimulates production of monocytes, not neutrophils.

11. **C** (epidermal Langerhans' cell) is correct. Poison ivy introduces a foreign antigen to the skin. Langerhans' cells function as the epidermal counterpart to dendritic reticular cells in the germinal centers of lymph nodules, since they are able to take up an antigen, process it, and present it to immunocompetent cells.

A (CD4 cell) is incorrect. The CD4 cell (T helper cell) can up-regulate antibody production by B cells by means of cytokine secretion. It participates in a secondary response to antigen exposure, rather than the primary response that occurs in the skin.
B (dendritic reticular cell) is incorrect. The dendritic reticular cell is found in lymph nodes and can trap, process, and present anti-

gens to immunocompetent cells. Since it is not found in the epidermis, it is not likely to participate in an immune response to poison ivy.

D (histiocytes in a cord of Billroth) is incorrect. Tissue macrophages or histiocytes can present an antigen after it has been phagocytosed and processed. A histiocyte in the spleen is not likely to be involved in an immune response to poison ivy exposure on the skin.

E (Kupffer cell) is incorrect. Kupffer cells are fixed macrophages (histiocytes) that line and/or bridge the hepatic sinusoids. Since they are not found in skin, they would not participate in an immune response to poison ivy.

12. *B* (chronic granulomatous disease of childhood) is correct. Chronic granulomatous disease of childhood is associated with a genetic defect that results in the failure of PMNs to produce hydrogen peroxide. As a result, bacteria that enter these cells are not killed by the cell. Instead, when the PMN dies, viable bacteria are released.

A (Chédiak-Higashi disease) is incorrect. Chédiak-Higashi disease is characterized by a lag in the initiation of the fusion of lysosomes with ingested bacteria (microbicidal defect). In this case, the cell is capable of destroying ingested bacteria, but may take longer to do so.

C (chronic inflammation) is incorrect. The term "chronic inflammation" is usually applied to a long-standing infection in connective tissue.

D (chronic myelogenous leukemia) is incorrect. CML is characterized by the appearance of undifferentiated hematopoietic cells in peripheral blood. In contrast, this patient's PMNs are fully functional (i.e., capable of killing phagocytosed bacteria). CML is more likely to occur in adults between the ages of 39 and 60 years.

13. *C* (loss of innervation of the superior tarsal muscle) is correct. Carcinoma in the apex of the left lung can destroy the superior cervical sympathetic ganglion, whose postganglionic sympathetic fibers innervate both the dilator muscle of the iris and Müller's muscle (the smooth muscle component of the levator palpebrae superioris muscle). Contraction of Müller's muscle raises the upper eyelid. Its function is overruled by contraction of the orbicularis oculi muscle. The activity of both muscles is seen during a blink.

B (destruction of the celiac ganglion) is incorrect. The celiac ganglion is a sympathetic ganglion located in the abdomen. Its postganglionic fibers do not innervate the eye.

C (destruction of postganglionic neurons in the ciliary ganglion) is incorrect. The ciliary ganglion is a parasympathetic ganglion. The clinical signs described for this patient strongly suggest a defect in sympathetic innervation of the eye, not parasympathetic innervation.

D (mesothelioma of the diaphragmatic surface of the left lung) is incorrect. Mesothelioma is a neoplasm that arises from the pleural mesothelium. A mesothelioma on the diaphragmatic surface of the lung would not be positioned correctly to destroy the superior sympathetic ganglion.

E (papilledema of the left optic disk) is incorrect. Papilledema of the optic disk indicates increased intracranial pressure, not a loss of sympathetic innervation to the dilator muscle and Müller's muscle of the eye.

14. *C* (megakaryocyte) is correct. The DNA in megakaryocytes undergoes several rounds of endoreduplication, which results in a cell with a multilobulated nucleus containing 16C, 32C, or 64C of DNA and a cytoplasm full of granules. Small islands of granule-containing cytoplasm are surrounded by membranes of the SER, often referred to as platelet demarcation membranes. Each island separates from the megakaryocyte to exist independently as a platelet.

A (basophilic erythroblast) is incorrect. Basophilic erythroblasts do not have a multilobulated nucleus. Also, their cytoplasm is full of free polysomes, not granules.

B (developing B lymphocyte) is incorrect. A developing B lymphocyte does not have a multilobulated nucleus. It has a small amount of cytoplasm that does not contain an SER or cytoplasmic granules.

D (neutrophil) is incorrect. Each PMN has a multilobulated nucleus and many cytoplasmic granules. However, these granules are of two distinct sizes (400 nm and 700 nm), unlike the uniform granules seen in platelets. Furthermore, a PMN would not show SER channels.

E (reticulocyte) is incorrect. Reticulocytes do not have a nucleus, and their cytoplasm contains only a few free polysomes.

15. *C* (stapedius muscle) is correct. The stapedius muscle controls the oscillatory stroke of the footplate of the stapes. Innervated by the facial nerve (CN VII), this muscle contracts in response to sudden, repetitive, loud noise and reduces the oscillatory response of the stapes. The stapedius muscle protects the structures of the inner ear from damage due to repetitive, loud noises.

A (oval window) is incorrect. The oval window passively responds to insult and has no protecting mechanism of its own.

B (round window) is incorrect. The round window responds passively to insult by bulging outward to relieve the pressure transferred to it by perilymph, which responds to the pressure induced by the movement of the footplate of the stapes against the oval window.

D (tectorial membrane) is incorrect. The tectorial membrane passively responds to insult. It does not have a protective mechanism of its own.

E   (vestibular membrane) is incorrect. The vestibular membrane passively responds to insult; it does not have a protective mechanism of its own.

16. *C*   (nonmineralized osteoid) is correct. The youngest part of a developing spicule of cancellous bone is along its outermost edge, which is composed of the fresh (nonmineralized) osteoid most recently synthesized by the layer of osteoblasts of the endosteum. Since vitamin D ensures an adequate supply of calcium to mineralize osteoid, this nonmineralized zone would be relatively thick in a patient lacking vitamin D.

A   (calcified cartilage) is incorrect. Calcified cartilage can be found in the center of spicules of bone formed by means of endochondral ossification. This would place the calcified cartilage farthest from the endosteal membrane.

B   (mineralized osteoid) is incorrect. Mineralized osteoid is the older osteoid in the bone spicule. It lies deep in the spicule, not close to the endosteal membrane.

D   (zone of hypertrophied chondrocytes) is incorrect. Hypertrophied chondrocytes are found in a specific layer of the epiphyseal plate. This layer does not have an endosteal surface.

17. *C*   (macrophages) is correct. The alveolar macrophage ("dust" cell) wanders over the alveolar surface, phagocytosing bacteria and other inhaled particles, including particles released from inhaled cigarette smoke. These cells digest the phagocytosed bacteria using lysosomal enzymes, which lack carbonase. Carbonase degrades carbon; thus this lack of carbonase causes the undigested particles of tar to remain in the cells for life.

A   (ciliated cuboidal cells) is incorrect. Ciliated cuboidal cells are found in higher (wider) segments of the respiratory tree (not in the alveoli).

B   (endothelial cells) is incorrect. Endothelial cells line the alveolar capillaries. Although they reside within the alveolar septum (respiratory membrane), they are not phagocytes. Therefore, they are unlikely to contain lung contaminants (including those introduced by inhaled cigarette smoke).

D   (type I pneumocytes) is incorrect. Type I pneumocytes lie within the alveolar septum and face the air in the alveolus. Because they are extremely thin structures, they are able to facilitate the passage of gas between air and blood. They are not phagocytes; therefore, they are unlikely to contain any lung contaminants (including those introduced by inhaled cigarette smoke).

E   (type II pneumocytes) is incorrect. Type II pneumocytes reside within the alveolar septum, where they synthesize and release surfactant. These are not phagocytic cells, and they are unlikely to contain any lung contaminants (including those introduced by inhaled cigarette smoke).

18. *B* (fully developed spermatozoa) is correct. The most advanced stage of spermatogenesis involves the production of mature spermatozoa. It takes about 62 days for spermatogonia to become spermatozoa. Spermatogenesis would result in the uptake of radioactive thymidine, and it would be found in all cells derived from exposed spermatogonia.

A (early spermatids), C (primary spermatocytes), D (secondary spermatocytes), and E (spermatogonia) are incorrect. The normal sequence of steps in spermatogenesis is spermatogonia, primary spermatocyte, secondary spermatocyte, and spermatid, which undergoes morphologic changes to become the mature sperm. The DNA of early spermatids, primary and secondary spermatocytes, and spermatogonia will contain labeled thymidine.

19. *B* (gastroesophageal junction) is correct. The stratified squamous wet epithelium of the esophagus changes abruptly to a simple columnar epithelium (as seen in the upper gastric region) at the gastroesophageal junction.

A (gastroduodenal junction) is incorrect. Both the stomach and duodenum are lined with a simple columnar epithelium.
C (lip) and D (lower anal canal and skin) are incorrect. The junction between the lip and surrounding skin marks a sharp transition from a stratified squamous wet epithelium to a stratified squamous dry epithelium. The same type of epithelial junction is seen between the lower anal canal and surrounding skin. Neither junction contains a simple epithelium.
E (oropharynx and esophagus) is incorrect. Both of these structures are lined with a stratified squamous nonkeratinized epithelium.

20. *C* (granulocyte-macrophage colony stimulating factor) is correct. GM-CSF facilitates the differentiation of a hematopoietic stem cell into the precursor of both the granulocyte and monocyte lines of cytodifferentiation, and it activates macrophages. GM-CSF has been used in clinical trials of patients with advanced stage malignant melanoma with encouraging results.

A (erythropoietin) is incorrect. EPO is produced by the kidney in response to low oxygen levels in blood. Its target is the red blood cell precursor in bone marrow, which causes it to become committed to erythrocytopoiesis.
B (granulocyte-colony stimulating factor) is incorrect. G-CSF enhances only granulocytopoiesis (not monocytopoiesis).
D (thrombopoietin) is incorrect. Thrombopoietin enhances thrombocytopoiesis. It does not induce monocytopoiesis or macrophage activity.

21. *A*   (alveolar macrophage) is correct. The alveolar macrophage (dust cell) wanders over the alveolar surface phagocytosing inhaled particles. This is the only place in the body where macrophages migrate over a surface area; elsewhere, they migrate within connective tissue. These cells are "free" and are located on the air surface of the respiratory membrane. As a result, they are easily captured by saline lavage of a pulmonary lobule or bronchopulmonary segment.

B   (endothelial cell) is incorrect. Endothelial cells line the walls of capillaries; they would not be exposed to the saline solution.
C   (goblet cell) is incorrect. Few, if any, goblet cells would appear in a lavage of a bronchopulmonary segment, because these cells are attached to their basal lamina.
D   (type I pneumocyte) and E (type II pneumocyte) are incorrect. Few (if any) type I and type II pneumocytes would appear in a lavage of a bronchopulmonary segment, because these cells are attached to their basal lamina.

22. *B*   (germinal centers of lymph nodes) is correct. The germinal centers in all lymph nodes are composed almost exclusively of B cells.

A   (deep cortex of lymph node) is incorrect. The deep cortex of a lymph node is composed mainly of T cells, not B cells.
C   (internodular connective tissue in the gastrointestinal tract) is incorrect. The connective tissue that lies between lymph nodules in the GI tract is composed mostly of T cells.
D   (parenchymal elements of the thymus) is incorrect. The parenchymal elements of the thymus are composed of T cells.
E   (white pulp surrounding a splenic artery) is incorrect. The white pulp that surrounds arteries in the spleen is composed mostly of T cells.

23. *B*   (Ehlers-Danlos syndrome) is correct. Ehlers-Danlos syndrome is a multitude of disorders caused by a defect in an autosomal recessive gene involved in the synthesis of collagen or collagen cross-linking events. At least 10 varieties of this disorder are known. This patient may have variant VI, which is characterized by decreased hydroxylation of lysyl residues in type I and type III collagen.

A   (cystic fibrosis) is incorrect. Cystic fibrosis is the most common lethal genetic disease affecting white children. It is caused by a defect in the function of all exocrine glands. The organs most likely to be seriously affected are the lungs and pancreas, because this disorder results in abnormally viscous secretions blocking the airways and the pancreatic ducts.
C   (familial hypercholesterolemia) is incorrect. Familial hypercholesterolemia is a genetic disease caused by mutations in the gene for receptor proteins. It results in defective catabolism and excessive biosynthesis of cholesterol. This patient's symptoms

suggest abnormal collagen formation; familial hypercholesterol-emia does not play a role in collagen formation.

D   (fragile X syndrome) is incorrect. Fragile X syndrome occurs in males and is characterized by mental retardation and macroor-chidism. It is identified by an abnormal banding pattern on the affected X chromosome, which represents the amplification of sets of three nucleotides and which disrupts the normal function of the gene.

E   (Marfan syndrome) is incorrect. Marfan syndrome is an auto-somal dominant disorder that results in a defect in the production of fibril, a structural glycoprotein secreted by fibroblasts that forms microfibrillar aggregates in the extracellular matrix. These aggregates serve as scaffolds for normal elastic fibers. The most serious clinical sign of Marfan syndrome is loss of elasticity in the tunica media of the aorta. This defect is the pathologic basis for aortic aneurysm, which can result in aortic dissection or rupture.

24. *C*   (extensive local blood supply) is correct. Endocrine glands have no duct system and secrete their product directly into the blood vessels that serve them. All endocrine glands are highly vascularized.

A   (dependence on autonomic innervation) is incorrect. Most en-docrine glands are influenced by pituitary factors or blood levels of the product they regulate. An exception is the adrenal medulla, which is influenced through direct innervation by the sympa-thetic division of the autonomic nervous system.

B   (dependence on pituitary stimulation) is incorrect. The activity of many endocrine glands is induced by factors released by the pituitary gland. The exceptions include the parathyroid gland (which is directly influenced by serum calcium levels) and the islets of Langerhans in the pancreas (which are directly influenced by the level of glucose in the blood).

D   (extensive smooth endoplasmic reticulum) is incorrect. Only endocrine cells that produce steroid hormones contain a well-developed SER.

E   (intracellular storage of large amounts of hormone) is incor-rect. Most endocrine glands store relatively small amounts of hormone; however, the thyroid gland stores large amounts of hormone extracellularly in colloid-filled follicles.

25. *E*   (thrombocytopenia) is correct: Thrombocytopenia is charac-terized by a thrombocyte count of $\leq 100,000$ platelets/mm^3. Clin-ically significant thrombocytopenia is the result of inadequate thrombocyte production in the red bone marrow or decreased thrombocyte survival in the blood. Thrombocytopenia is one of the most common findings in AIDS patients.

A   (leukocytosis) is incorrect. Leukocytosis is characterized by an abnormal increase in the WBC concentration in blood. The WBC concentration for this patient is within normal limits.

B   (neutropenia) is incorrect. Neutropenia is characterized by an abnormally low neutrophil count. The PMN concentration for this patient is within normal limits.

C   (poikilocytosis) is incorrect. Poikilocytosis is characterized by RBCs with abnormal shapes, but not necessarily by an abnormal number of RBCs.

D   (polycythemia) is incorrect. Polycythemia is characterized by an abnormal increase in the RBC concentration in blood. The RBC concentration for this patient is within normal limits.

26. *C*   (hyalomere microfilaments) is correct. The cytoskeleton of the thrombocyte is composed of microfilaments and microtubules. Most of these are found in the peripheral hyalomere (the clear zone) of the platelet.

A   (fibrinogen) is incorrect. Fibrinogen is a protein produced in the liver and is critical for blood clotting. It is not a component of the cytoskeleton of platelets, and thus does not contribute to the structural integrity of the platelet.

B   (glycogen) is incorrect. Glycogen is the intracellular storage form of glucose. It does not contribute to the structural integrity of the platelet.

D   (open canalicular system) is incorrect. The canalicular system is a set of cytoplasmic canaliculi that communicates with the exterior of the platelet. It is not a component of the cytoskeleton of the platelet, and therefore does not contribute to the structural integrity of the platelet.

E   (serotonin in the granulomere) is incorrect. Serotonin is stored in granules in the more centrally located granulomere region of a platelet. It does not play a role in maintaining the discoid shape of the platelets.

27. *C*   (nondisjunction of a sister pair of chromatids during a mitotic anaphase of embryogenesis) is correct. The failure of sister chromatids in a single chromosome to separate during early anaphase of mitosis results in one line of cells missing one chromosome and another line of cells having one extra chromosome.

A   (nondisjunction of a homologous pair of chromosomes [total of 4 chromatids] during anaphase I of meiosis) is incorrect. Nondisjunction during meiosis I can result in two different kinds of gametes: one with n + 1 chromosomes, and the other with n − 1 chromosomes. However, only one of these gametes would participate in fertilization with another normal (haploid) gamete. This would result in trisomy or monosomy, but not both.

B   (nondisjunction of a sister pair of chromatids at anaphase II of meiosis) is incorrect. When a pair of sister chromatids fails to separate during meiosis II, the result is two different kinds of gametes: one containing n + 1 and the other containing n − 1 chromosomes. Therefore fertilization of one of the abnormal gametes with a normal gamete would result in either trisomy or monosomy, but not both.

D (polygyny) is incorrect. Polygyny involving fertilization with a normal sperm results in triploidy (not aneuploidy).
E (polyspermy) is incorrect. Polyspermy involving fertilization with a normal oocyte results in triploidy.

28. *B* (apoptosis) is correct. Apoptosis (programmed cell death) occurs in several stages, which can be identified by light microscopy. During the first stage, pyknotic changes are indicated by the presence of one or more dark-staining masses on the inside of the nuclear membrane. During the second stage (karyorrhexis), nuclear material breaks into fragments. During the third stage (karyolysis), the nucleus breaks up into smaller membrane-bound bodies (apoptotic bodies), each of which contains some nuclear material. Eventually, this apoptotic debris will be scavenged by macrophages and lost to the luminal contents.

A (anaplasia) is incorrect. Anaplasia is a severe type of dysplasia characterized by marked pleomorphism, extreme hyperchromaticity of the nucleus, and a nucleus-cytoplasm ratio closer to 1.0 than the normal 1:5. It is not characterized by the changes described for this specimen.
C (dysplasia) is incorrect. Dysplasia is characterized by the loss of uniformity in cell size and a change in the shape and orientation of cells (pleomorphism). It does not result in degradation of the nucleus.
D (inflammation) is incorrect. Inflammation is characterized by a proliferation of immune cells: neutrophils (PMNs) during the acute phase; lymphocytes, macrophages, and plasma cells during the chronic phase. It is not characterized by the changes described for this specimen.

29. *D* (spherocyte) is correct. Poikilocytes are abnormally shaped red blood cells (RBCs). An example of a poikilocyte is a spherocyte, which is an RBC with an abnormal shape most likely due to a defect in the cytoskeletal protein spectrin. Lack of spectrin makes it impossible for the cell to maintain its normally biconcave shape.

A (erythrocyte <6 in diameter) is incorrect. An RBC <6 in diameter is a microcyte. Because it has a normal biconcave shape, it is not considered a poikilocyte.
B (erythrocyte >9 in diameter) is incorrect. An RBC >9 in diameter is a macrocyte. Macrocytes have a normal biconcave shape; thus they are not considered poikilocytes.
C (erythrocyte in a rouleaux formation) is incorrect. RBCs normally stack, forming a rouleaux; they must have a normal (biconcave) shape to do so.
E (stab eosinophil) is incorrect. The appearance of stab, or band, forms of neutrophils, basophils, and eosinophils is normal during the last step of cytodifferentiation, before the mature granulocyte is produced.

30. *E*   (type II pneumocyte) is correct. Type II pneumocytes (great alveolar cells) are located in the alveolar wall. They are large cells within myelin-like figures in their cytoplasm and produce surfactant in the alveolus.

A   (bronchiolar gland cell) is incorrect. Bronchiolar glands produce mucus, not surfactant.
B   (dust cell) is incorrect. Dust cells (alveolar macrophages with phagocytosed anthracotic pigment) are not involved in the production of surfactant.
C   (goblet cell) is incorrect. Goblet cells produce mucus, not surfactant.
D   (type I pneumocyte) is incorrect. Type I pneumocytes comprise the very thin surface lining of the alveolus. They are covered with surfactant, but they do not manufacture it.

31. *E*   (no change) is correct. A 0.9% NaCl solution is isotonic to red blood cells (RBCs). Therefore the cell will neither swell nor shrink, and nothing will happen to its intracellular contents.

A   (crenation) is incorrect. Crenation is the loss of water from the cell to the surrounding fluid. It occurs when a cell is placed into a hypertonic solution, such as a 1.5% NaCl. The solution would draw water out of the cell, leaving it dehydrated and shrunken (or crenated).
B   (hemolysis) is incorrect. Hemolysis of RBCs occurs when RBCs are placed in a hypotonic solution (e.g., 0.02% NaCl), which causes them to swell and burst.
C   (rise in oxyhemoglobin content) is incorrect. The blood sample being placed in a saline solution will have little or no effect on the oxyhemoglobin content of RBCs. If anything, the RBCs in solution would gradually lose oxygen and become progressively deoxygenated.
D   (spherocytosis) is incorrect. Spherocytosis is characterized by the presence of RBCs with an abnormal shape (round, not concave) due to a genetic defect in the cytoskeletal protein spectrin.

32. *A*   (CD4 T cell) is correct. The CD4 T cell (helper T cell) is one of the major targets for HIV (macrophages are also major HIV targets). Several years after the initial infection, the number of CD4 T cells declines. This results in the loss of a multitude of helper functions, which take place by means of the lymphokines that are normally secreted by these cells to enhance the activity of other immune cells. The patient will then become increasingly susceptible to infection by other organisms (opportunistic infections).

B   (CD8 T cell) is incorrect. The CD8 T cell is not a direct target of HIV infection. However, its ability to function is adversely affected when lymphokine production decreases as the number of CD4 cells decreases after an individual is infected with HIV.

C   (CD20 B cell) is incorrect. CD20 is a nonpolymorphic molecule expressed only on B cells. It can be used as a marker to classify lymphoid neoplasms immunologically. The B cell is not a common target of HIV.

D   (natural killer cell) is incorrect. The NK cell is not a direct target of the HIV virus. However, its ability to function is adversely affected by the decrease in lymphokine production that results from the loss of CD4 cells in individuals with HIV.

E   (plasma cell) is incorrect. Plasma cells are terminally differentiated B lymphocytes. They are not direct targets of HIV.

33. *C*   (natural killer cells) is correct. NK cells normally provide surveillance for the immune system. Their cytotoxic activity is triggered by exposure to transformed cells, including neoplastic cells. Immunosuppressive therapy, such as cyclosporin therapy, selectively suppresses NK cell activity, thereby increasing the patient's risk for cancer.

A   (basophils) is incorrect. The basophil is a granulocyte that takes part in immediate hypersensitivity reactions. Suppressing the hypersensitivity reaction does not induce cellular transformations that can result in a neoplasm.

B   (dendritic reticular cells) is incorrect. Dendritic reticular cells are found in the germinal centers of lymph nodules. These cells trap and present antigens to immunocompetent cells. Suppressing these normal functions does not induce cellular transformations that can result in a neoplasm.

D   (plasma cells) is incorrect. The plasma cell is a terminally differentiated B cell. It synthesizes antibodies, which target specific nonself entities and mark them for extinction. Suppressing plasma cell activity does not induce cellular transformations that can result in a neoplasm.

E   (T suppressor cells) is incorrect. T suppressor cells (CD8 T cells) down-regulate antibody production. Suppressing their activity does not induce cellular transformations that can result in a neoplasm.

34. *D*   (osteoporosis) is correct. Osteoporosis is a reduction in bone mass, which increases the risk for fracture after minimal trauma. Osteoporosis develops as a result of an imbalance between bone deposition and bone resorption. Women tend to be at greater risk for this condition as they age, because the life span and activity of osteoblasts decreases with the loss of estrogen after menopause. If the loss of osteoblast activity is not accompanied by a change in osteoclast activity, bone loss will continue, resulting in a detectable loss of bone mass over time.

A   (osteoclastoma) is incorrect. Osteoclastoma (giant cell neoplasm in bone) is a relatively common benign bone neoplasm and comprises 20% of benign bone neoplasms. It usually arises in the epiphyseal regions of the long bones of the extremities, and it is characterized by the presence of a large number of osteoclast-like cells. It has no effect on the life span of osteoblasts.

B   (osteomalacia) is incorrect. Osteomalacia is characterized by inadequate mineralization of bone matrix. It is associated with vitamin D deficiency, which reduces the rate of absorption of calcium across the lining of the intestines; this then reduces the amount of calcium available to mineralize bone matrix.

C   (osteopetrosis) is incorrect. Osteopetrosis is characterized by the production of excessive amounts of bone matrix. Patients with this condition develop brittle bones.

E   (scurvy) is incorrect. Scurvy is characterized by the inability of osteoblasts to manufacture normal amounts of bone matrix (collagen). Scurvy is often associated with hypovitaminosis C.

35. *B*   (corpora arenacea in the pineal gland) is correct. Calcified corpora arenacea (brain sand) is found in the normal pineal gland, which is located in the midline of the posterior portion of the third ventricle. It is often used as a marker for the midline of the brain.

A   (corpora amylacea in the pineal gland) is incorrect. Corpora amylacea are not found in the center of the brain.

C   (cupula of the crista ampullaris) is incorrect. The cupula of the crista ampullaris in the semicircular canal does not contain any material that would appear as radiopaque specks on an x-ray film.

D   (otoliths in the macula of the saccule) and E (otoliths in the macula of the utricle) are incorrect. Otoliths (ear stones) are found in the gelatinous mass in the macula of the utricle or saccule of the inner ear. They are too small to be detected by an x-ray film. Furthermore, they are components of the vestibular system in the ear; they are not located in the center of the brain.

36. *D*   (monocyte) is correct. Mononuclear phagocytes (monocytes and macrophages) respond to liposaccharides by releasing TNF, which causes endothelial cells to release interleukin 6 (IL-6) and IL-8.

A   (basophil) is incorrect. Basophils induce type I hypersensitivity reactions (anaphylaxis) by releasing a variety of vasoactive substances (e.g., histamine) and chemotactic factors for PMNs and eosinophils.

B   (endothelial) is incorrect. Endothelial cells respond to increased levels of TNF by releasing IL-6 and IL-8.

C   (eosinophil) is incorrect. Eosinophils play a role in immune responses to parasitic infections and immune responses mediated by IgE.

E   (platelet) is incorrect. Platelets are involved in homeostasis and in the production of platelet derived growth factor, which induces the proliferation and/or migration of monocytes, fibroblasts, and smooth muscle cells.

37. *C* (myeloblast) is correct. CML is characterized by the presence of granulocytic and erythroid cells at various stages of differentiation in the peripheral blood. In general, the younger (less differentiated) the cell, the larger its size and the more prominent its nucleoli. The myeloblast is the least differentiated of all the cell types listed. Therefore it would have the most prominent or largest nucleoli.

A (basophilic myelocyte) is incorrect. The myelocyte is the next to the least mature cell listed. Myelocytes usually show their nucleoli, but not as prominently as a promyelocyte or myeloblast.
B (mature neutrophil) is incorrect. Mature PMNs do not show nucleoli.
D (neutrophilic metamyelocyte) is incorrect. As a moderately differentiated cell with a bean-shaped nucleus, the metamyelocyte may or may not contain highly distinct nucleoli.
E (polychromatophilic normoblast) is incorrect. In the polychromatophilic normoblast, most of the nucleus is heterochromatized or pyknotic. As a result, its nucleoli would not be seen.

38. *D* (400) is correct. The G_2 cell contains four times the amount of DNA as the gamete. Therefore it will contain 400 copies of the ribosomal genes.

A (100) is incorrect. There are 100 ribosomal genes in a gamete.
B (200) is incorrect. There are 200 ribosomal genes present during the G_1 phase of the cell cycle.
C (300) is incorrect. There are 300 ribosomal genes in some cells during the early part of the S phase of the cell cycle.

39. *D* (non–carrier-mediated transport) is correct. When molecules cross the cell membrane without a carrier, they cannot move against their concentration gradient and energy is not required for their movement. Non–carrier-mediated movement is restricted to a class of molecules with similar physical properties (e.g., a high molecular weight).

A (active transport) is incorrect. Active transport requires energy.
B (carrier-facilitated diffusion) is incorrect. Carrier-facilitated diffusion involves the use of molecule-specific carriers.
C (exocytosis) is incorrect. Exocytosis is used to transport material in bulk out of the cell.

40. *A* (a nexus is found in the intercalated disk) is correct. Nexi (gap junctions) in the intercalated disk play an important role in the transmission of stimuli from one cardiac muscle fiber to the next.

B (each fiber is innervated by an individual nerve ending) is incorrect. Cardiac muscle fibers are not innervated separately.
C (it lacks myofibrils) is incorrect. Cardiac muscle fibers contain striated myofibrils.

D (T tubules are found at the A-I intercept) is incorrect. T tubules are located at the Z line.

41. *B* (a multinucleated cell results from the fusion of many single cells) is correct. The skeletal muscle cell is the result of the fusion of many myoblasts into a myotube.

A (a multinucleated cell is formed by repeated nuclear divisions in the absence of cytoplasmic division) is incorrect. The skeletal muscle cell is a result of the fusion of many myoblasts.
C (after puberty, muscle mass grows by an increase in cell number) is incorrect. Muscle grows in mass by an increase in cell size (hypertrophy), not cell number.
D (skeletal muscle is derived from epithelial ectodermal and endodermal layers) is incorrect. Skeletal muscle is derived from mesoderm.

42. *C* (endocytosis) is correct. Endocytosis is a mechanism for cellular uptake of macromolecules.

A (active transport) is incorrect. Active transport is a mechanism for carrying small molecules across a plasma cell membrane.
B (carrier-facilitated diffusion) is incorrect. Carrier-facilitated diffusion is a mechanism for the uptake of small molecules into the cell.
D (exocytosis) is incorrect. Exocytosis is a mechanism for moving material out of the cell.
E (non–carrier-mediated transport) is incorrect. Non–carrier-mediated transport is a mechanism for the uptake of small, uncharged molecules and lipid-soluble material into the cell.

43. *D* (loss of secondary constrictions) is correct. The nucleolar organizer contains the secondary constriction region. If the organizer is completely deleted, the secondary constriction region is also removed from the chromosome.

A (increased hybridization of DNA with 18S and 28S rRNA) is incorrect. If the nucleolar organizer is completely deleted from the cell, the genes that code for rRNA will be lost.
B (increased number of nucleoli) is incorrect. If the nucleolar organizer is completely deleted from the cell, no nucleoli will be formed in the cell.
C (increased synthesis of 45S RNA) is incorrect. If the nucleolar organizer is completely deleted, the cell will not be able to synthesize 45S (a precursor to rRNA).

44. *B* (mitochondria and vesicles containing neurotransmitters accumulate in the presynaptic area) is correct. Mitochondria and synaptic vesicles containing neurotransmitters are found in the presynaptic area of the neuron.

A (a myelin sheath must be present if synaptic transmission is to occur) is incorrect. Synapses occur between myelinated and non-myelinated axons.
C (most synapses exist between two dendritic processes) is incorrect. Most synapses occur between axons and dendrites.
D (occluding junctions hold the two neuronal processes together) is incorrect. Synapses do not contain occludens junctions.
E (satellite cells intervene between the neuronal processes) is incorrect. There are no intervening cells in a synapse.

45. *D* (presence of occluding junctions between capillary endothelial cells) is correct. The zona occludens is found between adjacent endothelial cells, and it plays a major role in the function of the blood-brain barrier.

A (accumulation of reactive astrocytes at the site of injury) is incorrect. Reactive astrocytes form at sites of injury. The blood-brain barrier is active in the uninjured brain.
B (association of the choroid plexus with pia mater cells) is incorrect. The choroid plexus plays an important role in the production of cerebrospinal fluid.
C (maintenance of the resting membrane potential) is incorrect. Membrane potentials are determined by the overall charge across the membrane of the nerve cell. They do not affect the blood-brain barrier.

46. *B* (resorption of water from the straight collecting tubules) is correct. A hypertonic interstitium in the area of the straight collecting tubules enhances the resorption of water in response to antidiuretic hormone.

A (resorption of water from the proximal convoluted tubule) and C (resorption of water from the thick ascending portion of Henle's loop) are incorrect. The resorption of water from these segments of the nephron is more strongly influenced by the movement of sodium, which is actively pumped out of each segment.

47. *C* (partial resorption of haversian systems by osteoclasts) is correct. During the remodeling of compact bone, osteoclasts resorb major regions of existing haversian systems, leaving some of the lamellae of these systems in place. Thus the resulting interstitial lamellae are the oldest lamellae in compact bone and have the highest degree of mineralization.

A (failure of haversian systems to form correctly) is incorrect. Interstitial lamellae are found in the remnants of remodeled haversian systems. After osteoclasts have ceased creating tunnels during the resorption process, the tunnels are filled by means of osteoblast activity to create a new haversian system. The haversian system must be normal for the remodeling process to occur.
B (inadequate intake of vitamin C) is incorrect. Vitamin C is necessary for the osteoblast to synthesize the collagen component of

osteoid. Hypovitaminosis C results in scurvy, which is characterized by thin spicules of bone, indicating that little or no collagen synthesis is occurring.

D (pulling apart of haversian systems by Sharpey's fibers) is incorrect. Sharpey's fibers are collagen fibers that run from the periosteum into compact bone, anchoring the periosteum firmly to the bone. Sharpey's fibers do not hold haversian systems together.

E (stimulation of periosteum by parathyroid hormone) is incorrect. PTH enhances the production and activity of osteoclasts. If anything, PTH activity would reduce the number of interstitial lamellae in compact bone.

48. *A* (decreased synthesis of androgen-binding protein) is correct. Removal of the anterior lobe of the pituitary would remove follicle-stimulating hormone (FSH) and lutein hormone (LH) and lead to decreased synthesis of androgen-binding protein by the Sertoli cells. Antigen-binding protein is the binding protein for sex hormones and has a higher binding affinity for testosterone than for estrogen.

B (increased production of testosterone) is incorrect. Removal of the anterior lobe of pituitary would end FSH and LH production and lead to a decrease in testosterone production.

C (increased spermatogenesis) is incorrect. Removal of the anterior lobe of pituitary would eliminate FSH and LH and lead to decreased spermatogenesis.

49. *D* (stomach) is correct. Every columnar cell on the surface of the gastric epithelium secretes an insoluble mucus, which plays an important role in protecting the stomach wall from being digested by its own highly acidic secretions.

A (duodenum) is incorrect. The duodenum is lined with both simple columnar absorptive cells (enterocytes) and goblet cells, which produce mucus. However, the goblet cells are interspersed among the duodenal enterocytes; therefore mucus is not produced by every surface cell.

B (esophagus) is incorrect. The esophagus is lined with a stratified squamous wet-type epithelium, which does not manufacture mucus.

C (lower anal canal) is incorrect. The lower anal canal is lined with stratified squamous wet-type epithelium, which does not secrete mucus.

E (transverse colon) is incorrect. Although the colonic epithelium contains a large number of goblet cells (which secrete mucus), these cells are interspersed among colonic enterocytes (water-absorbing cells). As a result, mucus is not secreted by every surface cell.

50. *D* (promyelocytic leukemia) is correct. The cell is a promyelocyte, which has a round nucleus containing several prominent nucleoli and a cytoplasm filled with small azurophilic

granules. Dominance of this type of cell in the blood smear suggests promyelocytic leukemia. This type of leukemia is a distinctive variant of chronic lymphocytic leukemia (CLL) of B-cell lineage, or B-CLL. It is characterized by massive splenomegaly, and the leukocyte count is markedly elevated. The disease is most common in elderly men; it is aggressive with a survival rate of 2 to 3 years.

A (acute lymphoblastic leukemia) is incorrect. ALL is characterized by a large number of lymphoblasts or immature lymphocytes. The cytoplasm of these cells is not filled with azurophilic granules. The peak age of incidence is childhood, and occurs twice as often in white as in blacks.
B (basophilic leukemia) is incorrect. Basophilic leukemia is a rare form of leukemia characterized by the presence of basophils in various stages of differentiation.
C (monoblastic leukemia) is incorrect. Monoblastic leukemia is characterized by an abundance of agranular monoblasts.
E (stem cell leukemia) is incorrect. Stem cell leukemia is characterized by an abundance of very immature cells. These cells have prominent nucleoli, but they are not differentiated well enough to show cytoplasmic granules. This type of leukemia is also known as *acute undifferentiated leukemia*.

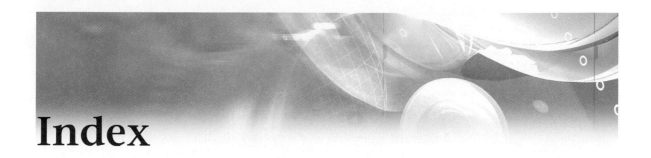

Index